REJUVENATE YOUR BRAIN NATURALLY

ROBERT DALE ROGERS (RH) AHG

DEDICATION

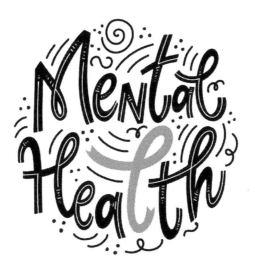

The writing of this book would not have been possible without the support and encouragement of my wife, and best friend, Laurie Szott-Rogers. Our 30 years together have been a remarkable journey of love, sharing and inspiration.

Her wonderful father Josef Szott and my mother Joyce Rogers both suffered from senile dementia (Alzheimer's disease) in their later years. Their love and legacy carry on.

I also dedicate this book to the millions of individuals and families struggling with mental health issues.

It is my hope this book provides inspiration and a pathway to follow. It is never too late to change your mind.

Robert June 2019.

Contents

INTRODUCTION

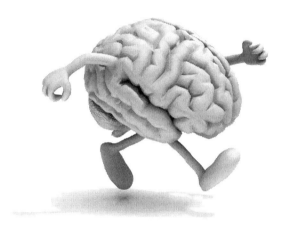

"Science advances one funeral at a time."

MAX PLANCK

"If people let the government decide what foods they eat and what medicines they take, their bodies will soon be in as sorry a state as the souls of those who live under tyranny."

THOMAS JEFFERSON

Why did I write a book on brain health?

I watched my own dear mother Joyce suffer the onset of Alzheimer's disease at 84 years of age, and for the next five years watched her painful, personal path of cognitive decline and lowered quality of life. I was re-assured in the later stages, that it was more painful for me, as she was no longer suffering. I am not sure that is true.

Around the same time, my beloved father-in-law, Joe, followed a similar path (from ages 84-89) created, in part, by the over-use of cortisone creams for his painful pustular psoriasis. This led to Roid Rage, and his quickened pathway to dementia.

This is largely why I feel the necessity to share the important information in this book.

We are living longer than ever, with longevity rates increasing over the past two centuries. This is due, in large part, to improved sanitation, reduction of infectious disease, and addressing malnutrition.

The last point is suggested, tongue in cheek, for during the last forty years we have witnessed a steep decline in the quality and nutritional content of food in our grocery store aisles.

Certainly, the movement to organic food by an increasing number of people is supporting this important ecological and environmental shift to wellness.

But are we really healthier than our great grandparents, even our parents? Or are we any happier?

There is a link between happiness and genes that influence brain serotonin metabolism. A study of 100 countries found residents of Denmark and the Netherlands have a mutation of the gene that helps support the high level of happiness. When researchers matched well-being of Americans to country of origin, the ancestral pattern, even several generations back, showed the same result.[1]

A recent study, in Denmark, looked at the amount of green space available during early childhood, and the later association with incidence of psychiatric disorders. Not surprisingly, a direct correlation of less green space and more mental health issues was observed in a number of categories, except for schizoaffective disorder.[2]

The reverse is also true. Epigenetics suggest our genetic code can be changed, and passed down to future generations. We are not prisoners of our genetic inheritance.

The pioneering work of Bruce Lipton, author of *The Biology of Belief*, has helped a whole generation understand how day-to-day influences of our mental, emotional and physical expressions either up-regulate or down-regulate our genetic codes.

The modification of gene expression allows nature and nurture to produce generational changes.

Brain neuroplasticity is becoming a well-known phrase to the general public. It suggests the brain adapts to internal and external stimuli and makes adjustments to optimize function.

Neuroplasticity is unfortunately, the latest trendy catch phrase in a variety of self-help marketing campaigns, but the idea is centuries old.

In the 1780s, a Swiss naturalist and Italian anatomist suggested mental exercise leads to brain growth.

The term "plasticity" came nearly a century later in the 1890 book *The Principles of Psychology* by William James.

He defined it as "the possession of a structure weak enough to yield to an influence, but strong enough not to yield all at once."

Brain health is related to a number of factors covered in this book, including both functional and structural plasticity.

We often hear we are only using ten percent of our brains. This is not exactly true. We use 10% for voluntary actions, but the other 90% is used for autonomic functions such as breathing, circulation, heart and digesting our food.

Why is this important? Because when the brain becomes impaired, it cannot activate the gastrointestinal tract and digestive problems begin. We will later explore in depth, the connection between a leaky gut and leaky brain.

The heart-brain-gut connection is vastly under-estimated but slowly accepting scientific recognition.

The brain has 100 billion neurons, while the gut has 500 million nerve cells, and 100 million neurons. This inter-connection is well-known, and will be examined more closely throughout the book.

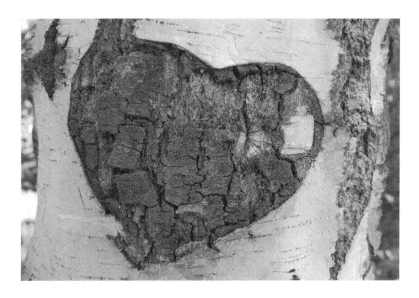

The heart contains about forty thousand neurons that can sense, feel, learn and remember. The connection is well known from brain to heart, and involves reactions of the sympathetic and parasympathetic nervous system to stress, or relaxation.

But recent work suggests the heart receives and processes information from our environment a few thousand milliseconds before the brain. It is these neurons in the heart that decide how we feel and react.

The heart generates its own compounds, including oxytocin, brain naturetic factor, norepinephrine and dopamine. These communicate with our gut brain and the hippocampus involved in learning and memory.

It is obvious that if negative emotions can harm your heart, positive emotions can heal. Scientists have found the amygdala is the site in the brain affected by the heart, and all three are connected by our vagus nerve.

All three brains offer us an aspect of human consciousness. The head helps us observe our world, dictating logic and reason and planning a future. The heart describes our inner life of emotion, visions, and dreams, while the gut provides instinct and intuition that is immediate and practical.

Grief and heartache harm the heart. Gut feelings help us avoid unpleasant or dangerous missteps. All three influence each other in a tri-directional manner.[3]

A broken heart or atrial fibrillation, also known as taktsubo cardiomyopathy, is present in those suffering acute anxiety, long-term stress and grief, moreso in post-menopausal women.

Acute stress gives us motivation, but chronic stress takes a great toll on our physical, mental and emotional health.

A recent Gallup poll found that 55% of Americans feel "stressed a lot of the day," compared to 35% in rest of the world.

Finding purpose in life, and confirming gratitude are important to our spiritual wellbeing. Studies have shown writing a journal and expressing gratitude increases our brain's neuroplasticity and expression of genes.

Anxiety affects about 18% of the American population.

Women suffer 70% more depression than men, but this may be more a statistic of those who ask for help. Overall, 12% of women suffer clinical depression over their lifetime, with over 80% of them, never receiving any treatment.

It is important to remind ourselves that anxiety and depression are not diseases, but symptoms associated with an underlying condition. Toxicity and inflammation are two major factors present in many cases.

Alzheimer's disease (AD), and senile dementia numbers are on the rise. It is predicted by the year 2050, over 15 million patients, in the United States alone, will be affected by this cruel mental condition.

Worldwide, it is estimated over 132 million people will be affected by various forms of dementia in the same timeframe.

It is a burgeoning global health epidemic.

But anxiety and AD are just the tip of the iceberg when it comes to brain health.

Various conditions, including Parkinson's disease (PD), depression, attention deficit and hyperactivity disorder (ADHD), obsessive-compulsive disorder, epilepsy, autism spectrum disorder (ASD), seasonal affective disorder, Asperger's disease, Huntington's disease (HD), multiple sclerosis, addictions, thyroid disorders and brain injury are exacting a huge toll on many people's lives.

And, in turn, this is increasingly straining a healthcare system overburdened with various other chronic conditions including cancer, cardiovascular disease, diabetes…and on and on.

I have been an herbalist for five decades, including nearly twenty years of clinical practice.

Presently, I am an assistant clinical professor in family medicine at the University of Alberta, and a faculty member in the Integrative Health Institute. For over a decade I first wrote, and then taught an introductory herbal course at Grant McEwan University, and now co-teach with my beautiful wife Laurie at *The Northern Star College of Mystical Studies*. The College name is deliberate as I have been privy to all sides of the biomedicine, complementary, alternative, and integrated health systems.

Some of my early training in plant medicine was with First Nations Cree healers of northern Canada, and shaman in Peru.

I therefore, have one foot in the traditional healing ways of Indigenous knowledge, and the other in the fascinating world of molecular science and biochemistry.

Anxiety and depression are today, most often treated with pharmaceutical drugs that mask the underlying issues.

Medical doctors are not trained to recognize or treat early stages of brain degeneration until it has progressed to a pathological stage. By the time memory loss is advanced, or Parkinson's tremor is really obvious, much brain damage has already occurred.

Numerous OTC medications including proton pump inhibitors (PPIs), anti-cholinergic medications and warfarin increase the risk of dementia.[4,5] PPIs deplete magnesium and B12, both of which induce proper production of neurotransmitters.

One of the strengths and weaknesses of large randomized clinical trials (RCTs) is they can easily test for one molecule, but not multiple variations. Evidence-based medicine (EBM) also has its limitations, as every individual has a specific physiology, with possible deficiencies and interactions.

A book I highly recommend to individuals experiencing opposition to natural approaches to health is *Tarnished Gold: The Sickness of Evidence-Based Medicine* by Hickey and Roberts. Among the many criticisms is that EBM avoids refutation, a critical part of the scientific method. A rational patient will reject EBM because it is inherently unscientific and impractical.

I believe the future is functional medicine, where patients are treated as unique individuals with specific health challenges.

This does not imply I am ignoring the vast pool of double-blind (DB), placebo-controlled (PC), randomized trials of the past half-dozen years. Far from it, but all studies must be critiqued for their bias. It is well known the observer influences the outcome of the experiment.

Also, we should never underestimate the power of belief.

"Research on placebo effects can help explain mechanistically how clinicians can be therapeutic agents in the ways they relate to their patients in connection with, and separate from, providing effective treatment interventions."[6]

This book is written from a holistic perspective focused on natural approaches that may help prevent and restore brain health.

One group of researchers estimated how long it would take to test seven possible treatments for Alzheimer's disease. We know that not one drug has passed Phase III clinical trials, but these researchers thought maybe combining different drugs affecting neurological pathways might be effective. Remember the triple cocktail for HIV treatment developed years ago?

They calculated the time to run 127 separate RCTs, with 63,500 patients, would take 286 years to complete.[7]

Individual nutritional and dietary needs are specific to your genetic requirements. The present professional training of dieticians is inadequate, as it is based on the premise we do not require vitamins and mineral supplementation; that our foods contain all the nutrients we require. This is utter nonsense.

7

Canada's Food Guide, released in 2019 is a start, but consider sitting down with a trained nutritionist to help plan a diet around your own individual requirements for preserving or restoring brain health.

It must be said that 80% of what we know today about the brain has been discovered in the past twenty years; and 80% of this information in the past five years. This book explores the latest science and puts a holistic spin on reclaiming your brain health.

If you are concerned about your own brain health or that of a loved one, join one of the support groups associated with their specific diagnosis. Share this book, and the names of experts found in the bibliography. The support of others with similar health issues, and a feeling of community is important. But so is the sharing of information about how there are other options other than surgery or pharmaceuticals.

Today we are quickly moving away, from a system of disease management to health creation and functional medicine. Part of this movement involves community-centered programs, for social isolation is more closely related with mortality than smoking, alcohol, poor diet and lack of exercise combined.

Social networking, comparing findings, and sharing success is empowering. If a local support group is not available or travel is unfeasible, there are numerous sites on the web.

Diet, supplementation, and lifestyle can make a dramatic difference in maintaining brain health. We will explore all these safe and sensible avenues so that you and your loved ones can achieve optimal brain function.

Dr. Dale Bredesen, author of *The End of Alzheimer's* writes. "If someone had told me a few decades ago that, as a research neurologist, I would be recommending protocols that involve meditation, yoga, laughter, music, joy, fasting, exercise, herbs, nutrition and sleep, I would have laughed. But I cannot argue with results, or with the conclusion of years of research."[8]

CHAPTER 1

WHAT A HEALTHY BRAIN NEEDS

"We are dealing with the best-educated generation in history. But they've got a brain dressed up with nowhere to go."

TIMOTHY LEARY

WHAT THE BRAIN DOES NEED

OXYGEN

It may seem obvious, but the two most important elements to brain health are clean air and water.

At one time, both of these critical, life resources were pure, plentiful and free. Early civilizations settled beside rivers and lakes, and abundant forests provided optimum oxygen.

Such is no longer the case on our increasingly urbanized planet.

Carbon dioxide levels are increasing worldwide, driven by fossil fuel consumption; and filling our air with thousands of chemicals, including known carcinogens.

Our brains require oxygen and restrictions associated with poor blood flow, including anemia, blood sugar dysregulation, apnea, low blood pressure, and hypothyroidism can lead to brain neuron death. Cold hands and feet are one good indicator the brain is starving for oxygenated blood.

It is well researched that nasal breathing influences cognition related to amygdala and hippocampal function.[9]

Physical exercise is imperative, even for sufferers of Parkinson's disease. A review of 1603 studies on exercise, found 29 randomized, controlled studies showed improved cognitive function in adults. Another trial found aerobic exercise, instituted for one year resulted in significant hippocampus enlargement. Even those who just walked a few days a week exhibited hippocampus enlargement, nine years after they began their exercise regime.[10]

Conscious breathing encourages relaxation and combined with meditation helps improve our brain plasticity and health.[11]

Air filters, in urban areas, are now a must for good brain health. Our homes trap all sources of harmful off-gases, mycotoxins and other respiratory and brain damaging compounds. Look for a good HEPA plus activated carbon filter unit with a CADAR of 300 or more. I live in northern Canada, and we are house bound for seven or eight months of the year.

Ozone may have application in some health issues, but generally, it is best to avoid inexpensive air filters with ozone generators.

While in clinical practice I witnessed several young mothers placing these filters near their new babies, creating respiratory distress. As soon as the low quality filters were removed from the room, everything normalized.

It is estimated over 100 million American structures contain deadly molds, largely associated with improperly maintained air conditioners. There are now available, probiotic sprays to help control this virulent assault on our immune systems.

Apnea deprives the brain of sleep, a time when cleansing and repair of the brain takes place. And yet, an estimated 75% of patients with sleep apnea remain undiagnosed. If snoring and hence breathing is interrupted at night, the brain is not getting the sleep it needs for neural restoration, and removal of toxins from the brain.

WATER

Water composes 80% of our brain and hydration is imperative for the prevention of neural dysfunction. When you are only 2% dehydrated, attention span, memory and physical strength diminishes.[12]

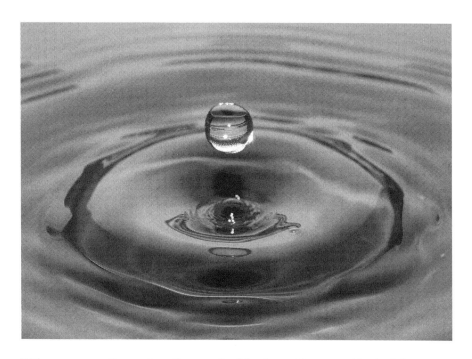

When young, the ratio of water inside the cell to outside is 1.2 to 1. By age 60 the ratio is 0.8 to 1, suggesting dehydration is a major problem.

Our waters are full of petrochemicals and pharmaceuticals, ingested directly, or found in the fish and animals we later consume. Birth control and anti-depressant residues are now found in wild Pacific coast salmon!

Over 90% of the tap water in America contains traces of plastic.

It is estimated the average human contains over 200 synthetic chemicals that are unnatural, residing in body tissue. Traces of 232 synthetic compounds have been recorded in the umbilical cord blood of infants at birth.[13]

In the United States, the National Toxicology Program lists 800 chemicals known to interfere with hormones (endocrine disruptors), and thousands of others identified we know little about.

In just the past 30 years more than three thousand cosmetic ingredients, nine thousand food additives and three thousand pharmaceutical drugs have been approved.

Six toxins of particular importance to avoid are:

1. PCBs (polychlorinated biphenyls) were banned decades ago but are still associated with impaired fetal brain development and found in farm-raised salmon. In 1976 the EPA (Environmental Protection Agency) enacted the Toxic Substance Control Act, and legally grandfathered sixty-two thousand chemicals safe to use. Since then, another twenty-three thousand additional compounds have been added to the list.

2. Pesticides. According to the EPA over 60% of herbicides, 90% of fungicides and 30% of insecticides are known carcinogens. These cause cancer, Parkinson's disease, and nerve damage. Pesticides are extremely toxic to our mitochondria, with numerous studies indicating disruption of hormones and brain health. This is one more reason to avoid GMO foods, due to their relationship to herbicides. In 2017, farmers applied 1.35 million metric tonnes of glyphosate to crops. Glyphosates inhibit cytochrome P450 enzymes produced by gut flora, and inhibit liver detoxification. They impair the function of vitamin D (see below), and the synthesis of tryptophan and tyrosine; important amino acids involved in neurotransmitter production. Bt (*Bacillus thuringiensis*) strains are found in over 180 registered pesticide products, with some approved for organic agriculture. In fact, some crops are engineered to produce the Bt toxin. This bacterium may disrupt the health of our sensitive microbiome, and contribute to leaky gut syndrome.

3. Dioxins are produced from combustion of municipal waste and burning coal and oil. A major source of dioxin exposure (95%) for humans is eating commercial animal fats. Magnetite, generated by coal-generated power plants, enters our olfactory bulb and amplifies the negative effects of EMFs mentioned below.

4. Chlorine (Chloroform) is in our air, drinking water and food. The chemical is related to bladder, breast and bowel cancers, birth defects, liver and kidney damage. The EPA has set

the safe level in drinking water at 4 ppm; and yet that level is high enough to kill a goldfish in your home aquarium. Fluoride is also problematic. Early exposure may raise the risk of future problems, including deposition in the human pineal gland. See Sunlight below.

5. The heavy metals lead, aluminum, mercury and cadmium; and toxic metals like arsenic, are related to various neurological disorders, including Alzheimer's disease, amyotrophic lateral sclerosis (ALS), Parkinson's disease (PD), hypo-parathyroidism and various neuromuscular disorders. Arsenic, for example, is found in antibiotics fed to chickens, and is present in 10% of all public drinking water systems in the United States. Use a water filter, or pure spring water whenever possible.

When I tested myself over 30 years ago, using hair analysis, I was shocked to discover sky-high levels of lead and arsenic in my body tissue. I had been a very conscientious eater and could not initially understand, nor even believe the results. I later read an article about spraying lead arsenate in apple orchards, and I immediately switched to an organic source of my favorite fruit.

In fact, one study found that concentrations of selected pesticide detected in urine samples decreased by 95% when families switched to organic foods for just two weeks.

For lists of high and lowest pesticide loads in foods go to www.ewg.org .

Consider having your amalgam (silver) fillings removed by a holistic dentist with equipment that protects you from mercury vapor. Sweden banned mercury in dental fillings over a century ago (1905), and yet it is still the material of choice for most dentists. Hot water drinks, brushing or grinding your teeth, and improper removal of mercury can attack your neurological and immune systems.

Fish such as tuna are heavily laden with mercury, as are other seafoods higher up the food chain.

One supplement that may help to move heavy metals from the body is Dimercaptosuccinic acid (DMSA). See Supplements. I would advise individuals with heavy metal toxicity to seek out the help of a health practitioner trained in the proper protocols of phase 1, 2 and 3 liver detoxification to ensure minimal harm associated with intravenous or oral chelation.

6. BPA (bisphenol-A) has been detected in the blood of 93% of North Americans. Originally produced in 1891 as a synthetic estrogen, it was initially given to women for nausea in pregnancy, and later used by farmers to promote cattle growth. It was banned in the 1950s and re-emerged in plastic. It is an endocrine disrupter in men and women, with uncertain action on gut flora. The bisphenol-S and bis-phenol F, now substituted for clear plastics, may be just as toxic.[14] Over 34 million tons are used annually, with nearly 20% reserved for lining food and beverage cans. Phthalates are widely found in a variety of cosmetic and soft plastic products, including baby bottles and pacifiers. Microwaving baby bottles leaches plastic, and alters the quality of milk. Glass is a better choice.

One study at Columbia University looked at the blood content of phthalates in 328 women in their 8th month of pregnancy, and divided the findings into four quadrants of exposure. The offspring, when seven years old, were tested for IQ and those children whose mothers tested in the highest phthalate group were deficient by 7 points. These children had reduced mental capacity from birth.

Another study found IgG antibodies to BPA in 13% of blood donors and IgM antibodies in 15%. Methylation is our only defense to break down and detoxify these toxins. Researchers have found BPA exposure *in utero*, creates a deficiency of the myelin protective coating around the hippocampus, which can later manifest as anxiety, depression, hyperactivity and ADHD.[15]

Both air and water filters can help our overall health. Spring water is my favorite choice, but in the urban environment this can be difficult, and/or expensive to access. Trace minerals and electrolytes are crucial to brain health. Dehydration is known to increase brain shrinkage, and yet over 40% of Americans report drinking less than four cups of water daily, about half the amount considered optimal for a 150 pound adult.

A good rule of thumb is to drink one-half ounce of water for each pound of weight.

A 3-4 percent decrease in water intake can cause fatigue, brain fog, reduced energy, headaches and mood swings.[16]

Research shows drinking 8 to 10 cups of water daily increases our brain performance by almost 30 percent.[17]

A glass of pure water first thing in the morning is recommended, but avoid drinking water with meals as this dilutes stomach acid, and may slow down digestion.

Distilled water, or so-called purified water is only recommended if trace minerals are added later. One exception may be the temporary treatment of hardening of the arteries, associated with a oral chelation program.

In our home, we use a Delphi system that is hooked up to the kitchen sink, with the filter replaced each year. We use Soda Stream to carbonate drinks, as metal cans are lined with BPA.

Chloride in drinking water disrupts production of B12, a high risk factor for dementia and depression.

There is no good science behind the alkaline water craze.

On the road, drink organic coconut water, which has twice the potassium of sports drinks, with low amounts of sugar. I remember one extremely hot day in Grenada, when Laurie and I were severely parched. We quickly downed the watery contents of several cold, refreshing coconuts, opened on the spot.

Organic fruits and vegetables contain up to 95% water, and are a good source of hydration.

SUNLIGHT and SLEEP

Sunbathing is healthy, but seasonally restricted in northern climates. Many ancient cultures used sun bathing to encourage healing.

Placing patients in a sunlit room after surgery, for example, significantly decreases their pain.

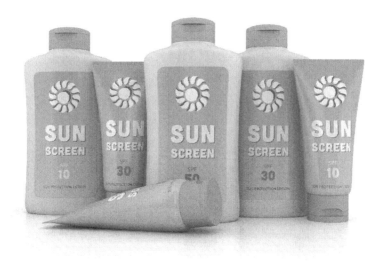

We all benefit from sunlight, and the plants that use the energy to produce our food. Sunburn skin damage is to be avoided, but so is the over-use of various chemical sunscreens. Oxybenzone, a common ingredient, found in the tissue of 96% of the American population, is a known endocrine disruptor. Nano-particled zinc oxide and titanium dioxide in sunscreen should be avoided. Retinyl palmitate (vitamin A derivative) increases growth of cancer cells by 21%. PABA and trolamine salicylate are not recommended. Of the 1400 plus sunscreens on the market, less than 5% pass the test for reduced chemical exposure.

The skin absorbs chemicals, and my rule of thumb is that if you cannot eat it, do not apply to your body.

Moderation of sun exposure is the key. Fifteen minutes of high noon sun exposure to arms or legs is all it takes to initiate sufficient vitamin D production.

Special cells known as melanocytes produce melanin from L-tyrosine, acting as a natural sunscreen for the skin. The more melanin, the less UVB rays penetrate, and the less vitamin D produced.

Medically, sunlight or visible blue light radiation is used for neonatal jaundice. This knowledge was used thousands of years ago by Greek and Roman physicians.

Psoriasis patients sometimes benefit from light therapy, often in conjunction with psoralen or drug that induces reaction on the skin.

My uncle Malcolm came home from the Korean War with tuberculosis, and spent several years in a sanatorium, where sunlight was part of his treatment.

And of course seasonal affective disorder (SAD) which is covered in chapter 7, is a winter depression helped by exposure to light from the sun, or full-spectrum artificial light.

L-tryptophan converts to serotonin and then melatonin in the pineal gland, secreted by a marked circadian rhythm. Melatonin receptors are found in the brain, the retina, the pituitary and elsewhere. Because tryptophan is found in foods with other amino acids, it is poorly absorbed, and best taken with small amount of carbohydrates several hours before bedtime.

Phases of light and dark affect our circadian rhythm, and poor sleep is associated with increased risk of depression, ADD and even schizophrenia disorder.

Insomnia affects over one-third of Americans, with 17% reporting sleep issues are a major problem. Nearly 12% rely on prescription (sedative hypnotic) drugs.

Individuals taking thirty or more sleeping pills per month have a 25% greater rate of mortality.

The World Health Organization classifies shift work as a "probable carcinogen."

But our natural body clock of day and night is controlled by some twenty thousand nerve cells in the hypothalamus, which receives its cue from special sensing cells, at the back of the eye.

Night-shift workers are out of sync with their hypothalamic clock.

Fluoride calcification of the pineal gland interferes with melatonin production and is associated with a variety of neural diseases.

Chronic exposure to fluoride in pregnancy and early infancy may impair Na^+, K^+, and $-ATPase$ activity implicated in neurodevelopment, neuropsychiatric and neurodegenerative disorders.[18]

Disruption of pineal gland function may explain, in part, brain health issues, including schizophrenia and bipolar disorder.

ELECTROMAGNETIC FIELDS

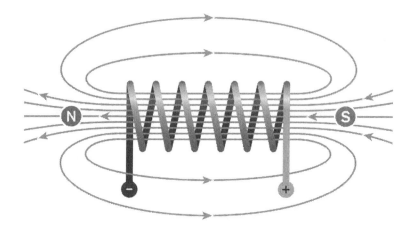

Our modern society has embraced the widespread use of computers, microwaves, and cell phones. I am writing this book on a computer at this moment.

All these devices emit strong electromagnetic fields (EMFs) that affect brain health.

One recent study found EMFs from cell phones may cause neurological ill effects, including cognitive dysfunction, emotional instability and even brain tumors.[19]

Microwave EMFs act via voltage-gated calcium channel activation, and produce neuropsychiatric issues including insomnia, headache, depression, fatigue, memory changes, anxiety, and attention dysfunction. Eighteen epidemiological studies provide substantial evidence of harm from cell/mobile phone bases stations, excess cell phone use and wireless smart meters.[20]

Children using a cell phone before the age of twenty have a fivefold increased risk of glioma, a malignant brain cancer.

Even more frightening, is that electromagnetic radiation can penetrate right through the entire brain of a five year old.

And there is an 80% increased risk of a child having behavioral issues if their mother used a cell phone during pregnancy.

Cell phones not only reduce sperm count and motility, but damage our DNA. EMFs may affect your prostate function and even promote cancer.[21]

If a cell phone is held just one inch from the body, it reduces the EMF penetration by two-thirds.

I stopped putting my cell phone in a pocket over my heart, due to my feeling a rhythm irregularity. This impression was later confirmed, for me, in a study.[22]

And this was with 3G. The world is now moving to 5G, which has greatly expanded capacity and penetration.

Thinking of taking them to court? In small print, iPhone documents read, "Carry iPhone at least 10 millimeters away from your body to ensure exposure levels remain at or below the as-tested levels." Instead get a radiation cover for your cell phone and avoid heavy use. Use a landline whenever possible.

In 2011, the World Health Organization (WHO) classified EMFs as 2B carcinogens, due to their ability to damage your DNA.

Exposure to EMFs can disrupt pineal gland function and circadian patterns of melatonin. One study of people using electric blankets found the low frequency electric or magnetic fields disrupted pineal gland function.[23]

EMF pollution is found in batteries, cars, trains, buses, planes, cellular and digital phones, computers, televisions, power lines, house wiring, microwave ovens, smart meters, wearable performance trackers, wireless baby monitors and wireless gaming consoles. It is all around us.

We have all seen the cartoons of people wearing aluminum hats to ward off radiation. The humor may be based in some degree of truth.

A study of 64 patients, with auto-immune conditions, involved wearing a silver-threaded cap to protect the brain and brain stem from EMFs. Ninety percent reported "definite" or "strong" changes in their disease symptoms, compared to the 3-5% rate reported for EMF sensitivity in the general population.[24]

Magnetite (Fe_3O_4) is found in the brains of bees, birds and human, acting as a form of internal compass. EMFS appear to excite these molecules, as beta amyloid peptides in the brains of AD patients show higher than average levels. They interact strongly with external magnetic fields.

This could be due in part to the use of coal for the generation of electricity; as well as other combustion-derived, iron-rich airborne released toxins.[25]

These magnetite particles are less than 200 nanometers in diameter and enter the brain directly via the olfactory bulb. Parkinson's disease, for example, is associated with high levels of iron in one part of the brain.

FATS

The water-rich brain is about 11% fat, not the 60% often cited if you google "brain fat".[26]

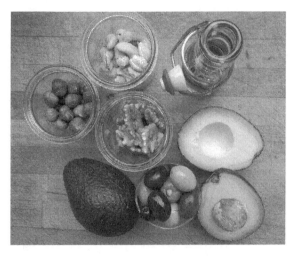

Phospholipids and sphingolipids account for nearly 70% of fat found in the brain.

Cholesterol-rich foods cannot enter the adult brain, except for butyric acid, found in whole milk and butter, and acids in coconut oil. Young children and adolescent brains require saturated fats when growing new brain cells, but this is shut down by early adulthood.

Brain cholesterol is produced by our glial cells, and smaller amounts by neurons. Conditions such as AD, PD, and Huntington's disease are linked to problems with metabolism of cholesterol in the brain.[27]

Mother's milk, for example, is 48% saturated, 33% monounsaturated and 16% polyunsaturated fat.

Butter is 52% saturated, 30% monounsaturated and 4% polyunsaturated fat. Notice the relative comparative levels.

Many health diet books suggest our mature brain needs saturated fats, but it can make what it needs, all by itself.

Polyunsaturated fats (PUFAs) are found in fatty fish, algae and some nuts and seeds. Omega-3 is the most well known and is the one fat our brain cannot manufacture on its own.

There are specific gateways for PUFAs located within the blood-brain barrier. As quickly as they arrive, they are consumed to form the phospholipids and sphingolipids mentioned above.

Omega-3 and Omega-6 are critical to immune health. The latter are pro-inflammatory and play a key role in helping us respond to bacterial, viral or fungal infections.

Too little Omega-6s can increase the risk of hemorrhage.

Omega-3s turn down this immune respond and are anti-inflammatory in nature.

Omega-3s help improve the diversity of your microbiome, boosting the numbers of *Lactobacillus* and *Bifidobacterium* species. See Chapter 2.

Possessing the correct balance helps maintain our optimal immune function, by modifying inflammation and yet being alert to fight infection.

A ratio of 2:1 (twice the omega-6 to omega-3) is considered an optimal ratio, although some experts cite 1:1, which is harder to achieve. Walnuts have an excellent ratio at 4:1.

We will cover the ratios of EPA (eicosapentaenoic acid) and DHA (docosahexaenoic acid); as well as GLA (gamma-linolenic acid) supplements for optimal benefit in various chapters. Evening primrose (9%) and borage oil (24%) are rich sources of GLA, and are helpful in liver enzyme deficient conditions.

Alas the average American diet contains twenty to thirty times more omega-6s, due to widespread consumption of various vegetable oils, often heated, refined, bleached and void of any nutrition. These harmful oils may be derived from corn, canola, soy, grape seed, peanut and sunflower seeds. Note the first three may be from GMO sources.

Presently, the *U.S. Food and Nutrition* board recommends ten times the omega-6 to omega-3, suggesting a pro-inflammatory response.[28]

Good sources of omega-6 oils include organic nuts and seeds, including walnuts, hazelnuts, pecans, brazil nuts; sunflower, sesame and pumpkin seeds. They should be raw, unroasted and refrigerated for optimal benefit to the body.

I remember my mother switching from butter to margarine at the insistence of her medical doctor in the 1970s. She listened to the "expert", instead of her herbalist son, much to my dismay.

Olive oil is one of my favorites for salads, as long as it is organic, cold-pressed and extra-virgin. There is a great deal of adulteration of olive oil, due to olive tree disease and greed, so research by the consumer is necessary to obtain a reliable source.

I enjoy avocado oil for sauté and light broiling, or stir-fries.

Both oils are monounsaturated. A study of those who consumed at least 24 grams of these fats daily had an 80% reduced risk of Alzheimer's compared to those consuming less than 15 grams.[29]

Inflammation in the body creates arthritis, atherosclerosis, auto-immune response and tumor growth, while in the brain leads to various neurological conditions such as Alzheimer's disease.

Alpha-linoleic acid (ALA) is derived from plant sources, including flaxseed, hemp, chia seeds, sunflowers, walnuts, and algae.

Unfortunately, ALA must be converted to EPA and DHA with nearly 75 percent of benefit lost in the process.

Omega-6 linoleic acid (LA) is converted to GLA, and arachidonic acid (AA) both of which are essential for brain health, hormone metabolism and modulating inflammation.

Again, rich sources of LA include walnuts, hazelnuts, pecans, pine nuts, Brazil nuts, and seeds from sunflower, sesame and pumpkin.

Arachiodonic acid (AA) is treated unfairly in many chemistry texts, suggesting it is responsible for pro-inflammatory conditions. This is partially true. It comprises some 12% of all brain fatty acids (similar to DHA) and research has found patients with autism, schizophrenia and bipolar disorder have low levels of AA in their system. Phospholipase A2 (PLA2), that releases AA from the cell membranes over-reacts and leaches it from the brain.

On the other hand, adequate amounts and activation may help preserve cognitive health in early stage Alzheimer's disease.[30]

When present in adequate amounts it helps maintain hippocampus cell membrane fluidity. Chronic inflammation activates PLA2, as do bio-toxins, heavy metals, aspartame and high levels of insulin. AA is adequately supplied by organic sources of meat, eggs and dairy products.

Omega-3 fatty acids include docosahexaenoic acid (DHA) and eicosapentaenoic acid (EPA) found in fish oils, such as cod, wild salmon, mackerel, herring and sardines. The roe (eggs) of various fish are our richest source of DHA. The optimal ratios of EPA/DHA for various brain-related conditions are covered later.

My grandfather Maxwell Webber lived his entire 92 years on the south shore of Nova Scotia. When I was a young child he often told me people living in the province were smarter because they ate a lot of fish. He was right!

As a young boy I was fed a teaspoon of cod liver oil each day during the winter months, and really disliked the taste. Not only does it provide a good combination of omega-3 fatty acids but vitamins A and D. Both of these fat-soluble vitamins show benefit in brain health, and the latter is very important for patients with multiple sclerosis.

Unlike fish oil it is produced strictly from the cod liver. One teaspoon (4.5 grams) contains 4500 IU of vitamin A, 450 IU of vitamin D, one gram each of saturated and polyunsaturated fatty acids and two grams of monounsaturated oil. The ratio is about 8:10 EPA to DHA, as opposed to a fish oil ratio of 3:2.

For several years I lived in northern Alberta in a log cabin without electricity, or running water. There was a freshwater fishing industry in the nearby small town, and I would go down on days they were gutting whitefish, pickerel and walleye, and take home five gallon pails of the caviar. Fish roe is a rich source of omega-3s, a whopping 579 mg/ 100 grams. Only cold liver oil at 570 mg/100g is close. In third place are fresh, organic egg yolks, at a respectable 424 mg/100g.

The fishermen were unwittingly tossing this valuable resource in the town dump. It was a major food source for me, and to this day I enjoy flying fish roe and salmon roe when out for sushi.

A number of epidemiological studies have found omega-3s the primary nutrient to protect from cognitive decline and dementia.

One study of 6000 participants (65 years and older) found that those consuming low amounts of omega-3s had a 70% higher risk of developing Alzheimer's.[31]

This is not to suggest you cannot enjoy the occasional steak. In fact, organic, grass-fed beef and bison are rich in omega-3s, as well as conjugated linolenic acid (CLA); and without the hormones and antibiotics present in commercial animals.

Another important way to nurture our brains is with phospholipid-rich foods, including fish, crustaceans and chicken eggs.

Organic, range-free chicken eggs may be one of your best bang for your buck, nutritious foods. Found in 100 grams of egg yolk is 230 mg of Omega-3s and over 10,000 mg of phospholipids.[32]

Eggs contain choline, complete protein (all essential amino acids), a variety of vitamins and minerals, including lutein. Studies show no association between eating eggs and cardiac risk. A recent study suggested a link between higher intake of cholesterol OR eggs and increased cardiovascular risk.[33] Poached eggs retain higher levels of the phospholipids and lecithin for better health. Folate-enriched eggs are highly stable and suffer little or no loss with storage and cooking.[34]

Phospholipids are present in sweet peas, cucumbers, oats, barley and sunflower seeds.

Excess saturated animal fat consumption can cause inflammation, and restrict oxygen uptake in the brain. A study of the 6000 elderly mentioned above, found those consuming 13 grams of saturated fat daily were almost twice as likely to develop cognitive decline. This would be the equivalent of three slices of bacon daily.

Organic meats and dairy can be part of a healthy brain diet. Organic dairy, including lactic-acid fermented kefir and yogurt provide us with a healthy ratio of unsaturated to saturated fats.

I am a big fan of organic butter. One study found that residents of New Zealand consume five times more butter than Americans, and yet have one-fifth the level of heart disease.

In clinical practice I suggested making better butter to clients; half, unsalted organic, grass-fed butter and half cold-pressed, organic flaxseed oil with lignins. After blending, it refrigerates well, with a soft texture. For those with dairy allergies, you can first make your own ghee that removes the allergenic milk proteins, casein and whey.

Butter contains butyrate, one of three short-chain fatty acids produced by healthy intestinal bacteria. Butryic acid is found in sweet potatoes, beans, nuts, and some fruits and vegetables, albeit in smaller amounts.

Coconut oil has become popularized in the past decade, for both ketogenic and vegan diets. Although a saturated fat, it does contain medium chain triglycerides (MCT) that are easily absorbed, metabolized by the liver, and can be converted to ketones. Ketone bodies are a source of alternative energy for the brain and thus useful for cognitive decline, including Alzheimer's disease (AD). It is suggested various cytokinins in coconut may prevent aggregation of amyloid-beta peptide involved in AD.[35]

I cannot recommend MCT derived from palm oil, partly due to the environmental damage caused by these plantations.

Saturated fats, from any source, are a problem when combined with simple sugars, carbohydrates and lack of fiber. You may choose to consume MCT for a few weeks and then switch to olive oil, nuts and avocados, if you like. This creates a mild ketosis and helps the conversion to a fat-based metabolism.

A prospective study on AD patients involved 40mL of coconut oil, taken daily for three weeks. Pre- and post-treatment test scores found positive improvement in memory.[36]

When broken down, coconut oil releases d-beta-hydroxybutyrate, a powerful anti-oxidant that stimulates the growth of new brain cells. Monolaurin and caprylic acid, in coconut oil, help dissolve pathogenic bacterial biofilm living on our gut lining. See Supplements for more information.

Lauric acid composes 50% of the fatty acids in coconut oil. This, in turn, is converted by the body into monolaurin.

Coconut oil and MCT oils may be helpful in Parkinson's disease (PD), ALS, Lewy body dementia, Huntington's disease (HD), autism, multiple sclerosis, myasthenia gravis, optic neuropathy, vascular dementia, and Down syndrome (trisomy 21).

However, there are a number of rare genetic disorders in which ketone dietary interventions are contraindicated. Individual research for your particular health concern will be useful.[37]

A recent study of 44 patients with AD found those given a coconut oil enriched Mediterranean diet for 21 days appeared to exhibit improved cognitive function.[38]

It is imperative that the oil be virgin, and never hydrogenated. Avoid coconut oil that has undergone any heat, solvent extraction or refining.

A low carbohydrate diet, supplemented with MCT (one teaspoon), or coconut oil (one teaspoon or more, three times daily) helps create mild ketosis. One helpful item is a ketone meter which measures ketone beta-hydroxybutryate. They can be easily purchased online.

I should include a brief mention about trans fats. They are convenient, toxic and cheap; and should be banned from commercial foods and all kitchens. Butter spreads contain trans fats, as present regulations allow foods containing 0.49 grams per serving to list zero on the food label. Avoid them whenever possible.

The brain, as I mentioned before, makes its own cholesterol. In fact, nearly all of it in the first few weeks of life with major help from nutrients in breast milk. It makes very small amounts in the adult brains, as the blood-brain barrier prevents its passage. Neurons do require cholesterol and depend upon LDL, or low-density lipoprotein to transport it to the brain. LDL is often called "bad cholesterol" but there is nothing bad about it. In fact it is not even a cholesterol molecule!

It is a myth that cholesterol-rich foods affect your brain function or cardiovascular health. What is true, however, is that low blood cholesterol levels have been noted in criminals with aggressive and violent personalities, people prone to suicide, and other anti-social behavior.[39]

Several studies, each with up to ten thousand patients, suggest hypercholesterolemia in midlife, increases chances of dementia, by up to three times, later in life. Even borderline high levels (220 mg/dL) nearly double the risk of Alzheimer's. This may be related to inflammation, causing plaquing and hardening of arteries that supply vital oxygen to the brain.

The Great Cholesterol Myth by J. Bowden and S. Sinatra is a worthwhile read, and one I recommend to my students.

Many people with "high cholesterol" do not have vascular issues, and people with normal levels may suffer serious cardiovascular disease. Vascular disease can cause vascular dementia associated with numerous small strokes.

The over-prescribing of statin drugs, to lower cholesterol levels, harms the brain by depleting our coenzyme Q10 and fat-soluble antioxidants. The drugs inhibit the production of low density lipoproteins and suppress neurotransmitter precursors. Crestor and Lipitor are small enough to cross the BBB and interfere with the brain's ability to make its own necessary cholesterol. And studies show they interfere with memory.[40]

Dale Bredesen writes. "So measuring total cholesterol to assess cardiovascular risk is like counting people in each home to estimate how many criminals there are: of course some homes will have only a few inhabitants, of whom most are criminals."[41]

Well said! See Chapter 5 for more specifics on fats and oils.

FOOD ALLERGIES AND SENSITIVITY

Tracking down specific food allergies can be difficult. There are a plethora of testing methods available that are both expensive and time consuming.

Suffice to say that when a suspected food is consumed, the body will respond with a histamine or mast cell response within thirty minutes. It may be subtle, and small signals are often ignored.

The Pulse test can help determine which foods to avoid in a quick and efficient manner. I used this in my own clinical practice with good success.

Write down your six favorite foods, ones that you could not imagine giving up. Avoid them for four days. Then take your sitting pulse rate, eat just one food raw or cooked, and take your pulse again in a half hour. If it goes up 10% you are allergic or sensitive to that food. If it rises 15%, you are highly affected and the food, and any derivatives, should be restricted until health improves. This does not mean the offending food can never be eaten again in a lifetime. As your gut and mental health improve, another test can be conducted in 2-3 months and re-assessed.

Remember, the test is free. You are running the show.

The top seven foods related to allergic or sensitivity responses in North America are dairy, wheat, soy, corn, eggs, peanuts, tree nuts and seafood.

One exception to dairy may be whey protein. Fermented soy may also be useful, but again, testing first for individual, allergic response is imperative.

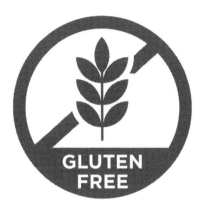

Gluten in grains, and casein in milk are poorly digested in people suffering brain health. Gluteomorphin and casomorphin peptides have been detected in the urine of patients with schizophrenia, autism, post-partum psychosis, ADHD, epilepsy, depression and Down's syndrome. The peptides travel through the leaky blood-brain barrier and block parts of the brain in a manner similar to morphine, heroin and other opioids.

A strict gluten-free diet may create withdrawal symptoms until the addiction is kicked.

Dr. Tom O'Bryan, in his excellent book *You Can Fix Your Brain*, suggests a few tips to lessen withdrawal symptoms.

Stay hydrated, stay calm and keep moving. He suggests seasoning your food with more sea salt than normal. Leg cramps are not unusual with gluten or dairy withdrawal, and a little extra salt, even tasting if on your tongue, can help. Of course, those on sodium-restricted diets for hypertension should consult their practitioner.

There are entire books written on gluten intolerance and cross-reactivity in the brain leading to autoimmunity with synapsin, located on neurons that regulate neurotransmitter release.[42]

Gluten can trigger immune reactivity to transglutaminase-6 (TG6), leading to destruction of brain and nervous tissue. TG2 is found in intestinal tissue in celiac disease, and TG3 is found in the skin, causing herpetic-like dermatitis.

Transglutaminase is widely used in the food processing industry, to tenderize meat, and is the "meat glue" or "pink slime" holding processed meats together. Some commercial beef patties contain up to 10% pink slime.

Glycoalkaloids in the Nightshade family of plant food over-stimulate our nervous system and should be tested for, and eliminated from the diet if an allergic concern. Tobacco is included in this list, as well as eggplant, potato, tomato, chili, gooseberry, goji berry and tomatillo.

When peptides of poorly digested food stick to your tissue they form neo-epitopes, which the immune system recognizes as an invader. It responds by producing antibodies; resulting in inflammation.

Agglutinins in potato, for example, form eno-epitopes to skin, thyroid and kidney tissue. Tomato develops eno-epitopes in the parietal cells of the stomach that produce hydrochloric acid, and the brush border of the intestinal lining.

However, solanidines, one of the glycoalkaloids, are the only plant food compounds known to inhibit both acetylcholine and butrylcholinesterase, both *in vitro* and *in vivo*. Some individuals stop eating nightshades without recognizing their potential benefit in AD and other cholinergic related conditions.

The potential interaction with other natural or pharmaceutical cholinesterase inhibitors remains to be considered.[43]

Lentils, peas and beans are excellent food for most people. They contain high protein, soluble fiber and a vast array of vitamins, minerals and nutrients. However, when poorly digested they can form neo-epitopes, and create immune response, antibodies and the resultant inflammatory conditions.

Soy bean agglutinin can bind to our skin, inside the mouth, parietal cells, brush border of intestine, thyroid, cartilage, liver, skeletal muscle, breast, and eye. Lentils react to tissue of the skin, mouth, lining of large intestine, connective tissue, thyroid, kidney, prostate and myelin of brain. Peas can trigger neo-epitopes in connective tissue, skeletal muscle and eyes. Kidney beans also exhibit a wide range of reactivity.

Use the Pulse test to determine your individual response.

PROTEIN

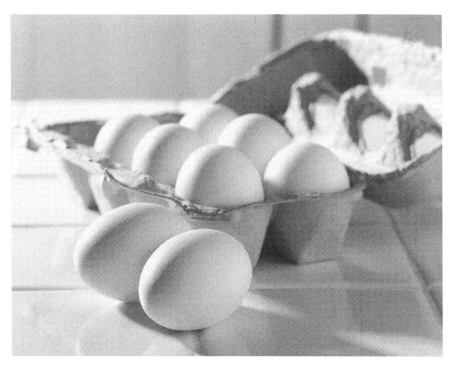

Protein is broken down to provide essential amino acids. So-called non-essential amino acids can be manufactured in the brain, whereas essential amino acids must be derived from our diet.

Our brain contains some 80 billion cells called neurons that do not touch each other, but have axons ending in synapses with a small gap. Each neuron has one thousand to ten thousand synapses, totaling 100 trillion in total.[44]

Neurotransmitters send electric impulses across these synapses. Some of the most important ones are serotonin, dopamine, GABA (gamma-aminobutyric acid) and its cousin glutamate; as well as acetylcholine. These neurotransmitters, and others, play a key role in memory and brain health. Each of them are discussed in detail, in chapter four.

Whey protein supplementation, if no allergic response, may be useful in Parkinson's disease. It is rich in cysteine and branched-chain amino acids that increase glutathione production and reduce homocysteine.[45]

Whey protein isolate (Immunocal®) helped ameliorate deficits in a mouse model study of schizophrenia.[46]

Unfermented soy, like other beans, peas and lentils, contain phytates that slow down absorption of nutrients. Many individuals react negatively to soy products due to early introduction in baby formulas. Unusually high glutamate foods include processed foods, casein, corn and soy protein, gelatin and the artificial sweetener aspartame.

Proteins exposed to sugar and charred, like crème brûlée or bbq chicken, form advanced glycation end products that tear openings in our gut and blood brain barrier (BBB).[47]

Your brain usually self repairs in four hours.[48] But if the assaults continue, then more macromolecules can enter, causing glial and microglial cells to over-react, create inflammation and then even larger antibodies can enter.

First comes a leaky gut, followed by leaky brain. Then a toxin, be it food, bacteria or chemical, stimulates a response from the immune system to protect you. These toxins look like your own tissue, so the antibodies attack, and things get progressively worse.

Two standard biomarker tests widely used in emergency rooms can help you identify BBB issues. They are called $S_{100}B$[9] and neuron-specific enolase (NSE). If elevated, you are leaking them into your bloodstream, and elevated antibodies to these markers indicate BBB defenses are compromised.

This can manifest symptoms in various neurological conditions including ADHD, seizures, anxiety, depression, schizophrenia, bipolar and unipolar disorder, dementia, Alzheimer's and Parkinson's disease.

CARBOHYDRATES

"Neurons are living cells with a metabolism. And they require glucose in order to function. Glucose is the fuel of the brain, just as gasoline is the fuel of your car."

DANIEL LEVITIN

Well maybe not, if you drive an electric vehicle.

Your brain needs glucose. At the same time, however, it is important to keep blood sugars level down, and this involves pancreatic production of insulin. Refined sugars, eaten over a period of time, exhaust our pancreas and decrease insulin sensitivity. Insulin resistance is the major reason for the present epidemic of type-two diabetes, where insulin is still produced, but blood sugar levels remain high.

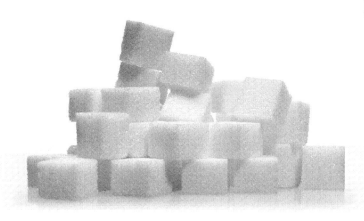

ALL REFINED SUGARS must be removed from your diet to attain optimal brain health. The average American consumes between 130-145 pounds of sugar and high-fructose corn syrup every year. There is a high correlation between sugar intake and depression.[49]

Complex carbohydrates, from grains and seeds such as brown rice, amaranth, quinoa, buckwheat and millet avoid gluten allergy issues, and provide a slow release of sugars that does not excessively spike insulin levels.

Insulin resistance sends too much glucose and insulin to the brain. This is why some health practitioners are calling Alzheimer's disease, "Type 3 diabetes."

In 2012, the *U.S. Department of Health and Human Services* estimated at least 86 million American adults over twenty years of age, suffer insulin resistance or pre-diabetes.[50]

Thirty years ago I taught courses at the University Hospital in my hometown, including the concept of pre-diabetes. On one occasion a MD challenged me that, suggesting there was no such thing; you were either diabetic or not! That was simply a reflection of the poor training MDs receive on nutrition. Today, many universities and medical schools cannot fit one day of nutritional training into a seven-year program. Hopefully, this will change.

But now, let's get back to glucose. Other sugars such as fructose and sucrose (white sugar); as well as lactose (milk) are transformed into glucose when needed.

The entry of glucose into our brain is tightly controlled. Glucose is quickly used, and any extra is stored as glycogen, which may create a one-day reserve at the very most.

If glucose levels are low, the brain turns to the liver to burn adipose fat and produce ketone bodies.

It may surprise you to find rich sources of glucose are readily available. One small beet contains 31% of all the glucose your brain requires for one day. Other great sources are green onions (one of my favorites), turnips and rutabaga, and kiwi fruit. Honey contains glucose and fructose, while maple syrup contains sucrose with some glucose and fructose. Raw, organic honey contains vitamin C, B3, folate and B6, and the minerals selenium and fluoride; but maple syrup supplies more minerals such as iron, zinc and manganese. I like to use both in moderation.

How much glucose does the brain need? A 150-pound adult needs about 62 grams of glucose over twenty-four hours. Three tablespoons of raw honey will do this, whereas it would take sixteen pounds of chocolate chips to achieve the same level.[51]

It is important to understand your food's glycemic index. This is a measure of how quickly food metabolizes into sugar. A low score indicates a low rise of blood sugar. Glycemic load looks at both sugar response and the amount of fiber a food contains.

Many years ago I worked as an herbal consultant for *New Era Nutrition*. They produce energy bars, and hit the right market by introducing SoLo bars, based on low glycemic effect. In my estimation, they are a great alternative to the plethora of high fructose/sucrose sugar bars on the market today.

Fructose, specifically high-fructose corn syrup (HFCS), is associated with blood sugar issues, insulin resistance, elevated cholesterol and hypertension. The effect is not immediate but problems develop over time. The average American consumes 80 grams of fructose daily, often in the form of HFCS.

Synthetic sugars are a significant detriment to gut flora, and hence our brain health. The bacteria found in the guts of humans that regularly consume sucralose, saccharin and aspartame are very different. The individuals weigh more, and exhibit higher fasting blood sugar levels. A French study of 66,000 women over twenty years, found the risk for diabetes more than doubled for those drinking artificial sweetened drinks, than those consuming sugar beverages.[52]

Long-term consumption of aspartame leads to an imbalance in anti-/pro-oxidant status of brain, via reduction of the antioxidant glutathione.[53] Aspartame (Equal, NutraSweet) breaks down into compounds such as phenylanine and formaldehyde. Sucrolose (Splenda) intake has been associated with leukemia, raises blood sugar levels and contributes to decreased insulin sensitivity. Sucrolose is metabolized like PCBs and dioxins, both of which have the potential of causing direct toxic effects. Sucrolose may induce glucose intolerance by affecting our gut flora.[54]

Splenda promotes the growth of harmful bacteria that increase weight gain, kill beneficial bacteria, and block absorption of prescription drugs.[55]

Saccharin (Sweet & Low) and Neotame should be avoided.

Aspartame and saccharin intake is linked to obesity, diabetes and cancer.

Stevia, extracted from the South American leaf, is 200-300 times sweeter than sugar and does not affect our blood sugar levels.

Stevia and Lakanto (made from erythritol and monk fruit) are considered two of our safer zero calorie sweeteners. Erythritol is readily absorbed and is not metabolized by gut flora.

I am not a fan of agave nectar. It measures low on the glycemic index due to its high levels of fructose, even more than high fructose corn syrup. Both sources are associated with onset of type 2 diabetes and non-alcoholic fatty liver.

Trehalose, a unique sugar derived from mushrooms and conifer saps, may be useful in treating Huntington's and Parkinson's disease.

NOTE: The current, and trendy, ketogenic or keto diet is rich in saturated fats, low in carbs and fiber, making the liver burn all available sugars before turning to fat to stabilize blood sugar levels. The brain can use ketones in place of glucose, but this is an exception not the rule.[56] This mechanism is meant for survival starvation situations, not to simply lose weight.

The research is incomplete but preliminary studies have found no significant benefit of a keto diet for Alzheimer's or Parkinson's disease.[57] Some animal models and pre-clinical studies suggest some benefit in the former, possibly due to lowered carbohydrate intake. The quality of the fats (Omega-3s) used in future, specific studies may show more promising results.

The brain needs glucose, as seen from cases of hypoglycemia.

VITAMINS

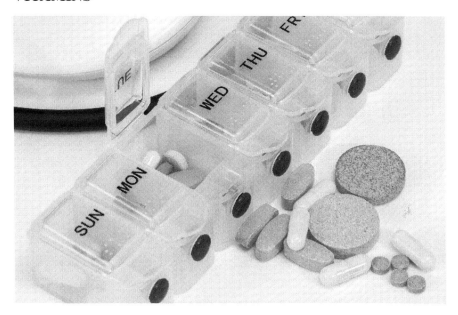

""Pop music is aspirin, and the blues are vitamins.""

PETER TORK

Vitamin supplementation, according to medical journals and popular media suggest they are not needed, are deadly in more than government recommended dosage, or more research is needed for your medical doctor to prescribe.

Unfortunately, this is all based on ignoring the past 75 years of laboratory and clinical studies on nutrient therapy.

There have been no recorded deaths from vitamin supplements over a 28 year period, despite over 60 billion doses of vitamins and mineral supplements taken each year.

Vitamin A is really a complex of various carotenoids and related yellow, orange fat-soluble products. High dose beta-carotene found in many multi-vitamin formulations was found to increase the risk of lung cancer in tobacco smokers.[58]

People with brain health issues cannot use synthetic forms of vitamin A efficiently. Cod liver oil source is preferred. Toxicity claims for vitamin A are greatly exaggerated. It would take 20 teaspoons of cod liver oil every day for weeks or months to create problems. One teaspoon daily is not a problem.

Various carotenoids, including beta-carotene, beta-cryptoxanthin lycopene, lutein, and zeaxanthin offer much value to brain and eye health.

Lutein and zeaxanthin show benefit in retinal health, and cognitive benefit in older adults. Forty-eight seniors were assigned 10 mg of lutein and 2 mg of zeaxanthin, or placebo, for one year. The supplements facilitated the aging brain's capacity for compensation by enhancing integration between networks that tend to be functionally segregated earlier in lifespan.[59]

Zinc, it should be noted, is critical for retinol-binding protein (retinol to retinal), necessary for vitamin A transport.

Both ADHD and autism spectrum disorder individuals may suffer convergence insufficiency, and may benefit from a neuro-visual optometrist. This correction in vision can improve attention, energy and mood.

A previous study found the two phyto-nutrients influence white matter integrity, especially in regions vulnerable to age-related decline.[60]

Lutein is found in spinach, kale, and egg yolk, as well as supplements derived from marigold flowers.

It helps protect dopaminergic neurons, suggesting benefit in the treatment of PD.[61]

Lycopene, particularly rich in cooked tomato products, but also papaya and watermelon, prevents neurotoxicity induced by MSG, methyl mercury and cadmium. It has prophylatic and/or therapeutic benefit in AD, PD, HD, epilepsy and depression. Lycopene may also be beneficial for alcohol addiction.[62]

The fat-soluble vitamins A, D, E and K should be taken with meals, containing good oils, for their optimal absorption.

Micellized A, D and E are water-soluble forms especially useful for mal-absorption problems, including celiac disease. In the intestine, micelle formation occurs via bile salts to allow absorption of fat-soluble vitamins.

I found micellized vitamins particularly useful in clinical practice, especially for intestinal and liver insufficiency.

Synthetic vitamin A palmitate is found in dairy products and commercial foods. Fish oil A is preferred, as it contains balanced vitamin D. Beta-carotene may be taken with vitamin A, as carotenoids only convert to vitamin A when body stores are low.

Generally speaking, most people benefit from a good quality B complex vitamin regime.

One study has found cognitive benefit of B vitamins dependent upon higher plasma levels of omega-3 fatty acids.

This ten year systematic review of randomized controlled trials identified four studies linking vitamin B supplementation to benefit in cognition.[63]

The water-soluble B vitamins, especially B1, B2, B3, B5, B6, B12 and folate, are important for brain health.

A complete B complex supplement; along with Omega-3s, is a great start to preventing brain aging and dementia.

Elevated homeocysteine levels, related to cardiovascular health, are significantly reduced by water-soluble B vitamins. Many studies suggest B vitamins protect against age-related dementia. One randomized, double-blind, placebo-controlled trial of high B supplementation in 85 patients with mild cognitive impairment was conducted over two years. At the end, homocysteine levels were normalized, and there was a 53% reduction in brain shrinkage.

Folic acid was added to processed food in 1998.

B1 was the first vitamin discovered, while biotin (below) did not receive a recommended intake until 1980, forty years after its discovery.

Thiamine, B1 plays a key role in the production of acetylcholine and GABA in the brain. Thiamine needs increase with smoking, alcohol consumption and age.

B1 deficiency has been linked to diabetes since 1940, in work by Kaufman. Benfotiamine is a synthetic, fat-soluble version that is 3.6 times more bioavailable and helps alleviate neuropathy in type 2 diabetes. Thiamine absorption is decreased by thiaminase 1 enzyme, found in sushi, alcohol, tea and coffee.

Riboflavin (B2) is equally important. Recent studies have found individuals with MTHFR and elevated homocysteine, also exhibit riboflavin deficiency. Vitamin B2 deficiency is considered rare. And yet a recent UK study found 75% of boys, 87% of girls, and 41% of adults showed blood markers of poor riboflavin status.

Older tricyclic antidepressants deplete B2.

Organ meats such as organic liver, kidney and heart are major sources, as are almonds, and lesser amounts are found in eggs, mushrooms, sesame seeds and seaweed. Make sure your multi-B contains adequate amounts.

Niacin (B3) is critical to our nervous system, and mitochondria production of energy. Under stress, we use up niacin and if not available our body makes it from tryptophan at a high cost, by converting 60 mg into 1 mg of niacin.

Mitochondrial cellular death is involved in PD, multiple sclerosis (MS) and dementia.[64]

Niacin supplementation may be useful in AD and has shown promise in the treatment of MS.

Tryptophan is used to make serotonin so a deficiency can greatly affect mood and brain function.

Niacin helps regeneration of glutathione and vitamin C, and supports glutamate metabolism. It is involved in over 500 biochemical processes in the human body.

Diuretics, tetracycline, alcohol, and anti-depressants increase niacin deficiency. Niacinamide does not cause the uncomfortable flush induced by niacin; is important in energy metabolism, and produces a calming effect. Niacinamide protects the brain neurons.

Dr. Hoffer recommended niacin be taken immediately after a meal. The uncomfortable niacin flush is a sign of its benefit. The more you can take without flushing, suggested a greater need. For some schizophrenia patients the range may be from 1500 to 6000 mg daily in three divided doses. A good health practitioner can assist in the proper dosage, especially in those with history of excessive alcohol abuse, liver conditions, diabetes or pregnancy. One randomized controlled trial found niacin was effective in benzodiazepine withdrawal.

Pantothenic acid (B5) possesses strong anti-histamine effect, making it indispensable for under-methylated autistic children, with IgE allergies, including asthma, eczema, itchy eyes, runny nose and dark circles under the eyes.

One subset of ASD children suffer from adrenal hypofunction, and B5 helps support adrenal cortisol function. It combines well with vitamin C and quercitin for anti-histamine and allergy support.

NOTE- B5 interferes with the efficacy of tetracycline, and is depleted by alcohol and diuretics. A recent study suggested B5 increases beta-amyloid in 49 AD patients with subjective and mild cognitive impairment. However, this was based on a food frequency questionnaire making the observation highly debatable.[65]

Vitamin B6 (pyridoxine) is essential for the production of neurotransmitters serotonin, dopamine and GABA, and must be consumed on a daily basis for optimal benefit. It absorbs best when taken with magnesium.

In 1965, Dr. Bernard Rimland promoted B6 therapy for autism, despite much ridicule from segments of the scientific community. Sadly, it often takes a minimum of one generation for science to be integrated into medical practice.

B6 is crucial to enable glutamate decarboxylase to convert glutamate into calming GABA. This imbalance is found in autism and children with ADHD.

Rich sources include pistachio and sunflower seeds, various animal proteins and fish (especially tuna), garlic and various cabbage family choices.

There are six forms of B6, found in grains, vegetables and fruit, but in a combination that reduces bioavailability.

Pyridoxine-5-phosphate is a more active form, affecting more than 100 enzymes. Caution is advised in patients with phenol sensitivity or intolerance due to defective sulphation, or hypermethylation, which can cause irritability.

It is best taken with magnesium, and should be taken along with a complete B complex.

In clinical practice I found B6 useful for depression in peri-menopausal women and in PMS, especially those women suffering chin line acne before menstruation.

Biotin is the forgotten B vitamin. And yet it is important for maintaining healthy gut flora, neurological function, and preventing behavioral disorders, learning disabilities, seizures, skin conditions that look like dermatitis or eczema, and unusual facial fat distribution on the face (biotin-deficient facies).

Repeated courses of antibiotics deplete biotin-producing flora leading to candida and fungal overgrowth.

In clinical practice I recommended biotin in cases of yeast overgrowth and intestinal dysbiosis, due to its ability to strengthen leaky gut walls; and keep yeast in a less invasive form. This helps eradicate the overgrowth more easily.

NOTE- in some rare cases, biotin deficiency is associated with digestive enzyme deficiency, but the use of antibiotics, valproic acid (epilepsy), and lack of magnesium and B5, all aggravate biotin deficiency.

Methylcobalamin (B12) contains cobalt and plays a critical role in the methylation folate cycle, converting homocysteine to methionine. Deficiencies may result from low stomach acid, celiac disease, pernicious anemia, a lack of intrinsic factor (absorption), overgrowth of anaerobic bacteria in the gut, antacids, diuretics, anti-seizure medications, neomycin or hormone therapy.

Symptoms of deficiency include neurological symptoms, fatigue, memory loss, mood disorders, depression, and low monocyte levels.

Since under-methylation is found in 95% of ASD, supplementation is vital. One subset of ASD involves lymphonodular ileal hyperplasia, affecting the lining of the small intestine. In this case, B12 deficiency is even more prevalent.

Vegans and vegetarians exhibit more B12 deficiency compared to omnivores.[66] This can easily be determined by a simple blood test. Supplementation of B12, due to decreased levels of homocysteine, may help delay progression of multiple sclerosis.[67]

NOTE- Methylcobalamin is better for supplementation than cyanocobalamin, the most common form in many B complex formulas. Why would anyone choose to take a cyanide-based vitamin?

Sublingual forms are well absorbed. If not, then subcutaneous injections may be required. Best to be taken in the morning.

Many B-complex vitamins contain folic acid. This synthetic form is not only poorly used, but amounts above 400 mcg can actually shut down the critical folate cycle. There are several natural forms of folate available in supplement form; folinic acid, and 5-methyltetra-hydrofolate (5-MTHF). Up to 40% of individuals with a MTHFR genetic variant, are not able to utilize even these forms, and it should be introduced very slowly. Folinic acid is a better choice for addressing this genetic variant that can only be identified with a DNA test. Without folate, the methylation cycle cannot be completed and brain health will suffer.

Methylation is a critical process, turning on or off gene expression, developing neurotransmitters, building flexible cell membranes, and producing creatine for energy.

Supplementation of processed foods containing folic acid is problematic. Without adequate B12, the conversion to methyltetrahydrofolate does not happen. Too much folic acid in the body and not enough B12 is linked to birth defects in babies, and memory problems in elders.[68]

Hypo-methylation occurs in more than 95% of people with autism, more than 99% in people with ADHD (with an oppositional defiant presentation), and 20-30% of other ADHD individuals. In autism (and to a lesser degree in ADHD), it is not uncommon to find a gene mutation MTHF reductase that makes individuals dependent upon therapeutic doses of these nutrients.[69]

The active metabolite of folate (5-MTHF), or folinic acid, re-methylates homocysteine, creating methionone, and then SAMe. It enhances production of tetrahydrobiopterin, an essential cofactor in monoamine (MAO) neurotransmitter biosynthesis.

Folate antagonists include alcohol, anti-seizure medication, diuretics, antacids, and tetracycline.

Sulfation, the addition of sulphur and amino acid, synthesizes glutathione (anti-oxidant) from homocysteine, helping repair gut walls, supporting mitochondrial function, and promoting T cell formation in the immune system.

When methylation stalls out, so does sulfation, which breaks down neurotransmitters when appropriate, and helps the liver with phase one and two detoxification. Hence the importance of sulfur rich foods in the diet, especially from the onion, legume and cabbage families. Magnesium (including Epsom salts- magnesium sulfate), alpha lipoic acid, selenium, zinc, N-acetyl cysteine, taurine and vitamins B2 and B3, all support sulfation and glutathione metabolism.

Phenol sulfotransferase enzymes metabolize phenols in healthy foods, but not the excessive phenolics in artificial colors, additives and salicylate medications. If the toxic load is more than the system can handle, your brain health will suffer.

Selenium is a trace mineral that requires methylation for metabolism, but is unique in that it substitutes for sulfur in cysteine, creating selenocysteine. This is important for metabolism, formation of glutathione, detoxification and methionine metal metabolism (zinc, copper and cadmium). It is depleted by the presence of heavy metals.

Low sulfation conditions are common in autism and to some degree in patients with ADHD.

A study of 502 patients, who added L-methylfolate to their anti-depressants, and 52 treated with the supplement only, found both groups achieved improvement in their symptoms.[70]

Depressed individuals with low serum folate do not respond well to SSRI drugs.[71]

L-methylfolate as an adjunctive therapy for SSRI-resistant major depression, showed benefit in two randomized, DB, parallel sequential trials.[72]

The presence of this gene may raise homocysteine levels, resulting in migraines. A recent study found folate, and vitamins B6 and B12, useful for migraine patients, particularly those suffering from migraine with aura.[73]

Fortunately, many leafy greens contain large amounts of folate, as well as legumes, eggs, beets and members of cabbage family. Spearmint, rosemary, basil, cilantro, marjoram and sage are herbs/spices rich in folates.

NOTE- Homocysteine levels should be less than 6 micromoles/liter.

Folate levels range from 2-20 nanograms/mL, with optimal greater than 3 ng/mL.

B12 normal levels range from 211-946 picograms/mL. Optimal levels are in mid-range of 500-600 or higher. Some practitioners recommend 1000-2000 due to high folic acid supplementation in processed foods, or difficulty with methylation.

Look for a product containing methylcobalamin, or hydroxycobalamin (1 mg daily) with a liposomal coating if available. B vitamin absorption is hindered by antacids, especially proton pump inhibitors.

The addition of trimethylglucine (glycine betaine) can be helpful if homocysteine levels remain high after following these steps.

We need Vitamin C on a daily basis and it is not produced in the human body. Fruits and vegetables are, of course, a rich source of ascorbic acid. Linus Pauling, a two time Nobel Prize recipient, was an advocate of large doses, due in part, to its water-soluble nature. He personally took 18 grams daily.

One study shows growing evidence of the importance of ascorbic acid in the prevention of AD, by reducing inflammation, inhibiting acetylcholinesterase, suppressing amyloid-beta peptide formation, and chelating iron, copper and zinc.[74]

Ascorbic acid is essential for increasing hippocampus neurogenesis, and improving memory function, critical to the aging brain.[75]

In the absence of vitamin C, nitrites and nitrates in preserved meats convert to nitrosamines. We all eat a sub or sandwich on the road once in a while, so pop a chewable vitamin C twenty minutes before eating and prevent the formation of this carcinogen in the gut.

Vitamin C is necessary for the manufacture of serotonin and dopamine. One hospital study found supplementing vitamins C and D helped ill patients, with a 71% reduction in mood disturbance and a 51% reduction in feeling distressed.[76]

Vitamin C is best taken as a time-released product so that small amounts are delivered over a twelve-hour time frame.

NOTE- nearly all vitamin C supplements derive from corn. It there is a corn allergy, try and find one derived from sugar beets (preferably not from GMO). Vitamin C supplementation is contraindicated in hemochromatosis (excess iron storage) and in G6PD deficiency associated with favism, an inherited disorder of red blood cells.

Vitamin D is not really a vitamin, but an active neurosteroid that plays a crucial protective role in the developing brain, immune modulation, and the regulation of neurotransmission.

We utilize sunlight to produce the precursor, from LDL cholesterol in our skin, which goes to the liver for conversion into active D3.

Ten minutes of sunlight exposure a day, on your arms and legs is all that is needed.

Vitamin D is generally taken for bone health but it has receptors through the entire nervous system, including brain neurons and glial cells. It regulates brain enzymes involved in neurotransmitters, stimulating nerve growth and reducing inflammation. When vitamin D enters a cell nucleus, it turns on over 900 genes.

Only two substances have receptor sites in every cell of your body; the thyroid hormone and vitamin D.

It influences the HPA axis, responsible for adaptation to stress.

A recent, 12 week, randomized, double-blind, placebo-controlled trial of sixty diabetics with coronary heart disease found vitamin D and probiotic supplementation improved blood sugar, cholesterol levels and showed a significant improvement on depression.[77] This includes seasonal affective disorder (SAD).

Prenatal deficiency is linked to autism, including a review of 11 studies.[78,79]

As well as ADHD.[80] This suggests that women considering getting pregnant be tested for vitamin D levels, and take a supplement if levels are low.

Vitamin D serum levels are lower during relapses in multiple sclerosis patients, suggesting supplementation is useful.[81]

Omega-3 fatty oils and vitamin D deficiency can lead to dysfunctional serotonin activation and may be one mechanism that leads to neuropsychiatric disorders, ADHD, bipolar disorder, schizophrenia, impulsive behavior and depression.[82]

Patients with vitamin D deficiency have been found to exhibit more than double the risk of getting Alzheimer's disease.[83]

Vitamin D modulates dendritic cell function that plays a key role in immune response, and auto-immune disease. Work at the University of Edinburgh found vitamin D helps regulate T cell formation associated with either fighting infection, or inappropriately attacking our own body tissue.

Vitamin D affects cognition, but taking high doses may be problematic. A DB randomized control trial of postmenopausal women found supplementation of 2000 IU daily for one year improved learning and memory, whereas those taking 4000 IU showed slower reaction times, than the group taking just 600 IUs daily.[84]

Health Canada and the Institute of Medicine in the United States have set 4000 IU as the upper intake level for adults and children over nine years of age. This is the amount you can take without supervision or blood tests. This amount may be on the low side.

I remember giving a lecture to third year medical students many years ago, and was roundly chastised by the professor at the time for suggesting everyone should take 800 IU daily. How times have changed!

Recently have we found vitamin D works through its regulation on gut flora. Our bacteria interact with vitamin D receptors to up or down regulate activity. Synthetic vitamin D is derived via a seven-step process from lanolin, obtained via sheep's wool. Vegans may choose vitamin D derived from medicinal mushrooms. Studies have found blood serum levels in humans the same, whether derived from mushrooms, or sheep lanolin. Cod liver oil is a rich source of vitamin D.

Fermented cod liver oil is preferred, due to industrial processing by many companies that use heat, pressure, solvents, bleaching and deodorization.

NOTE- Pharmaceuticals, including phenobarbial, dilantin, antacids, steroids and laxatives decrease vitamin D availability or absorption. A micellized D may be more useful in such cases.

One noticeable sign of deficiency is a painful scalp when you brush your hair.

VITAMIN E

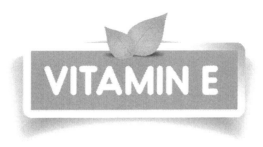

Vitamin E is beneficial in Parkinson's disease (PD). A mixed ratio of alpha, beta, gamma and delta tocopherols and tocotrienols is the preferred source. Many multi-vitamins contain alpha-tocopherol, which is a not representative of its full brain health potential. To avoid synthetic E look for l' or dl' prefix.

For too long researchers have considered alpha tocopherol the only form of vitamin E, worthy of study. Using only this form interferes with gamma-tocopherol, which is a better anti-oxidant against neurodegenerative disorders, and scavenges reactive nitrogen as well as oxygen species.

In autism, a combination of vitamin E with omega-3s shows benefit in promoting speech, and reducing excitotoxicity.

One study in Finland looked at patients 80 years and older, and found individuals with the highest blood serum levels of all 8 forms of vitamin E, also had the lowest risk of cognitive impairment.[85]

Natural sources include wheat germ, sunflowers, almonds, hazelnuts, peanuts, mangoes, spinach, broccoli and tomatoes.

VITAMIN K

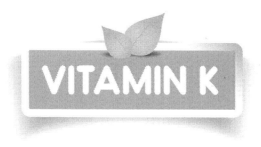

Vitamin K is a fat-soluble nutrient discovered in 1935. It plays a key role in blood coagulation and is unfortunately depleted by the use of warfarin, Coumadin and related blood-thinners.

Vitamin K affects sphinolipids metabolism that regulate proliferation, differentiation and survival of brain cells.[86]

Both vitamin K and D enhance the production of brain sulfatides during re-myelation of the nervous system; in an animal model of multiple sclerosis.[87]

A study of elderly patients found those with the highest dietary intake of vitamin K had the lowest levels of depression.[88]

WHAT THE BRAIN DOES NOT NEED

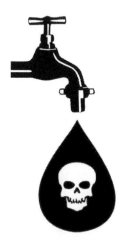

The brain loves minerals. Numerous toxic and heavy metals can interfere with the uptake of important minerals such as magnesium, zinc, iodine, selenium, manganese and potassium. Some minerals, such as iron, and copper are necessary, but when taken in larger amounts are contraindicated. Generally, adult males should avoid iron supplementation, as they do not have monthly cycles of bleeding that eliminate excess buildup.

In Supplement Chapter (15), we will look at magnesium, zinc and other minerals vital to our brain health. When our food was grown in mineral rich soils, this was not such an important issue. Trace minerals are not required for modern agriculture, and thus we are more likely to be deficient in these as well.

Copper reduces the brain's ability to clear toxic amyloid proteins before they form plaque associated with Alzheimer's. Even worse, research shows when diets are high in copper, as well as saturated and trans fats, people suffer roughly nineteen additional years of aging.[89] Copper water pipes are the most common source via our drinking water, but many multi-vitamin/mineral supplements contain high levels of copper and iron. Oral contraceptives increase copper and iron levels in women, creating zinc deficiencies. Small amounts of copper are necessary to balance zinc levels. Your red blood cell zinc should be 12-14 mg/dL.

However, with age comes lower zinc levels and those with AD often have very low zinc levels, making them more sensitive to harmful mercury and mycotoxins.

Zinc picolinate, alpha lipoic acid, vitamin C, B6 and avoidance of multi-vitamin/minerals with copper may be appropriate if tests show a copper overload.

Aluminum is widely found in everyday items such as baking powder, antacids, buffered aspirin, table salt, non-dairy creamers, baked goods, vaccines, antiperspirants, lipstick, cosmetics and various medications for depression and diarrhea.

It is widely used in cooking pots and pans, ensuring a daily amount is liberated and consumed.

The average adult consumes roughly 7-9 mg of aluminum per day in their food.[90] Levels are significantly higher in the brains of Alzheimer's disease patients and in the brains of those suffering Autism spectrum disorder.[91] The authors of these studies have been largely ignored or shunned by the larger scientific community. The aluminum theory and its association with AD has not yet been proven, but why take a chance.

Other problematic heavy metals include lead, cadmium, arsenic, chromium and mercury. Both cadmium and lead are linked to neuro-degeneration and learning disabilities, as well as violent behavior. Mercury has been linked to ADD, as well as memory and motor dysfunction. Fish at the top of food chain, dental fillings, fungicides, pesticides, and some vaccines contain mercury. A fetus can absorb mercury from its mother's blood and have concentrations 40% higher, with most coming from mom's inorganic mercury dental fillings. Methylmercury (organic mercury) destroys glutathione the body uses to reduce free radical damage.

Cadmium depresses the immune system and is found in traditional and electronic cigarettes, old water pipes, white bread and white rice. It acts with lead and arsenic to increase Alzheimer's-type changes in brain.

Arsenic is found in chicken (less in organic chicken), and groundwater. It affects the HPAA (hypothalamic-pituitary-adrenal axis) involved in various endocrine and hormonal issues, as well as AD.

Lead impairs cognitive function and leads to age-related cognitive decline.[92] Leaded gasoline and lead paints have been removed from the market, but other sources remain.

Mitochondria supply energy to our cells. They are descendants of bacteria that invaded our cells over a billion years ago. Numerous chemicals damage the ability of these powerhouses to convert energy and oxygen into ATP. The word *mitochondria* is derived from the Greek meaning "little granular thread". Antibiotics, statin drugs, L-DOPA, griseofulvin (anti-fungal), acetaminophen and other NSAIDs including aspirin and ibuprofen, cocaine, methamphetamine and AZT all damage our mitochondria.

MIND/BODY

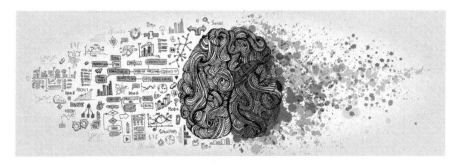

A number of studies suggest various mindful practices help reverse the expression of genes involved with inflammation, associated with stress. Yoga, Tai Chi, Qigong, breathing and related modalities down-regulate the nuclear factor kappa B pathway, the opposite of the effect of chronic stress.[93]

Drumming, for example, has been found in clinical studies to be helpful in those suffering anxiety, depression or symptoms of Parkinson's disease.[94]

Conscious trance states, induced by drumming, breathing, fasting, singing and psychoactive plants and mushrooms help us tune into subconscious or supraconscious states of mind. These practices help to increase brain plasticity and health.

A highly recommended book is *The Brain's Way of Healing* by Norman Doidge. It contains a plethora of remarkable natural therapies that can assist in making use of our brain's neuroplasticity.

HYPOTHALMIC-PITUITARY-ADRENAL AXIS

There are a plethora of books and health practitioners who suggest stress and anxiety are a major issue in brain health. I agree.

Constant complaining actually re-wires the brain for anxiety and depression.

Thyroid, adrenal and gonadal health play a critical role in supporting synaptic maintenance. Both under-functioning and over-reacting glandular dysfunctions occur throughout the entire endocrine and hormonal system.

Over 40% of women suffer from hyper- or hypothyroid function, especially during or after menopause. Tyrosine plus iodine (in small, but adequate amounts, produces thyroxin. Liver health will dictate to a large degree the conversion of T4 to T3, the active form the body requires.

Adrenal stress and exhaustion are often cited as the reason for fatigue, due to insomnia, long work hours, two-parent working lifestyle and other factors.

But the adrenals simply produce cortisol in response to the brain.

When elevated, blood sugar and insulin levels rise. Serotonin drops, leading to anxiety and depression. Chronic exposure to stress hormones kills hippocampus cells, especially when DHEA levels are low.

Stimulants such as coffee or caffeinated drinks in the morning, and alcohol, cannabis or medication to relax at night, exact their toll on adrenal health.

Many of the adaptogenic herbs, such as ashwaganda, rhodiola and holy basil impact the brain and hypothalamic-pituitary-adrenal axis (HPAA) and reduce the chronic production of cortisol that leads to exhaustion. See Medicinal Herbs chapter.

CHAPTER 2

THE MICROBIOME

"Am I simply a vehicle for numerous bacteria that inhabit my microbiome? Or are they hosting me?"

TIMOTHY MORTON

Only twenty years ago, it was widely believed there was little, or no relationship between our intestine and brain. *The Second Brain*[95] revelations opened my eyes to looking at the intestine in an entirely different way, and re-examining our mind-gut relationship.

This complex ecosystem contains trillions of bacteria, thousands of different species, and has evolved over time as a mutualistic relationship.

In fact, if you look at the tube running from our mouth to rectum, it resembles the hole in a donut. It is part of us, but is entirely separate for a number of reasons.

This microbiota-gut-vagus-brain axis involves bidirectional signaling that modulates behavior and influences mental disorders.[96]

Without the vagus nerve, various neurotransmitters would not make it to our brain. Unless, that is, the blood brain barrier is compromised.

Our brain communicates with the enteric nervous system (ENS) via the vagus nerve. The word is derived from the Latin meaning "wandering", which it does to all organs of the body. It carries information from the brain, to brainstem and then to ENS and vice-versa.

Microbiome health influences our immune and endocrine systems, the hypothalamic-pituitary-adrenal (HPA) axis, and neurotransmitter pathways.

As the brain loses health, digestion is first affected and then our bowel and bladder. Seniors requiring diapers, later in life, is a good example. This is also true in babies, where the gut-brain axis is not fully developed at birth, and they cannot control bowel and bladder until their digestive functions develop.[97]

An impaired vagus nerve can be related to a leaky gut, leading to poor absorption of nutrients, but permitting the passage of undigested proteins, as well as bacteria, fungus and other pathogens into the bloodstream.

The vagus nerve raises the uvula, the dangling tissue at the back of our throat. When your doctor opens your mouth, they are looking for it to rise, and if the vagus nerve is weak, the rise is little or none. However, very few MDs use this important indication to strengthen digestion and brain function.

Dr. Kharrazian recommends a few exercises to help strengthen our vagus nerve. Gargle with four large glasses of healthy water. Sing loudly, or use tongue depressors to stimulate the gag reflex. "Gag reflexes are like doing push-ups for the vagus, while gargling and singing loudly are like doing sprints," he writes.[98]

Nine times more information travels from the gut to the brain, than in the opposite direction. And the food we eat can have a profound effect on messaging, the very same day.

The blood-brain barrier (BBB) was believed, not that long ago, to prevent pathogens entering the brain. Meningitis was dismissed as a rare exception, and syphilis and Lyme disease (spirochetes) cause severe brain damage and cognitive impairment.

We are already aware HIV-1 related to AIDS can create a form of dementia, with symptoms that mimic Alzheimer's. The *herpes simplex* virus causing cold sores can trigger brain encephalitis.

We now understand various bacteria exist in the human brain, based on recent work by Roberts et al.[99]

Glial cells are extremely important for brain health. They are the non-neuronal cells of the nervous system, outnumbering neurons by 10:1. When first discovered, they were believed to form structure, hence *glia* meaning, "glue". They play a key role in information processing in our brain and spinal cord.

Microglia protect brain cells by sending inflammatory cytokines to destroy pathogens and cellular debris. This inflammation causes oxidative stress and damages neurons. They are our brain's immune cells, providing the first line of defense against pathogens and injury. When called upon, they move to damaged sites and surround and internalize them in a process known as *phagocytosis* meaning, "cell eating". Complement proteins tag unwanted neural-synaptic connections. The microglia take this as a signal to eat them. Synaptic pruning is useful in the developing and adult brain, getting rid of no longer desired synaptic connections.

Oligodendrocytes coat our connector neurons (axons) with myelin, a protective coating. These are highly susceptible to oxidative stress.

Astrocytes make up majority of our glial cells and form part of the BBB, process sensory information, supply nutrients and glutathione to neurons, and both release, and destroy excitotoxic glutamate. An excess of glutamate, and insufficient calming GABA, can result when our astrocytes are overwhelmed by toxins.

Each astrocyte has small branches that contact hundreds of dendrites and up to 150,000 individual synapses.

Our gut bacteria play a key role in how we feel and think. Conditions such as anxiety and depression are very much influenced by the presence of friendly, or not so friendly bacteria.

But why do bacteria produce neurotransmitters? What is in it for them? Do they want to control our food cravings?

Streptococcus bacteria, for example, love sugar and when you indulge in a sweet treat, they produce dopamine. We humans then connect sugar to happiness, and develop a craving.

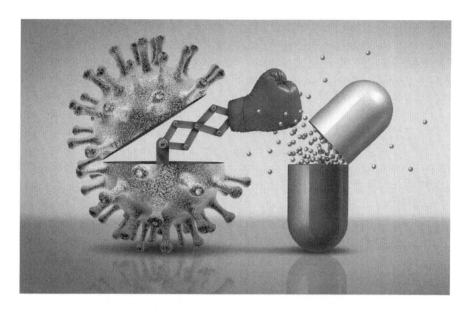

Various drugs have a significant negative effect on our gut flora.

Topping the list are antibiotics (meaning anti-life). Over 80% of the antibiotics produced in North America are not prescriptions for humans, but used to fatten livestock. In 2011, nearly thirty million pounds were fed to animals that later turn up on our plates.[100]

By the time the average American child turns eighteen, they have been prescribed ten to twenty courses of antibiotics. Studies show two years after a single dose of antibiotics our microbiomes are not yet back to normal.

In children, the number of antibiotics taken before age 5 shows a direct effect on intelligence (IQ).[101]

Antibiotics are widely prescribed before dental procedures. The long held myth patients with hip and knee replacements must always take them as a prophylactic, is not based on science. However, it may be prudent for patients in cases of prior infective endocarditis, prosthetic cardiac valves, congenital heart defects, shunts and other devices, and heart transplants.

Organic applesauce, chicken, fish, beef and bison bone broth, as well as pomegranate juice help heal the gut damage caused by antibiotics, and encourage the microbiome to rebuild healthy bacterial colonies.

The birth control pill depletes B6, a cofactor for the production of serotonin and GABA. Scientists have linked long-term use (over five years) to increased risk of Crohn's disease, by changing the permeability of our intestinal wall. One study of 233,000 women, conducted from 1976 to 2008, found a three-fold increased risk of this debilitating condition.[102]

Other factors that decrease healthy gut flora are proton pump inhibitors, steroids, NSAIDs, artificial and refined sugars, pesticides, alcohol, radiation, stress and high intensity exercise.[103]

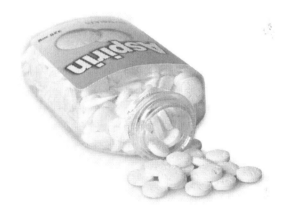

Two aspirin, for example, can cause a leaky gut.[104] In 2019, the American Heart Association withdrew their support of one-a-day 81 mg aspirin to prevent heart attacks, based on the science. One study found no obvious benefit to healthy people over 70 years old, but did find evidence of harm from bleeding and leaks of the stomach and brain. In brain scans of one thousand people taking aspirin, 70% had a higher chance of a brain bleed. Leaky gut and leaky brain create numerous brain health issues.

One study of 88,000 nurses found those who took two or more aspirins a week for twenty years had a 58% higher risk of pancreatic cancer. Those taking two or more daily had an 86% greater risk of this rare, but deadly cancer.[105]

Emulsifiers, such as carboxy-methylcellulose and polysorbate 80, thin gut mucosa and reduce the diversity of our microbiome.

Thinning the gut wall leads to leaky gut. Unfortunately, these two culprits are used in gluten-free foods, meaning celiac individuals are exposed to further damage.

In fact, only 8% of people with celiac disease heal completely on a gluten-free diet, and 65% feel better but still suffer inflammation of the intestine and permeability problems even on a gluten-free regime.[106]

Food companies producing gluten-free products should be held accountable for their use of these harmful emulsifiers.

Both prebiotic and probiotic foods help restore a healthy gut microbiome.

Prebiotics such as fructo-oligosaccharides (FOS) and galacto-oligosaccharides (GOS) act as fuel for healthy bacteria, by encouraging their growth.

Examples of prebiotics include onions, artichokes, asparagus, jicama, Jerusalem artichokes, garlic, beets, fennel root, beans, lentils, endive, leeks, radishes, bananas and oats. The latter contain 1,4 beta glucans, that nourish healthy bacteria, and optimize our immune system.

Leeks are rich in folate and B6, and decrease homocysteine.

Radishes are one of my personal favorites. They are rich in magnesium and manganese, as well as B6. I wash and eat the radish leaves in salads. Why? Because they are rich in erucamide, a potent acetylcholinesterase inhibitor that may help prevent memory loss related to Alzheimer's disease.[107] Erucamide is a fatty acid amide, similar to the endocannabinoid analogue oleoylethanolamide. It regulates the HPA axis, and has a positive influence on depression and anxiety.[108]

The consumption of prebiotic foods is no small matter. It is estimated for every 100 grams of prebiotics consumed, 30 grams of healthy bacteria are produced.[109] This is very important as the life span of a gut microbe is only about twenty minutes.

Fortunately, there are an estimated 100 trillion bacteria in our gut, composed of at least 500 species.

Other examples of pre-biotic rich herbs include chicory, dandelion and burdock root. They are rich in inulin, an invert sugar that feeds healthy bacteria, but not the more harmful ones. Inulin helps us absorb calcium and magnesium, and in animal studies inhibits colon cancer.

Larch bark is rich in arabinogalactans that feed healthy bacteria, and modulate the immune system.

Fermented food, or more accurately, lactic acid fermentation, occurs when good bacteria convert sugar into lactic acid. This protects the fermented food from attack by harmful bacteria, due, in part, to lowered pH.

Nutrients from green leafy vegetables, just one serving per day, help slow cognitive decline.[110]

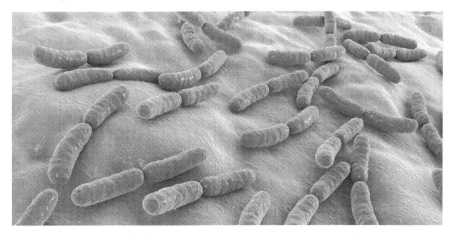

Lactobacillus and *Bifidobacterium* species play an important role in gut health.

They help maintain integrity of our gut lining, are natural antibiotics, anti-virals, and anti-fungals, control inflammation, and suppress the growth of pathogenic bacteria. Healthy bacteria help to produce short chain fatty acids and increase the availability of vitamins.

The three main short-chain fatty acids produced in the gut are acetate (60%), propionate (25%) and butyrate (15%). Propionate, when it propagates in an unhealthy microbiome, crosses the blood-brain barrier and is toxic to tissue.

Propionic acid, for example, induces autistic-like behavior in rats.[111] Both propionic and acetic acids are associated with elevated anxiety in irritable bowel syndrome (IBS).[112]

Butter contains butyrate, both words derived from the Latin *butyrum*. Butyrate is involved in immune modulation, the repair of our intestinal barrier; and reduces inflammation of colon mucosa. It may influence microbiome behavior via social communication.[113]

Of course, the right pre-biotics help increase butyrate levels, which improves insulin sensitivity.

Bifidobacterium produce butyrates that feed and heal the lining of your gut. Some butyrate makes its way to the brain where it reduces inflammation, induces good mood, and the production of brain growth hormones.

Root vegetables contain high levels of insoluble fiber that help encourage butyrate formation.

Butyrate inhibits histone deacetylases (HDACs) associated with various neurological disorders, including depression, neuro-degenerative diseases and mental cognition.

Butyrate-producing *Faecalibacterium* and *Coprococcus* bacteria are consistently associated with higher quality of life and lower levels of depression.[114]

Unhealthy gut flora allows *Actinomyces*, pathogenic *E. coli*, *Mycobacterium* and *Corynebacterium* species to thrive. These iron-loving organisms consume iron supplements, preventing benefit in cases of anemia; and actually make the microbiome health worse.[115]

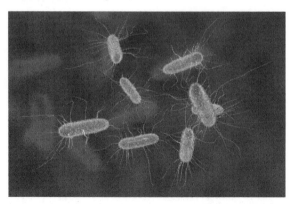

Not all forms of *E. coli* are harmful. In the colon this bacteria and *Streptococcus* produce serotonin, a major neurotransmitter. Serotonin dictates peristalsis of the bowel, which is why people taking SSRI medication, in low doses, suffer less constipation.

Clostridia species, especially *C. botulinum* and *C. difficile* thrive in a damaged microbiome, producing toxins similar to tetanus. These neurotoxins affect the brain and nervous system, causing sensitivity to light and noise; typical tetanus symptoms. Autism, schizophrenia, psychosis and dyslexia patients exhibit an abnormality of muscle tonus. Autistic spectrum children will walk on tiptoes or self-stimulate by stretching arms, fingers and legs in odd positions.[116]

Research at the University of Reading found high levels of *Clostridia* in the gut of 150 autistic children.[117]

Some Clostridia species, such as *Faecalibacterium prausnnitzii* are benign, eating oligosaccharides and producing butyrate fatty acid. It helps soothe Crohn's by muting an immune response.

Before introducing pre- and probiotics into our gut, it is important to heal the leaky lining. Taking probiotics prematurely lends itself to fragments entering the blood stream; and increasing inflammation.

Live cultured yogurts, kefir, tempeh, miso, beet kvass, kim chi and sauerkraut, pickled fruits and vegetables as well as cultured condiments are some of my personal favorites. Fermented foods are considered functional foods that alter gut physiology and impact anxiety and depression.[118]

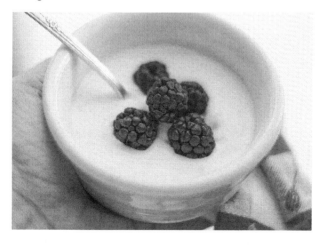

Fermented foods and beverages balance intestinal permeability and barrier function, influencing our moods, behavior, hormone balance, food cravings and brain health.[119]

A questionnaire of over 26,000 individuals aged 19 to 64 years old, assessed the relationship between probiotic food consumption and self-reported clinical depression. The results suggest they are beneficial for everyone, particularly men.[120]

Cultured dairy has been recommended for over a century for melancholia associated with intestinal distress. The introduction of *Lactobacillus bulgaricus* into the diet of psychiatric patients from England, helped alleviate their depression.

By 1917, there were 30 different probiotics on the U.S. market and by 1923, *Acidophilus* was recommended for psychoses.

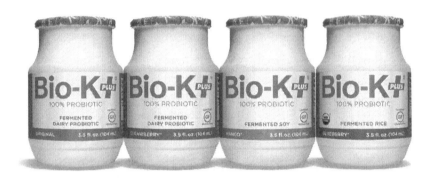

While in clinical practice in the 1990s, my probiotic of choice was Bio-K, a fermented, refrigerated product that comes in packs of 6 or 15. It is an excellent product, and contains *L. acidophilus*, *L. casei* group and closely related *L. rhamnosus*.

The latter has been found to interfere with the hyphal formation and adhesion to epithelial cells associated with Candida overgrowth.[121]

This product reduces incidences of antibiotic diarrhea and *Clostridium difficile* infection in human clinical trials.[122]

Spores of the latter bacterium are able to survive laundering in commercial washer extractors and may contribute to sporadic outbreaks, based on one UK study in 2018.

Today, a large variety of lactobacilli (Lacto) and bifidobacterium (Bifido) products are on the market; some especially useful for brain health. Over 200 species of *Lactobacillus* have so far been discovered. Vitamin D, it should be noted, enhances the benefit of active microbes in yogurt.

Fat-free yogurts do not contribute health benefit. In a study of 14,500 Spanish university studies, only a whole fat yogurt helped lower levels of depression.[123]

NOTE: A number of products on the market are unreliable. One study found only 4 of 13 probiotic products contained the strains claimed on the label. Well-formulated mixtures of Lacto and Bifido can be synergistic, while other strains can be competitive, reducing any benefit. Personal research is your best bet.

An excellent book, *The Psychobiotic Revolution*, shares a list of brands recommended by two world-renowned researchers working at the *APC Microbiome Institute*.[124]

LACTOBACILLUS

In some studies of individuals suffering irritable bowel syndrome, various Lactobacillus manipulate the opioid and cannabinoid receptors in the brain, acting like a shot of relaxing morphine.

Lactobacillus acidophilus is found in beneficial yogurts, and helps restore balance in women suffering yeast infections such as *Candida albicans*. It contains baceriocin that attacks pathogenic bacteria, reducing their small intestinal overgrowth.

It increases opioid and cannabinoid receptors, reducing gut pain.[125] It helps produce the neurotransmitters GABA and acetylcholine in the transverse colon.

Lactobacillus bacteria in the ileum produce B12, a deficiency of which can lead to mental health problems. It competes against the pathogenic *Campylobacter jejuni*, associated with gastric upset, by preventing its ability to stick to and infect the gut lining.[126] In turn, this reduces associated anxiety. This bacterium is one of the most common sources of food poisoning, resulting from undercooked chicken, and contaminated water.

It can be fatal in young children, the elderly and in immune-compromised people.

Lactobacillus acidophilus L-92 shows promise in relieving hay-fever and seasonal pollen allergies.[127]

L. acidophilus is present in yogurt, sauerkraut and kefir.

Lactobacillus brevis lives in sauerkraut and fermented pickles. It increases immunity and is most useful for vaginosis, a bacterial vaginal infection, as compared to the anti-yeast *L. acidophilis*. The bacterium increases levels of brain-derived neurotrophic factor (BDNF), helping increase our brain health. One cup of sauerkraut contains up to 10 million CFUs of *Lactobacillus* species.

In our transverse colon, this microbe helps produce tyramine, phenylethylamine, lactic acid, ethanol and GABA.

Lactobacillus bulgaricus (*L. delbrueckii*) now (*L. helveticus*) is found in yogurt and kefir, very often combined with other Lacto and Bifido species. It ferments lactose, helping individuals with dairy intolerance. The bacterium is added to cheese cultures, and helps reduce hypertension[128], depression and anxiety, by lowering inflammation and improved serotonin signaling.

Human studies show it enhances nutrient absorption, reduces allergens and fights pathogenic bacteria.[129]

In the transverse colon it helps produce tryptamine, GABA and acetylcholine.

Lactobacillus casei is found in cheese and yogurt products, and prevents antibiotic-induced diarrhea and *C. difficile* infections. Human studies show improvement in depressive moods in only ten days, after consumption of yogurt containing *L. casei*.[130] It increases microbiome Bifido levels, as well.

The bacterium reduces anxiety and improves gut health in patients suffering chronic fatigue syndrome;[131] and produces GABA and acetylcholine in the transverse colon.

The microbe helps relieve constipation and improve the quality of life in patients with Parkinson's disease.[132]

Lactobacillus fermentum ME-3 helps increase the production of glutathione, an extremely important anti-oxidant.

Lactobacillus paracasei helps alleviate intestinal distress associated with antibiotics and reduces liver damage resulting from chronic alcoholism.[133]

Lactobacillus plantarum is found in kimchi, sauerkraut, brined olives, and cultured vegetables. It can survive in the stomach for considerable time, and helps regulate immunity and reduce gut inflammation. It strengthens our gut lining, especially when combined with L-glutamate, reducing permeability associated with leaky gut, and reducing the pain of IBS. It helps digest protein, so particles cannot enter the bloodstream and create food allergies. It helps to absorb omega-3 fatty acids and in animal studies showed benefit in symptoms associated with multiple sclerosis.

The *L. plantarum* strain 229v, or placebo, were given to 79 patients taking an SSRI for major depression. This DB, PC study found improved cognitive function in the probiotic group.[134]

A larger, 12 week, randomized DB, PC study of 111 stressed patients found the *L. plantarum* DR7 group had reduced cortisol levels, enhanced serotonin, and stabilized dopamine pathways. Increased levels of anti-inflammatory IL10, improved attention, emotional cognition, and memory function were observed in this group compared to placebo.[135]

In humans, it has been shown to attenuate soy allergies.

L. plantarum C-29 fermented soybean supplement may help those with mild cognitive impairment. One hundred individuals took the product or placebo in this DB, PC randomized trial for 12 weeks. Changes in serum brain-derived neurotropic levels and cognitive performance showed improvement, especially in attention. Once again this suggests the importance of the gut-brain axis in cognitive deficits.[136]

It competes with pathogenic *Clostridia* and *Enterococcus* species, and helps produce GABA and acetylcholine in the transverse colon.

Lactobacillus reuteri is a potent probiotic that colonizes quickly, lowering inflammation and increasing oxytocin, associated with bonding, in mice and humans.[137]

It decreases ghrelin, the hunger hormone, and increases leptin, the satiety hormone, suggestive of benefit in weight loss programs. It helps lower LDL (unhealthy cholesterol) and reduces cardiac risk.[138] The microbe helps produce GABA, acetylcholine and serotonin in the transverse colon.

Furthermore, the bacterium helps reduce intestinal pain, and in turn anxiety, whether the bacterium is dead or alive.[139] Garlic and black pepper appear to encourage growth of this friendly bacterium, and inhibit pathogenic *E. coli*. Bananas, apples and oranges enhance its survival and growth.

Lactobacillus rhamnosus is mentioned very briefly above. A thirty-year review cites its benefit in irritable and inflammatory bowel disease, allergies, non-alcoholic fatty liver disease, cystic fibrosis and cancer. [140]

Various studies suggest its benefit in treating dermatitis, diarrhea, obesity and peanut allergies.

A DB, PC trial of pregnant women given this probiotic at 14-16 weeks of gestation until six months postpartum, found the probiotic group suffered significantly lower incidences of anxiety and depression. This may be due to increased levels of GABA. The bacterium produces histamine and acetylcholine.

In one study, it produced results similar to Prozac, without the side effects.

In a mouse study, it alleviated obsessive-compulsive disorder, and reduced stress-induced corticosterone, anxiety and depression-related behavior. When the vagus nerve was severed these effects disappeared, suggesting a communication pathway between gut bacteria and brain.[141]

A study in Finland found an association between ingestion of this bacterium for the first six months of life and a follow-up at age 13. Those kids taking placebo had a 17% rate of ADHD and/

or Aspberger's, compared to the supplement group exhibiting no evidence of either.[142]

It is found in yogurt, Parmigiano-Reggiano cheese, kefir, fermented sausage and soy cheese. Bananas, apples and oranges enhance its growth.

NOTE- Use with caution if the immune system is impaired, such as in HIV or lupus, as it may possibly trigger sepsis.

Various Lacto and Bifido bacteria help produce intestinal GABA.

Up to 98% of bacteria in newborns are *Bifidobacteria*, and in the adult are seven times more numerous than *Lactobacilli*.

Bifido species help create amino acids, proteins, B vitamins, and assist in the absorption of iron, calcium and vitamin D.

Bifidobacterium bifidum is normally picked up when babies pass through the birth canal. When combined in a capsule with *L. acidophilus* and *L. casei* for eight weeks, it has shown benefit in people suffering major depression.[143] This microbe produces GABA in both the ileum and colon.

Bifidobacterium lactis (*B. animalis lactis*) is commonly found in healthy yogurt. It destroys pathogenic salmonella and enhances our immunity. The bacterium has a proven record of helping bring relief to individuals with ulcerative colitis,[144] and improve constipation and diarrhea associated with irritable bowel syndrome.[145] This microbe assists production of GABA in the colon.

The bacterium is not competitive with other Bifido and Lacto species. Bananas, apples and oranges enhance its growth.

Bifidobacterium longum (*B. infantis*) is one of the first colonizers after birth. In lab mice it reduced anxiety, and increased BDNF production. It lives in the large intestine and helps prevent and/or treat colon cancers. It helps reduce lactose intolerance and food allergies. Via the neuroendocrine system and vagus nerve, it reduces anxiety and cortisol levels.[146] It may improve our cognition and reduce depression, by boosting the amount of available tryptophan, the precursor of serotonin.

B. longum 1714 reduced the perception of stress and morning cortisol levels, and improved memory in one human study.[147]

A randomized, DB, PC trial of the same strain on 40 healthy volunteers, found it altered neural oscillation after social stress, by increasing theta and alpha band waves.[148]

Both this strain and *Lactobacillus helveticus* occur naturally in yogurt, kefir and sauerkraut.

B. infantis microbes encourage production of GABA and tryptophan in the colon.

Bifidobacterium breve helps prevent the growth of *E. coli* and *Candida albicans*, and relieves allergies, diarrhea and irritable bowel syndrome. It has been found to improve the microbiome of premature babies,[149] and those birthed by caesarean.

It is similar to *B. longum*, but appears to have greater benifit on anxiety, rather than depression, and alleviates problems associated with antibiotics.[150] The microbe produces GABA in the colon.

Bifidobacterium cell walls contain muramyl dipeptide, which activates the production of lymphocytes, and may play a key role in genetic factors involving Crohn's and other inflammatory bowel diseases.

Vaginal douching and rectal enemas with Bifido and Lacto bacterium can be extremely beneficial for those who educate themselves in the proper procedure. Morning is the best time for implantation, after a bowel movement. It is not for everyone, but this procedure can produce much quicker results.

Saccharomyces boulardii is a non-pathogenic yeast resistant to stomach acid, bile and pancreatic enzymes. First discovered in 1920, growing on lychee fruit, the supplement inoculates both our upper and lower gastrointestinal tracts. Antibiotics do not impact its growth so the two can be taken concurrently for diarrhea, irritable bowel syndrome, inflammatory bowel disease, Crohn's, and ulcerative colitis.[151] There are more than 200 scientific papers published on the benefits of this probiotic. It helps produce the enzyme protease in our ileum and colon.

NOTE- it is a yeast, and may not be suitable for those with *Candida albicans* overgrowth and sensitivity. Do not take concurrently, with anti-fungal medications.

One alternative to antibiotics is Phage therapy, involving viruses that live inside bacteria. *Bacillus subtilis* is one such bacterium with phage capacity. The increasing incidence of antibiotic-resistant super bugs is a growing epidemic. One product, containing five species of *Bacillus* is MegaSporeBiotic™. The product reduced intestinal permeability by 60% in just 30 days, in a human clinical trial.

Also look at the wide range of Medicinal Herbs in Chapter 16 for specific indications involving microbiome health.

Medicinal mushrooms, which I have researched and written about for some twenty years, contain 1,3 and 1,6 beta glucans. These compounds help to nourish healthy flora, reduce inflammation and modulate the immune system.[152] Read more about the fungal pharmacy in its own chapter (17).

Our gut has its own immune system, sometimes called the "gut-associated lymphatic system", or GALT. It represents up to 80% of our entire body's immune system. This will be discussed in the next chapter under our immune system and inflammation. If fortunate, our first exposure to bacteria is on the descent through a mother's birth canal. One study found infants born vaginally, obtained *Lactobacillus johnsonii* bacteria from their mother's vaginal microbiome, whereas those born through C-section acquired bacteria associated with the skin surface, such as *Staphylococcus*.[153]

Lactobacillus creates a slightly acidic environment in gut, thwarting the growth of more unfriendly organisms. *L. johnsonii* bacteria grow from the lactose in breast milk and immunity is provided by valuable colostrum in our first few days. They receive more *Bifidobacteria*, which helps mature the gut lining more efficiently. Mother's milk contains oligosaccharides (prebiotics) that help nurture a healthy microbiome.

In clinical practice I suggested colostrum powders and/or capsules, especially in young children deprived of breast milk.

Orthodox obstetrics make it a regular practice to give C-section women antibiotics, adding to the problem. It is estimated by 2020, fully half of the babies born in the United States will be delivered by this schedule-convenient manner.

Studies show a five-fold increased risk of allergies, triple the risk of ADHD, twice the risk of autism, 80% increased risk of celiac disease, 50% increased risk of obesity, and 70% increased risk of type-1 diabetes.[154]

If C-section is necessary or chosen, you may wish to use the "gauze technique", to collect birth canal bacteria and transfer it to the newborn baby's mouth and nose.

Your entire gastrointestinal tract, from esophagus to rectum, is lined with a single layer of epithelial cells. These are coated with a mucous membrane for protection. Nutrients move through these cells, and keep out harmful matter. When permeability is compromised, a "leaky gut" sets up an inflammatory state that can result in irritable bowel, celiac, autism, auto-immune conditions, and later set the stage for Alzheimer's and Parkinson's disease.

In turn, a leaky gut can lead to a leaky brain allowing various proteins, viruses and bacteria to move through the blood-brain barrier.

One test for leaky gut is to ingest the sugars lactulose and mannitol. The latter pass through the gut normally, but lactulose will not, unless the gut is leaky. This will show up in your urine.

Gluten sensitivity, for example, makes this barrier more permeable due to the protein gliadin.

It should be noted gluten sensitivity, with or without celiac, increases the production of gut cytokines, creating inflammation affecting intestinal and brain health. There are numerous studies confirming the link between gluten sensitivity and neurological dysfunction.[155]

Gram-negative bacteria possess a fat and sugar coating called lipopolysaccharide (LPS) on their cell wall. Up to 70% of our intestinal flora are coated with LPS to protect them from aggressive bile salts. Unfortunately, a leaky gut allows the large molecular size LPS to enter our bloodstream as an endotoxin, and cause inflammation in the brain, by forming neo-epitopes. LPS is found in the brains of people suffering from AD, PD and schizophrenia.

Our body produces LDL cholesterol to neutralize this bloodstream toxin, and later cascades into blood vessel swelling and constriction. LDL is blamed as "bad cholesterol", but is really the hero if viewed from this perspective.

LPS is a serious problem, and the entire immune system reacts. High levels of LPS can create sepsis, leading to organ failure and death.

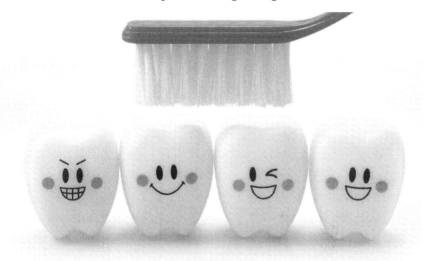

Dental health and periodontal disease affects brain health. In one study, 100% of people with a single root canal tested positive for LPS in their bloodstream.[156] Sepsis is the leading cause of death in hospitals, killing 258,000 Americans each year.

Porphyromonas gingivalis (gingivitis) is implicated in gum disease. It releases a potent toxin that disrupts the microbiome, causing leaky gut. A one-minute coconut oil oral swish or pull can help reduce bacteria and viruses in our oral cavity.

And don't forget the nose, throat and sinus routes to the brain.

Chronic sinusitis and rhinitis often result from bacterial, mold and fungal biofilms resistant to medications. These pathogens emit toxins that can access a leaky brain. There are natural nasal sprays that will help restore this harmful imbalance.

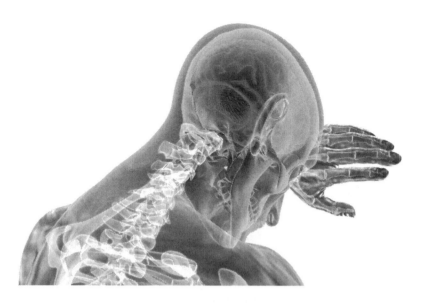

Brain and gut inflammation do not cause pain, as neither the brain nor mucus lining of the intestines have pain receptors. Chronic inflammation caused by leaky gut does make the immune system overactive, leading to confusion between undigested food, bacteria, and the body's own tissue. Auto-immune conditions of the pancreas or thyroid, as well as brain tissue destruction, can result.

"According to Harvard's Dr. Alessio Fasano, exposure to the gliadin protein in particular increases gut permeability in all of us."[157] This suggests wheat, rye and barley be avoided, even in their whole, complex carbohydrate form, especially if mental issues are a concern.

Studies suggest elevated LPS may contribute to increased beta-amyloid in the brain. Alzheimer's and ALS patients have three fold levels of LPS in their blood, compared to healthy controls.[158]

Celiacs, for example, react to gluten by triggering zonulin, a protein that opens up the tight intestinal wall, as well as the blood-brain barrier. Some researchers believe gluten (gliadin) widens the gaps in everyone's intestinal barrier.

A functional medicine practitioner can test for anti-bodies to zonulin, actin, LPS, S100B and neuron-specific enolase. Other antibodies involved in brain tissue disease, which can be tested for, are transglutaminase 2 and 6, gangliosides, *herpes simplex* (See Alzheimer's), *Chlamydia pneumoniae*, gliofibrillar acid protein, myelin basic protein (multiple sclerosis), glutamic acid decarboxylase, alpha and beta tubulin, and synapsin. The tests are expensive, but can give a clearer picture of a direction towards restoring brain health.

Studies on Parkinson's disease have found a direct correlation to gut permeability.

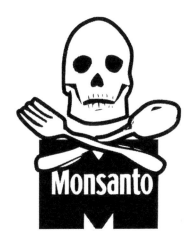

The use of Roundup® (glyphosate) to ripen wheat (bigger, better yields) suggests many individuals suffering with irritable bowel syndromes, may suffer a disruption of their gut flora, causing a two-pronged attack on the microbiome. In 2017, farmers sprayed 1.35 million metric tons of glyphosate on food crops.

In fact, when you compare the levels of celiac and use of glyphosate over past 25 years, a direct correlation pattern appears.[159] I have been living on the planet too long to believe in coincidences. Roundup disrupts the shikimate pathway in our gut bacteria, interfering with the precursors of serotonin and dopamine.

L-glutamine (see Supplements) and zinc can help heal your leaky, inflamed gut.

Tea, coffee and chocolate all contain polyphenols, which reduce inflammation and increase colonies of healthy bacteria. Black and green tea increase gut bifidobacterium, and reduce clostridial species.

Cocoa ingestion increases bifidobacteria and lactobacilli species, and reduces C-reactive protein, a marker of inflammation.

One study found elderly patients suffering from mild cognitive impairment, and consuming cocoa and chocolate (sugar-free), improved insulin sensitivity, lowered blood pressure, reduced free radical damage, and exhibited improved cognition.[160]

Chocolate consumption is associated with protection of middle-aged people suffering tinnitus and hearing loss. Over 3500 people took part in this review. Severe hearing loss was inversely correlated with frequency of chocolate consumption.[161]

One final thought on our microbiome. Digestive enzymes can be useful for those with food sensitivities, especially pertaining to casein, gluten and soy. In both autism and ADHD, these proteins are not completely digested and enter the blood stream through the leaky gut. In turn, they cross the BBB and block neurotransmission, trigger brain inflammation, and create opiate-like doping effect.

Digestive enzymes help reduce this load while clients are moving toward an elimination diet. Dipeptidyl peptidase-IV helps digest the opioid peptides found in gluten, dairy and possibly soy; helping relieve brain fog, and irritability. They are best taken at the beginning of each meal.

DOSE- Follow the recommendations for various age categories keeping in mind that die-off of unhealthy yeast and bacteria can create headaches, flu-like symptoms, irritability and behavioral regression. Activated charcoal can alleviate the side effects to some extent, but lowering probiotic dosage and increasing their introduction slowly is the best approach.

CHAPTER 3

OUR IMMUNE SYSTEM AND INFLAMMATION

"Even if all the experts agree, they may well be mistaken."

Bertrand Russell

Neurodegenerative conditions are estimated to affect some 90 million people in the 65+ age group, by the year 2050.[162]

I personally observed my own mother's suffering through a half decade of declining cognitive ability; possibly related to Alzheimer's disease (AD).

Incidence of Parkinson's disease (PD), multiple sclerosis, myasthenia gravis and numerous other auto-immune conditions are dramatically on the rise.

There is a strongly established correlation between the widely used anti-cholinergic drugs and dementia. This means that medicines taken by millions of people for depression, asthma, and allergies may be affecting brain metabolism and atrophy.[163]

Antihistamines, anti-depressants, cardiovascular medications, heartburn medications, anti-Parkinson's drugs, muscle relaxants, motion sickness remedies, and medications for urinary incontinence are among the more than one hundred over-the-counter and prescription drugs that utilize anti-cholinergic pathways.

One study looked at the brains of 451 men and women, with 60 taking one or more anti-cholinergic medicines. Researchers found those taking one of the medicines "were four times more likely to develop either mild cognitive impairment or dementia", than those not taking these medicines, according to the lead author Dr. Shannon Risacher.

This followed an earlier retrospective cohort study examining the long-term use of anticholinergic drugs in 3690 older adults, and finding a significant correlation with cognitive impairment and dementia.[164] Over 800 developed dementia, and if the drugs were taken for three years or more, there was a 54% higher dementia risk than taking them for only three months.

Benzodiazepine use has been linked to AD. A team of researchers in France and Quebec looked at nearly two thousand men and women over the age of 65 diagnosed with AD. They then randomly selected seven thousand other seniors, without AD, who were matched for age and sex, and looked at their drug prescriptions for five to six years before diagnosis.

Those individuals taking drugs such as Ativan, Serex, Xanax, Elavil, Serzone, Halcion and other anti-anxiety/anti-depression/ insomnia medications for three to six months had a 32% greater risk of AD, and those taking only one for more than six months, had an 84% greater risk than those who took none.

This makes sense when you remember these medications block the transmission of acetylcholine, or boost GABA (gamma-aminobutyric acid) in the brain.

Proton pump inhibitors (PPIs) used by people aged 75 years or older, produce a 44% greater risk of developing dementia, including AD.[165] This seven-year study involved 74,000 participants.

Suppressing hydrochloric acid production allows unhealthy bacteria to dominate our microbiome, and induce vitamin B12 deficiency.

An earlier study examined cognitive effects of short-term use in sixty, otherwise healthy, young adults, aged 20-26 years.[166] Six groups received a different PPI or placebo for seven days. All the drug groups had a statistically and clinically significant impairment in cognitive function. In just one week! Imagine the implications of their long-term use.

Studies show that PPIs and H2 blockers are related to small intestinal bacterial overgrowth, one possible cause of irritable bowel syndrome, with its attendant anxiety and depression. In fact, studies suggest those patients suffering mental distress, get less relief from ingesting PPIs, suggesting the dysbiosis mitigates the effects.[167]

While in clinical practice, I observed that nearly 80% of my clients using Tums, Rolaids and other antacids, actually suffered from a deficiency of hydrochloric acid. The symptoms of heartburn, gas, bloating and discomfort are due to the inability of food to move out of the stomach to the small intestine, in a timely manner.

The herb Queen of the Meadow (*Filipendula ulmaria*) helps regulate and balance stomach acid production, either high or low. This herbal medicine helped many of my clients stop taking antacids and PPIs, and later restore their own hydrochloric acid production.

A pathogen in chronic periodontitis, *Porphyromonas gingivalis*, has been identified in the brain of Alzheimer's patients. It is common in patients with gingivitis and periodontal infection, but also is found at low levels in 25% of healthy individuals with no oral disease.[168]

Gingipains, and toxic proteases, may contribute to neurotoxicity and building of amyloid plaque. Previous work on this bacterium showed a link with atherosclerosis. Various compounds in early harvest, organic, cold-pressed, extra virgin olive oil, including maslinic and oleanolic acid, show significant inhibition. Swish a teaspoon in the mouth for one minute and spit.

The immune system involves T-cell helpers type one and two.

Th1 involves cell-mediated immunity and fights bacterial and viral infections in the mucus membranes, preventing pathogens from doing harm.

Immunoglobulin A (IgA), interleukin-2 (IL-2), IL-12 and gamma interferon are involved. When gut flora is compromised, this side of immunity becomes less efficient and activates Th2 associated with our humoral immunity. IL-4, 5, 6 and 10, immunoglobulin E, and alpha interferon then become more active.

A Th-2 stimulated immune system protects us from parasites and worms, and helps produce antibodies against pathogens. The dark side of Th-2 dominance creates a predisposition to allergies and asthma. Most people are Th-1 dominant and these cytokines protect us against viruses, cancer and certain mycoplasma bacteria that attack our cells. The bad side of this dominance is that it can launch an attack against your own cells, and create auto-immune responses, organ transplant rejection and even fetal rejection.

In fact, women will automatically switch from Th-1 dominance to Th-2 dominance during pregnancy.

Underactive Th1, and overactive Th2 immune response is found in viral infections, chronic fatigue syndrome, allergies and autism.

In countries with good hygiene, vaccination and antibiotics, a low level of Th-1 stimulation results in an increase in Th-2. This triggers an exaggerated mucus production and contraction of muscles in the airways that can cause allergies and asthma. In the reverse scenario, where pathogens are abundant and vaccination and antibiotic use is low, Th2 responses are activated, leading to repeated cycles of infection and inflammation; the latter countered with natural anti-allergic reactions. It is as if Th-2 has learned to recognize an innocuous but foreign substance and respond but not produce a panicked response, with swollen tissue and dripping glands. Hence the large amount of anti-histamines and anti-cholinergic drugs on our pharmacy shelves.

An excess of histamine is known as histadelia. The condition was discovered by Dr. Carl Pfeifer, in many people with depression, schizophrenia, addictions and autism. Anti-histamine drugs are prescribed, by some psychiatrists to treat schizophrenia.[169]

Zinc supplementation supports Th-1 but diminishes protection against worms and parasites. Insufficient zinc and poor nutrition means worm defenses flourish and our defense against pathogens, such as viruses, grows weaker.

Herbs that stimulate Th1 immune direction are Echinacea, astragalus, lemon balm, and maitake mushrooms.

Th2, on the other hand, is stimulated by pine bark extract (*Pycnogenol*), grape seed extract, acai berry and green tea.

These are only a few examples.

Vitamin A supports Th2, boosting protection against parasites and decreasing our cell-entry defense.

Another aspect of the immune system involves Th3, loaded with opioid receptors, and involving dampened auto-immunity. The high, experienced by runners, involves this response, but when over-done, exercise training activates IL-6, which in turn, activates Th17 and promotes auto-immunity. The key is balance, just pushing yourself at the end of your exercise, but no longer.

Positive mental attitude, including love and self-esteem promote natural opioid release. Negative thoughts, internal stress, violence and unhealthy relationships promote IL-6 and activate Th17. External stressors such as a bad job, unrealistic expectations or chemical exposure can also precipitate this destructive cascade.[170]

But perhaps the real answer to our increased levels of chronic neuro-degenerative disease, lies in roles played by our immune system and levels of inflammation.

There are no pharmaceutical drugs that will improve immune response, and reduce inflammation at the same time. That is, the drug cortisone reduces inflammation, but suppresses our immune system.

Auto-immune conditions respond well to medicinal mushrooms due to their ability to up-regulate the immune system when deficient, or down-regulate it, whenever there is inflammation and destruction of tissue.

The optimizing of immune function and reduction of inflammation in the body may be one key to longevity, and increased quality of brain health. Thus my continuing interest in the health benefits of medicinal mushrooms.

The immune system "listens" to microbe-brain communication stemming from the gut, via the vagus nerve, to several parts of the nervous system.

Stress slows down antibody reactivity to pathogens, which is a good thing in the short term. Chronic stress, however, contributes to a leaky gut, and other inflammation, that creates a nasty feedback loop of dis-ease, or lack of ease.

A fascinating book by Michal Schwartz explores the relationship between our immune system and brain.[171]

She previously published a paper proposing immune cells keep our brain healthy, and how they do it.

Not many years ago, scientists believed immune cells did not exist in the brain. Early studies into multiple sclerosis, for example, looked at how immune cells attack the nerve tissue. But maybe we have not been looking at the issue correctly.

Her work suggested immune cells control formation of our brain's stem cells, shape cognitive performance, and affect our mood and ability to cope with stress.

This all happens at a special border of the brain, so that when called upon, the immune cells assist via molecules delivered to the brain, or by controlled entry, help repair the damaged, or diseased brain.

Sir Frank Macfarlane Burnet was awarded the Nobel Prize in 1960 for his work on auto-immune cells. Since that time, scientists have considered such cells to be associated with auto-immune disease, but such is not the case.

In fact, these cells are not only harmless, but are essential for the re-generation of nerve cells and the preservation of learning and memory.

Michal calls them, "the immune cells of wisdom". Her research team found that immune cells communicate with the brain from a site located at the border between our brain and circulating blood. This is a thick layer of epithelial cells called the choroid plexus.

This area controls the access of immune cells to brain tissue when called upon. It filters our blood of compounds needed to keep the brain healthy, and creates our cerebrospinal fluid. In fact, it was believed for decades, its only role was the production of this fluid.

Immune cells interact with a healthy brain without actually entering the tissue, but under certain conditions this site acts as a gate that selects and shapes the immune cells allowed entry to the brain.

Our blood brain barrier (BBB) remains sealed to immune cells under most conditions, and if by-passed, results in pathological inflammation.

In turn, the chronic inflammation is cited and treated with immune suppressing drugs.

"While it begins as a defense process, physiological inflammation can soon become pathological inflammation. The belief of clinical researchers that we can break such a vicious cycle by suppressing the immune system outside the brain has turned out to be an illusion," she writes.[172]

Physiological inflammation, if not resolved, can lead to pathological inflammation, which biomedical health practitioners attempt to shut down. This is a mistake.

This approach denies a diseased brain the immune assistance it needs from the blood. Suppressing the immune system outside of the brain to reduce chronic inflammation within the brain tissue does not work, as it denies the damaged brain the assistance it requires from the immune system, including blood-borne immune cells. In turn, the suppression prevents the immune system from resolving pro-inflammatory response, as it senses it is under attack.

Both Parkinson's disease (AD) and multiple sclerosis (MS) patients show high levels of T cells in the ventral mid-brain. Recent studies suggest the cells may be auto-reactive, recognizing disease-altered self-proteins as foreign antigens; creating an auto-immune response to alpha-synuclein. Thus, the inflammation associated with PD may be both protective and pathogenic.[173]

The creation of inflammation in the body is connected to heat, pain and discomfort. Acute inflammation, such as the raising of body temperature to fight a viral, bacterial or fungal infection, is a natural process. In fact, it is the body's only mechanism of dealing with invasive pathogens.

A fever increases the production of immune cells from the bone marrow, and creates production of receptor proteins, that direct them to the site of inflammation. The raised temperature optimizes production of macrophages, B cells and dendritic cells that initiate T cell production. This is all good.

Aspirin, as an example, reduces fever by stopping the production of prostaglandin E2, triggered by the detection of invasive pathogens.

When our temperature reaches 41° Celsius, the replication of viruses in our body, decreases 200 fold.

The Ukrainian biologist Élie Metchnikoff emphasized, against the common wisdom of the day, the health benefits of inflammation in fighting pathogens, repairing tissue, and maintaining a healthy body. He was awarded the Nobel Prize in 1908 for his work on natural immune cells.

A variety of over-the-counter and prescription drugs are widely available to anyone wishing to suppress these inflammatory conditions.

But there is a cost. By continuing to suppress the ability of body tissue to throw off toxins, more chronic states of inflammation result. As the body attempts to move from a chronic state to an acute state and restored homeostasis, there is, again, fever, pain, and inflammation.

By supporting our body through this period of time, the acute state will abide and the body continues its natural state of well-being and balance.

It is the pathway of disease and healing crisis I teach my herbal students at The Northern Star College of Mystical Studies.

But if the symptoms are suppressed repeatedly, the vicious cycle continues. This is one reason why anti-inflammatory drugs fail to treat neurodegenerative disorders.

Tens of millions of people take sleep medications with acetaminophen on a nightly basis.

Over-the-counter (OTC) sales of anti-inflammatory drugs are staggering. In 2015, a total of 2.9 billion retail trips were made to purchase OTC drugs. The average American consumer makes 26 trips a year to purchase OTC products, and yet they visit their physician, an average of three times per year. Acetaminophen is the most commonly used children's medication for reducing fever and pain. Benadryl, Dimetapp and Palgic, for allergies and colds, contain anti-cholinergics.

A recent DB, PC study found acetaminophen reduces empathy for other people's suffering.[174]

This may explain, in part, the increased levels of anti-social, them vs. us attitudes and behavior, prevalent today.

Twenty-three percent of American adults use acetaminophen on any given week.[175] Some epidemiological and laboratory studies suggested NSAIDs (non-steroidal anti-inflammatory drugs) reduce the risk of AD, by lowering levels of inflammation. Work by Szekely et al, however, found acetaminophen and ibuprofen do not lower the risk of dementia or AD.[176]

Using a drug that indiscriminately shuts down our immune response, reduces the physiological inflammation required for healing.

Stronger anti-inflammatory medications reduce inflammation, but at the cost of suppressing the choroid plexus and its interaction between the immune system and the brain.

In only the past few years lymphatic tissue was discovered in the brain. It was widely accepted our central nervous system is under constant immune surveillance within the meningeal tissue, but the entrance and exit of immune cells was poorly understood. The discovery in 2015 of functional lymphatic vessels lining our dural sinus tissue, shed new light on the connection between neuroinflammation and neurodegeneration associated with immune system dysfunction.[177]

It was widely assumed the blood-brain barrier (BBB) would not permit movement of nutrients and waste via this system.

The system has been re-named the glymphatic system and in order for neurotoxic wastes, including beta-amyloid, to be removed, our brain must sleep. Unfortunately, this system is suppressed in various neurodegenerative conditions.[178]

The term glymphatic relates to the involvement of glial cells, and astroglial cells that form channels along the blood vessels into the brain. This system moves cerebrospinal fluid surrounding the brain and spinal cord; deeper inside the brain bringing glucose, immune cells and nutrients in, and moving dead cells and waste products like beta amyloid out. This, in turn, connects to the lymphatic system, where waste can be eliminated. It must be noted both systems do not have a pump but rely on exercise, lymphatic drainage or cranio-sacral manipulation to move the fluids.

People with brain problems suffer exhaustion and sleep poorly. This exacerbates health issues as during sleep the glia open up special channels that allow waste and toxic buildup, including proteins of dementia, to be discharged through the cerebral spinal fluid bathing our brain. This channel is ten times more active in the sleeping brain than in its waking state.

A study of ten men and ten women measured the levels of beta-amyloid plaque in their brains after only one night of restless sleep. A 5% burden of plaque was found in the hippocampus.[179]

Sleep deprivation suppresses glymphatic activity, and it appears that slow-wave sleep, the deepest phase of non-REM sleep when dreaming, takes place and is associated with enhanced memory consolidation.

The optic nerve, incidently, is surrounded by cerebrospinal fluid along its entire length. Research suggests that glaucoma may indicate impaired fluid dynamics and reduced clearing of beta-amyloid via this glymphatic system.[180]

CHAPTER 4

OUR NEUROTRANSMITTERS

"Tears come from the heart and not from the brain."
LEONARDO DA VINCI

The healthy brain requires adequate levels of four major neurotransmitters for optimal function.

As a child, we have an estimated 10 quadrillion synapses firing at any time, and by late adulthood this diminishes from 50-90%.

Neuronal communication is complex, and involves more than simply adjusting diet and taking supplements. Healthy thoughts, positive mood and personality are a large part of how we view the world, and dictates our response to human interaction.

Tinnitus, for example, has multiple factors, but one variable is brain neurons too easily triggered. Some people are overly sensitive to strong light, sound and scents, and react to any stimulation, with more fatigue.

Levels of serotonin, dopamine, GABA (gamma-aminobutryic acid), its counterpart glutamate, as well as acetylcholine, influence anxiety, depression, attention deficit hyperactivity disorder (ADHD) seasonal affective disorder (SAD), obsessive-compulsive disorder (OCD); as well as Alzheimer's and Parkinson's disease.

Each of these brain related conditions are discussed in their own chapter, with special attention to the consequence of low or high levels of various neurotransmitters.

In chapter 2, we discussed the production of neurotransmitters, and how they are manufactured by a healthy microbiome.

It is important to add our enteric nervous system (ENS) to the discussion at this point. The ENS operates independently of the brain and spinal cord, but it does receive and act on information received from the central nervous system via the vagus nerve (parasympathetic) and prevertebral ganglia (sympathetic). It is often called the "second brain" due to some one hundred million neurons, similar in number to those found in our spinal cord.

The ENS is embedded in the gastro-intestinal lining and is involved in more than 30 neurotransmitters, including acetylcholine, dopamine and serotonin. In fact, more than 90% of the body's serotonin and 50% of the body's dopamine is produced in our gut.

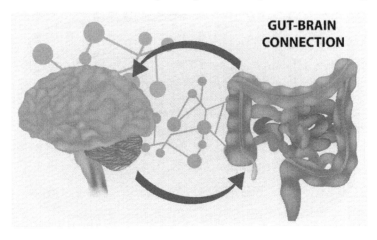

GUT-BRAIN CONNECTION

The corpus callosum helps connect the left and right hemispheres of our brain. It has been suggested left-brained individuals are more analytical, thinking and rely on practical skills. They are well organized and see things as part of patterns or sequences. Left brainers tend to be GABA dominant, and make sure that everything is in good working order, and right-side up.

Right-brained individuals tend to focus on feelings, intuition and are more socially active, spontaneous, and empathic. They are dominated by acetylcholine, controlling creativity and speed. They are very sensitive to feelings of others and are pleasant to be around.

At one time, not long ago, it was believed that neurons created and then released only one neurotransmitter classifying them as dopaminergic, or GABAnergic etc. We now understand some neurons use more than one transmitter, and in fact, more mature neurons can change which transmitter they choose to use. That is, a previously excitatory synapse can convert to inhibitory, and vice versa.[181]

SEROTONIN

> "Dave was a confirmed serotonin junkie. Any day of the year, he chose a good book, a hot cupper and air-conditioning over jeopardy to life and limb."
>
> DAN SOFER

> "A person's mood is like a symphony, and serotonin is like the conductor's baton."
>
> JAMES STOCKARD

Serotonin is an ancient neurotransmitter found in the venom of amphibians, wasps and scorpions, and in the nervous system of flatworms, crickets and lobsters. It is widely distributed in plants and fungi, playing a key role in communication.

Delta waves are related to the production of serotonin and our occipital lobes that control the visual process. Serotonin provides a soothing, nourishing feeling and when levels are adequate, sleep is deep and peaceful, food is enjoyable and thought patterns are appropriate. When out of balance, depression, hormonal imbalances, including PMS, as well as eating and sleeping disorders are present. About 17% of the population is a serotonin type. They exhibit great eye-hand coordination when in balance, but can become risk takers when deficient. A distain for order and structure and a love of independence can create, in them, undue hardship. Delta waves, mentioned above, occur at one to four cycles per second. Infants one to two years old are in a predominantly delta-theta state, when the mind and body are in harmony.

Depression and moodiness associated with seasonal affective disorder (SAD), anger, OCD, migraines, tinnitus, bipolar and anxiety disorders are related to serotonin deficiencies.

Too much of this excitatory neurotransmitter can create extreme nervousness, making you vulnerable to criticism, afraid of being disliked, or become hesitant or distracted. At the opposite extreme, one can feel extremely shy and withdrawn, suffering issues of self worth, sadness and a desperate need for interpersonal relationships, but retaining the fear of initiation.

Extreme serotonin production may be associated with estrogen excess, especially associated with the use of oral contraceptives or hormone replacement therapy.

Anorexia and bulimia are related to serotonin deficiency. Too little serotonin will produce insomnia, and night sweats. It is important to remember our serotonin receptors, particularly 5-HT2$_a$ are not just found in the central nervous system, but our platelets, cardiovascular system, our enteric nervous system, mast cells, fibroblasts, neurons of the peripheral nervous system, and human monocytes.

In the human body, 90% of serotonin production is found in the neurons of our gut, and released to determine bone growth or shrinkage. Another 8% is found in blood inside platelets and mast cells. It was initially found in blood serum, and determined to have a tonic (constricting) affect on the vascular system, hence its name (serum tonic). A small percentage is found in the brain, in the same location as every other vertebrate brain, suggesting its presence on earth some 500 million years ago.

The 5HT-1A serotonin receptor is receiving a lot of research attention. The number of serotonin receptors in our brain is inversely correlated with self-ratings of religiosity and spirituality.

People who respond negatively (anxiety/depression) to the challenges of everyday life, possess fewer receptors and are more likely to find comfort in religious faith and practice.

Certain serotonin receptor profile individuals suffer more from social anxiety, including extreme fear that other people are thinking bad things about them.

Fortunately, these individuals respond more positively to placebos and affirmations. Afformations, discussed under Addictions (Chapter 14), may be more useful.

Serotonin helps us feel happy, and relaxed. Low levels in the brain can reduce the frequency of happy thoughts, resulting in depression and anxiety.

Estrogen levels in women, and testosterone levels in men, keep our receptor sites sensitive to serotonin.

However, women synthesize brain serotonin at half the rate of men, perhaps explaining in part, why women are more prone to depression.

Sixty-five year old brains have 60% fewer serotonin receptors than those at age 30.

Serotonin is well-known for its role in sleep via its conversion to melatonin. However, one of its main roles is memory, associated with aging and dementia.

In order to produce serotonin, the body requires the essential amino acid tryptophan. Many plant and animal foods are rich in

tryptophan, but less than ten percent can be used to make serotonin.

It is a common myth, associated with Thanksgiving dinner, that turkey is a rich source of the amino acid. The drowsiness is more likely due to an insulin spike, from over-eating.

Chia (*Salvia hispanica*) seeds are a rich source of tryptophan (One tablespoon equals 100 mg), as well as high levels of omega-3 fatty acids.

Other rich sources include raw chocolate, spirulina, pumpkin and sesame seeds, salmon, tuna, and organic, unsweetened yogurt. We do not lack tryptophan foods, even in the SAD (Standard American Diet). The issue is getting the precursors to the brain. The transport protein that carries tryptophan across the blood-brain barrier is called the "large neutral amino acid transporter." Insulin spikes will disrupt this transport.

Tryptophan is found in many foods, but low amounts of protein in the diet can cause deficiency, especially individuals on a vegan or low animal protein regime. High protein meals taken at same time diminishes the absorption of tryptophan. For optimal benefit, it is best to eat a complex carbohydrate meal at supper, with your tryptophan supplement.

Iron is required for conversion of tryptophan to serotonin. Even slight anemia can be problematic.

Foods that help increase serotonin production include sweet potatoes, apples, blueberries, carrots, chickpeas, avocados, eggplant, plums, walnuts, and steel-cut oatmeal.

Rich sources of serotonin precursors are oats, angelica, burdock, dandelion, ginger, wild yam, black cohosh, St. John's wort, and cannabis. *Griffonia simplifolia* seeds contain high levels of 5-HTP. See Medicinal Herbs Chapter 16.

Other supplements helping ensure transport and absorption of tryptophan are SAMe, B6, B3, B12, methyl folate, iron, and magnesium.

Serotonin is converted to melatonin in the brain's pineal gland. The adrenal hormone norepinephrine is involved in this process, explaining why adrenal exhaustion from chronic stress can block conversion. High cortisol levels can affect conversion, as people with insulin resistance may suffer low cortisol levels in the morning, and then high levels at night, the opposite of a healthy situation.

Melatonin helps initiate sleep cycles. HEV (blue) light from electronic devices suppresses melatonin production, leading to memory loss, insomnia, lower cognition, increased mood swings, and low energy. When you rise in the morning and expose yourself to a half hour of sunlight, you will naturally produce melatonin 14 hours later. A thirty minute walk, three times a week helps alleviate depressive states, by pushing larger amino acids toward muscles, and allowing the smaller tryptophan to get to your brain.

Exposure to EMFs, such as cell phones, televisions, and Wifi, even living close to power lines, can suppress your melatonin production. Prozac lowers blood melatonin levels. Aspirin, ibuprofen and acetaminophen may reduce prostaglandin production, which suppresses melatonin levels and affects circadian rhythm.

A deficiency of melatonin can result in anxiety and mood disorders, insomnia, and immune suppression. Excess melatonin production is associated with seasonal affective disorder (SAD), low thyroid and adrenal function. Since full spectrum lighting reduces melatonin production, light therapy can help patients suffering SAD.

Decreased melatonin levels are associated with depression and some cases of psychosis.[182]

A study of 232 ICU patients found the group given melatonin significantly decreased the occurrence of delirium.[183]

And when melatonin levels decline, an exacerbation of multiple sclerosis symptoms has been found.[184]

Melatonin supplementation that assists sleep suggests an issue with serotonin production, and a disruption of our normal circadian rhythm.

A combination of L-theanine, 5-HTP and melatonin may be helpful for some people. Start with 3-5 mg of melatonin at least one hour before bedtime and add 5-HTP (100 mg) and 200 mg of L-theanine just before going to bed. Cut back to the minimum that allows you to enjoy a good sleep.

NOTE: In 1989, a rare disorder- eosinophilia-myalgia syndrome (EMS) occurred in 1500 people taking L-tryptophan, including twenty-eight deaths. The problem was traced to a contaminated GMO bacteria-based product from Japan and it was banned from the North American market. Since then, the FDA has approved its sale.

5-HTP may increase drowsiness, digestive issues, or sexual dysfunction. It should not be taken with SSRI or MAO inhibitor drugs. It may cause problems in Parkinson's disease in those taking carbidopa (L-dopa) and has been linked to seizures in Down syndrome. Discontinue 5-HTP for at least two weeks before any surgery.

Individuals coming off SSRIs after taking them for a long period of time, will be deficient in methyl donors and B6 (pyridoxal-5-phosphate). Birth control and estrogen creams also deplete these methyl donors.

In utero exposure to SSRIs reveals a statistically significant association with ASD, ADHD and mental disorders in children.[185]

OCD individuals with low serotonin activity may find 5-HTP makes their symptoms worse.

CAUTION- Do not take L-tryptophan or 5-HTP if you have carcinoid tumor or are already taking an SSRI such as Prozac or Zoloft. Excess levels of serotonin may be dangerous in cases of coronary artery disease.

SSRI medications are associated with bone loss and increased risk of fracture. A cross-sectional study of 85 subjects found the drugs, taken at therapeutic dosage, reduced bone formation.[186]

DOPAMINE

> "What draws us into a story and keeps us there is the firing of our dopamine neurons, signaling that intriguing information is on the way."
>
> LISA CRON

Dopamine is involved in our reward/motivation response.

The neurotransmitter was only discovered in 1957, and initially thought to be a way for the body to produce norepinephrine (adrenaline in the brain). Only 0.0005% of our brain cells produce dopamine. That is, our brain contains millions of serotonergic neurons and only about ten thousand dopaminergic neurons.

Dopamine is our gas pedal of pleasure. Anti-psychotic drugs that antagonize its function, reduce our ability to experience pleasure. It is the molecule of love, the molecule of anticipation.

This is different from the influence of serotonin and endocannabinoids, which give us pleasure from sensation and emotion.[187]

Unlike serotonin-deficient people who cannot seem to enjoy life, dopamine-deficient people can find enjoyment but are not motivated to do anything.

Both types suffer depression, but look very different.

People with low dopamine still enjoy things, but their mood is low in general, and they find it difficult to do things. They may suffer low libido, poor self-esteem, have a short fuse and crave stimulants and carbohydrates.

They often feel worthless or hopeless, which is not always the case with low serotonin. Of course, some people suffer from a deficiency of both!

Dopamine helps our frontal lobes process information faster. ADHD is most often identified in children, because the frontal lobes of the brain develop last, and this is where control dopamine acts. When control dopamine is weak, people go after things they want without regard to any long-term consequences.

Ritalin, given to ADD and ADHD classified children improves their school performance but creates other issues.

The FDA schedules Ritalin and other amphetamines in the same class as opioids, including morphine and Oxycontin. Biochemists they are not.

Ritalin affects the brain dopamine system in a similar manner to cocaine. When addicts stimulate their dopamine system it demands more. Nicotine, discussed in the Addictions chapter, stimulates additional dopamine release, but is cheaper and easy to access.[188]

Many over the counter anti-histamine drugs block the reuptake of dopamine, in a manner very similar to cocaine.

Marion Sigman writes. "We can think of dopamine as the water that makes clay more pliable, and the sensory stimulus as the tool that marks a groove in that damp clay. Neither can transform the material on its own. Working with dry clay is a waste of time. Wetting it if you aren't going to sculpt it is as well."[189]

Beta brain waves, associated with alertness, occur in the frontal lobe, when dopamine is present. Dopamine works like a natural amphetamine and controls energy, excitement, motivation, and our bodily functions including blood pressure, metabolism and digestion.

It helps generate the electricity that controls voluntary movement, intelligence, abstract thought, our long-term planning and personality traits.

The beta brain state begins to predominate at about the age of thirteen, and is associated with reason and analysis. This helps us to express ourselves, and give our intuition direction and form.

It should be noted those individuals dominated by beta waves have a mental pattern of constant, low-power chatter. It is a state of questioning rather than action, and not being tuned into your intuition. Low amplitude beta states lead to living your life according to belief systems.

Its by-product is adrenaline. A lack of dopamine can lead to addictive behavior, obesity, exhaustion, and of course, Parkinson's disease. When deficient, the body naturally increases levels of cortisol, produced by the adrenal glands. Low levels then lead to depression, social anxiety and anhedonia, the inability to experience pleasure. These individuals may function well sexually, but experience no pleasure in sex and intimacy.[190]

When dopamine is present in excessive amounts, violent controlled behavior including reckless driving, sexual assault and other criminal activity may occur. Excessive amounts are associated with psychosis, schizophrenia, and high libido.

Cocaine attaches itself to dopamine transporters, preventing re-absorption. Crack cocaine, on the other hand, targets the ventral tegmental area of the brain. Dopamine types represent about 17% of the population, and they tend to crave carbohydrates.

Parkinson's disease, ADHD, drug addiction, and schizophrenia are influenced by levels of dopamine. That is, levels of this neurotransmitter, either too high, or too low, are problematic.

Dopamine stimulates luteinizing hormone (LH) in both women and men, affecting progesterone and testosterone levels.

Just as estrogen is necessary for serotonin uptake, dopamine uptake requires healthy levels of these two hormones.

Degeneration of dopamine receptors leads to progression and symptoms associated with Parkinson's disease (PD).

Drugs used to treat PD are dopamine agonists, meaning they enhance dopamine activity.

Drugs that interfere with dopamine's normal function (anti-psychotic drugs) resemble the symptoms of Parkinson's.

Other pathways near the substantia nigra go to areas of our brain associated with emotion, and another to the frontal lobes.

Production of dopamine and norepinephrine begins with tyrosine, the amino acid. In turn, it is converted to levodopa, or L-DOPA, by an enzyme. An important co-factor is iron, suggesting the close relationship of anemia and depression.

Tyrosine is affected by the enzyme tyrosinase and converted to a dark pigment vulnerable to genetic mutation. Albinism and vitiligo are associated dysfunctions. Tyrosine and iodine help produce thyroxine for thyroid health, and both progesterone and thyroid hormones sensitize receptor sites to dopamine.[191]

Faba bean is rich in L-DOPA and thus useful in Parkinson's.

Vitamin C and copper are required for a third enzyme pathway, preventing oxidation.

Serotonin and dopamine levels need to be balanced in a healthy brain; and compete with each other for influence.

Tyrosine, a non-essential amino acid, is useful for thyroid health, and production of DOPA (dihydroxy-phenylanine).

In our diet, tyrosine is produced in the liver from the essential amino acid, phenylalanine. Patients with a history of hepatitis, or fatty liver will have difficulty with this conversion. Insulin resistance prevents its proper transport across the blood-brain barrier. Iron and folate deficiency will prevent the conversion of L-tyrosine to L-dopa.

Phenylalanine (amino acid) is found in high protein animal products including organic sources of chicken, beef, fish and eggs, as well as cheese (cheddar and parmesan), avocados and yogurt. Chia, sesame and pumpkin seeds, almonds and legumes, including lima beans, are also rich sources. However, consumption of these foods is generally not that effective, except when plentiful in vegan and vegetarian diets.

Supplementation of D, L-phenylalanine is sometimes indicated. The D form produces PEA, and the L form is converted to dopamine.

Beta-phenylethylamine (PEA) easily crosses the blood-brain barrier and stimulates and modulates the release of dopamine. It improves attention, relieves depression and influences endorphins, helping with feelings of pleasure.[192]

DL-phenylalanine and especially D-phenylalanine may help quell endorphin deficiency.

Chocolate is a rich source of PEA, explaining our healthy "addiction" when the brain is fatigued.

Other supplements required for dopamine production are magnesium, selenium, vitamin B6, N-acetyl-tyrosine (see supplements), iron, and the B vitamin folate. Reducing brain inflammation with glutathione precursors such as NAC and alpha lipoic acid is highly recommended.

Tetrahydrobiopterin (THB) is produced from folate foods or supplements by our gut flora. B6, for example, is depleted by regular alcohol consumption.

Sources of dopamine precursors are found in medicinal herbs such as ginseng, nettles, red clover, milk thistle, fenugreek, dandelion, peppermint and beets. Velvet Bean and Faba Bean contain very rich sources of L-dopa.

Falling in love will, of course, boost your dopamine levels.

NOTE: Patient compliance may be an issue for low dopamine patients. Those coming off SSRIs or dopamine selective reuptake inhibitors (DRIs) become deficient in methyl donors including B6. This is also true of those taking birth control pills or using estrogen creams.

CAUTION- Use extreme caution with L-tyrosine, L-phenylalanine or DL-phenylalanine if you are prone to migraines, taking anti-depressants, L-Dopa medication, suffer hypertension or bipolar disorders, are pregnant, or diagnosed with melanoma, or suffer phenylalanine hydroxylase deficiency, an autosomal recessive disorder with intolerance to the amino acid.

This affects about one in fifteen thousand people. Proper diagnosis and diet help in the prevention of brain related disorders.

GLUTAMATE AND GABA

> "If you want to know if your food contains gluten, aspartame, high fructose corn syrup, trans-fats or MSG, you simply read the ingredients listed on the label."
>
> BERNIE SANDERS

Theta brain waves are associated with drowsiness, and related to GABA (gamma-aminobutyric acid), produced in the temporal lobes. They help balance frontal lobes that govern personality, and the parietal lobes, controlling thinking and acting. GABA is the brain's natural tranquilizer, giving calmness to our mind, body and spirit. There are about ten known types of GABA receptors in the brain.

Theta waves are involved in the production of endorphins, the feel good hormone associated with a "runner's high". They are produced during exercise and sexual intercourse. Any imbalance can lead to headaches, hypertension, heart palpitations, low sex drive, and seizures.

Almost 50% of the world's population is a GABA type. This is a good thing, as GABA in balance is stable, consistent, social and concerned with the wellbeing of others. They are team players, and rarely exhibit broad swings of emotions or outbursts of anger. GABA deficiency can result in frequent bowel movements, due to its effect on the peristalsis or rhythm of the intestinal tract.

Gamma brain waves relate to GABA, improving well-being, memory recall and focus, and increased happiness. Meditation, for example, increases gamma wave production.

Poor GABA activity may create anxiety and a sense of dread, or a feeling of being overwhelmed. Deficient GABA individuals tend to worry, with restless minds that cannot shut off.

When suffering chronic pain, the deficient GABA type may turn to cannabis, alcohol or narcotics. In the hippocampus, it helps one orientate with time and space. They tend to fall asleep watching television, or are constantly late for appointments.

When present in excess, it can lead to people expending energy seeking love. Or they seek opportunities to take care of others, at the neglect of their own health. Too little GABA can leave one feeling tired throughout the day. The theta state generally occurs at four to seven cycles per second and predominates from birth until about seven years of age. This is the time children have the greatest capacity to express themselves uniquely, because they do not have enough reasoning power to question themselves. Theta is a non-judgmental state, with little editing of what is observed and experienced. Our brain, of course, records everything happening in its environment.

Glutamate plays a key role in the entry of calcium ions for neuron health.

Your brain uses glutamate from food to prune synapses that have become unnecessary. The young brain requires it, but later as an adult it allows the brain to be more "plastic", and molding responses to our environment increases our chance of survival.

It has two faces, like the Roman god Janus. One is for early brain development and function, and then brain pruning in later life.

Traumatic memories formed through its action can haunt us as in post-traumatic stress disorder (PTSD), due to its amazing efficacy in forming long lasting impressions on the brain.

Glutamates can over-excite the brain neurons. The book *Excitotoxins* describes the negative symptoms and effects of monosodium glutamate (MSG) and its plethora of misleading descriptors in food products.

A few drugs of abuse clinically target glutamate receptors. PCP, also known as Angel Dust, and ketamine, antagonize the NMDA type of glutamate receptor. As they block this excitation, they depress the brain's level of anxiety, slowing down the flow of information further and further.

PCP was once used as an anesthetic, with unfortunate consequences, such as losing the ability to breath, becoming delirious, slipping into a coma and dying.

Xanax®, an anti-anxiety drug works on GABA pathways by increasing their receptor site sensitivity.

Scientists believe the brain makes its own endogenous PCP-like molecule, now called angeldustin.

Reduced function of angeldustin may contribute to mania.

Lithium chloride does not involve glutamate neuron function but slows the manic brain in another manner.

It may induce the birth of new GABA releasing neurons, which are more deficient in the brain of bipolar patients.

However, we all need some of glutamate's excitatory action to learn, and pay attention.

One way to slow down the brain is to stimulate the function of our GABA (gamma-aminobutyric acid) neurons.

In order for glutamate to convert to GABA an enzyme is required, utilizing B6 as a cofactor.

GABA is useful in treating anxiety and insomnia. The receptors are widely distributed throughout the brain, and GABA is almost always inhibitory. Ironically, low serotonin levels are involved, as a positive regulator of GABA-GABA receptor interaction.

Eating or ingesting GABA containing substances does not help, as the ingested GABA becomes electrically charged and cannot pass the blood brain barrier. Or so it was once thought.

One DB, PC randomized trial found GABA improved temporal, but not spatial visual attention.[193]

There is controversy over whether oral GABA can actually cross the blood-brain barrier, or works via the enteric nervous system.

Taking a few hundred milligrams of GABA may not, theoretically, reduce anxiety or help you sleep.

Because of the molecular size, only nano-particles should be able to pass the BBB. GABA does not possess a blood-brain barrier (BBB) transport protein, so technically, it should not be able to cross. But if you take GABA and notice an effect, it may be due to a leaky BBB.

The supplement is widely available and unfortunately many people believe it is the cure and not a symptom of a leaky brain.

Take 800-1000 mg of GABA between 6 p.m. and 9 p.m. so you can sleep. If it sedates and you feel calmer or more relaxed, you may suffer a leaky brain-barrier and/or neuronal inflammation may be present.

If it does work don't take it regularly, or you may shut down your receptor sites.

If it causes you anxiety, or irritability or panic this may also indicate a permeable blood-brain barrier, and is temporarily remedied by eating some protein.

Feeling no change is a sign your blood-brain barrier is intact.[194]

Early work used various salts of halide bromine to reduce brain activity. Taking a Bromo, often seen in old movies, to tame a headache was a common remedy.

The drugs, however, were toxic to kidneys and later removed from the market.

Alcohol was probably our first anti-anxiety agent.

Alcohol enhances the action of GABA, and inhibits the excitatory glutamate.

This explains, in part, the classic blackout and memory loss associated with intoxication.

Normally, your brain's vomit control center will activate at 0.12% blood alcohol. But slow and steady drinking will sneak up on the neurons, and allow a chronic drinker to bypass this step.

Barbiturates were introduced at end of 19th century. Equally unsafe benzodiazepines were first synthesized in 1947 and sold commercially as Librium in 1960. Diazepam, sold as Valium followed soon after and became the most prescribed anti-anxiety drug in the western world.

These and newer, more lipid soluble products only work in the presence of GABA at its receptor sites.

The brain contains its own valium-like compounds- the beta carbolines. These antagonize or enhance GABA function, but they all inhibit destruction of dopamine, norepinephrine and serotonin. Taken together, they produce mild, relaxed euphoria.

Some research suggests the brains of those suffering anxiety may produce too many of these chemicals, which are derived from the diet.

Coffee produces beta-carbolines, and alcohol can be converted by *Helicobacter pylori* in the gut to produce beta-carbolines.

The brain possesses both exhibitory and inhibitory neurotransmitters. Glutamate (glutamic acid) excites our entire nervous system, including the brain. In fact, over 90% of all brain synapses are geared to the release of glutamate. One specific version is called N-methyl-D-aspartate (NMDA). This plays a key role in opening the gates and permitting information to flow.

Glutamate is used to make GABA, the main inhibitor of the nervous system. GABA exerts influence through ionotropic ($GABA_A$) and metabotropic ($GABA_B$) receptors.

Both receptors play a role in producing anxiety, epilepsy, insomnia, spasticity, and aggressive behavior.[195]

And here is where the use of medicinal herbs for anxiety gets tricky. Various herbs will interact with either glutamic-acid decarboxylase (GAD), or GABA transminase.[196]

Valerian root (*Valeriana officinalis*) and Gotu kola (*Centella asiatica*) stimulate GAD, whereas German chamomile (*Matricaria chamomilla*) and Hops (*Humulus lupulus*) show significant inhibition of GAD activity, related to symptoms of anxiety.

The former herbs may be useful in Parkinson's disease[197], and possibly in schizophrenia and bipolar disorder.[198]

Autistic brains contain reduced GAD protein (both 65kDa and 67kDa) by 50% or more. This may account for increases of glutamate in the blood and platelets of autistic subjects.[199]

On the other hand, Lemon Balm (*Melissa officinalis*) infusions exhibit high inhibition of GABA transminase.

The active form of B6 (pyridoxal-5'-phosphate) further reduces the degradation of GABA, making for a great combination.

All these plants are covered in more depth in the Medicinal Herb chapter.

NOTE: A common GAD auto-immune reaction is associated with celiac, gluten intolerance, Hashimoto's hypothyroidism, type 1 diabetes and other conditions. Glucose plays a role in GABA production, while hypoglycemia, insulin resistance and diabetes all lower glucose in the brain.

Auto-immune thyroid conditions create insomnia, anxiety and a racing heart, looking very similar to a GABA deficiency.

When we eat, our bodies convert glutaminic acid to glutamate, and the GAD enzyme converts it to GABA. If you have a wheat allergy, for example, you create an antibody to GAD that inhibits the enzyme from working.

If you have elevated antibodies to casein (protein in milk), both antibodies to myelin basic protein, and myelin oligo-glycoproteins are elevated. These are markers associated with multiple sclerosis.

When this autoimmune/antibody reaction to the enzyme occurs, conversion to GABA suffers, and too much excitatory glutamate remains between neurons.

This may result in individuals being more prone to OCD, facial tics, and "stiff man syndrome" a progressive severe disease. Autism, and especially severe temper tantrums in children may be related.[200]

People with positive GAD antibodies should avoid artificial glutamates including MSG. Lab tests can confirm the presence of this antibody.

Huntington's patients have certain glutamate receptors that are overly sensitive. Blocking glutamate receptors or reducing the amount of glutamate released by other cells is one approach to reducing symptoms in this difficult disease. Trehalose, derived from sunflower seeds and mushrooms helps block brain cell destruction.

Acetaminophen is used to lower fever and inflammation mediated by $GABA_A$ receptors. This is discussed in more detail in chapter 3 on inflammation.[201]

Therefore this amino acid helps excite, sedate and form long term memory. Glutamate is a non-essential amino acid, meaning the brain can produce its own from glucose.

Glutamate as an amino acid or in free form constitutes up to 8-10% of amino acid content in human diet, with an average of 10-20 grams daily. It is an important fuel for intestinal tissue.

Your muscle tissue produces about 90% of the synthesis of glutamine; again emphasizing the importance of regular exercise. Supplementation of L-glutamine can help support regeneration and repair of intestinal lining, increasing the number of cells in small intestine and number of villi, and height of villi on the gut lining. It reduces the permeability of a leaky gut.[202]

NOTE- The synthetic monosodium glutamate (MSG) is problematic, despite disclaimers from the manufacturers, and recent publications.[203] It is suggested that glutamate is restricted by the blood-brain barrier, but in clinical practice I observed numerous cases of brain and muscle excitability decrease simply by eliminating this questionable additive.

Systemic levels of glutamate rise when high doses of MSG are ingested and normalize within two hours. It does however act as a signaling molecule in our enteric nervous system.

The book *Excitotoxins: The Taste that Kills*[204] looks at MSG, aspartame (Nutrasweet), cysteine and aspartic acid. It cites over 500 scientific studies linking brain health to these food additives. MSG is often hidden on food labels. Examples of misnomers include hydrolyzed, autolyzed or textured protein; yeast extract, protein isolate, maltodextrin, hydrolyzed vegetable protein and others. Some health practitioners suggest glutamate supplementation be avoided in many nervous system disorders.

Bone broth, gelatin, tofu and collagen supplements are rich in natural glutamate. One of our richest vegetable sources is red cabbage, particularly when fermented as sauerkraut.

Other high glutamate foods to avoid include processed foods, casein, corn and soy protein, and aspartame.

Glutamate stimulates histamine release, and may play a role in the aggravation of food sensitivities.

Ingestion of MSG should be curtailed at the onset of dementia, and progression of any brain health issues.[205]

L-theanine, from green tea, is a glutamate antagonist, and therefore calming for some people. It increases GABA and dopamine levels in the brain. See Green Tea in Chapter 16.

Other supplements enhancing GABA production are valerian root, passion flower, lithium orotate, taurine, B6, magnesium, zinc and manganese.

Lithium orotate may be useful in bipolar disorder, but also appears to work by increasing GABA receptor site sensitivity.[206]

NOTE: Some individuals have a genetic disorder involving glutamic acid transminase, and thus have lifelong GABA deficiency. How do you know? If one purchases alpha-ketoglutaric acid, a glutamate precursor, and takes three to four milligrams, on an empty stomach, nothing much will happen. In those with a genetic expression, the surge of glutamate will create nervousness, anxiety and excitability. These individuals will find GABA and precursors a useful life-long support.[207]

CAUTION- Phenibut (beta-phenyl-gamma-aminobutryic acid) is a receptor type B agonist. It is a nootropic widely available via the internet. I do not recommend its use, due to its unpredictable side effects. Do not supplement L-glutamine if you have cancer.

Do not ingest GABA or taurine if you have very low blood pressure.

GABA is best taken on an empty stomach. Do not use concurrently with benzodiazepines, barbiturates, narcotics or gabapentin.

ACETYLCHOLINE

> "Happiness is nothing more than good health and a bad memory."

ALBERT SCHWEITZER

Acetylcholine is one of our main brain neurotransmitters; involved in memory and learning, as well as arousal/reward.

Alpha brain waves help our brain understand, and react to sensory input. The waves are produced in the parietal lobes, and associated with acetylcholine, controlling our brain speed. In a sense, acetylcholine is a lubricant, helping act as a building block for the myelin sheath that surrounds the neurons, similar to how plastic or rubber insulates an electrical wire. This insulation makes sure the signal does not lose strength until it reaches its destination.

By the age of seven, the alpha wave state begins to predominate, and children become indoctrinated into the expectations of their family and society. Alpha waves operate at seven to thirteen cycles per second. Alpha is a state through which the subconscious mind interprets information and experiences, which occurred before birth and during infancy. These may include phobias, complexes and positive affirmations. This state influences how information from other sources, including transpersonal self, are interpreted and expressed. As a child moves to age thirteen, theta becomes less dominant and the body changes to a form less capable of expressing functions of our higher self. The neurotransmitter is involved in the conversion of short-term memory to long-term, which happens in the hippocampus region of the brain.

Symptoms of deficiency include loss of visual memory, forgetting what is just read, or poor verbal memory involving words. It involves our sense of direction and spatial orientation.

Acetylcholine helps facilitate good digestion, and relaxation of breathing and cardiovascular health, due to its connection with the parasympathetic nervous system.

Acetylcholine out of balance can lead to language disorders, childhood learning disabilities, and later, senile dementia and Alzheimer's disease. In deficient states, these individuals tend to crave rich, and fatty foods, or may binge on sweets and caffeine.

Phosphatidylserine (PS) is a helpful supplement for deficient states. See Chapter 15.

When the brain needs acetylcholine and cannot get enough building blocks from dietary fats, it will break down brain tissue for PS and phosphotidylcholine.

In excess, the acetylcholine type gives too much of themselves to the point of being masochistic. They may feel as if the world is taking advantage of them, or they experience paranoia and choose isolation.

Acetylcholine types make up about 17% of the population.

Acetylcholine affects either muscarinic or nicotinic receptors.

Most of the receptors in our brain are the former, with less than 10% nicotinic type.

Both forms of receptors have been found in earthworms, and early peanut worms that lived 500 million years ago.

The brain cannot produce its own, and about ten percent of total choline in the body is produced by a healthy liver. The other ninety percent comes from our diet; the same number of Americans suffering deficiency. The low fat diet craze, thankfully now dispelled, is partially to blame. The consumption of hydrogenated and trans-fats is also implicated.

Blood sugar dysregulation and oxygen deficiency affect our acetylcholine production.

Acetylcholine is produced by *Lactobacillus* species in our healthy microbiome. Stimulating the vagus nerve produces this neurotransmitter, which tells immune cells to stop over-reacting to microbes.

Foods are a rich source of choline, including egg yolks, fish roe, sardines, salmon, milk, shrimp, nutritional yeast, beef liver and shiitake mushrooms. Marmite, a popular product from brewer's yeast is very popular in kitchens in Great Britain and Australia; and a great source of choline.

Lecithin is a good source of phosphtydlcholine, but most is produced from soy; an allergenic for some people. Fortunately sunflower lecithin is a rich source of choline and phosphatidylinositol. It is available as powder that can be added by the tablespoon to foods, including smoothies.

Choline is the precursor of membrane phospholipids such as phosphatidylcholine (PA), the neurotransmitter acetylcholine, and via betaine, the methyl group donor S-adenosylmethionine (SamE). Adequate amounts during pregnancy and early childhood may improve cognitive function in children and adults. PA prevents age-related memory decline in senile dementia, and helps repair neurological damage in epilepsy, fetal alcohol syndrome, as well as Down and Rett syndromes.

Choline rich foods may influence cognition via an effect on PA containing EPA and DHA; as low levels are found in brains of AD patients.[208]

NAC (N-acetyl L-carnitine) supports acetylcholine activity.

L-alpha glycerylphosphorycholine, also known as choline alfoscerate, is a form of choline found naturally in our brains.

It is a parasympathomimetic acetylcholine precursor that delivers choline across the blood-brain barrier (BBB).

It helps mental recovery after cerebral ischemic attacks.[209] This is well absorbed, crosses our BBB easily, and is then converted into acetylcholine.

It improves cognitive capacity in AD, and may help prevent or delay its progression.[210]

DMAE (dimethylaminoethanol) is found in sardines, and increases acetylcholine levels in the brain. The supplement should be taken in consultation with your healthcare provider. It should, however, not be taken in cases of bipolar, convulsions or anyone with a history of epilepsy.

Pantothenic acid (B5) helps the synthesis of coenzyme A involved in the transport of carbon atoms to make acetylcholine.[211] B6 (pyridoxine-5-phosphate), B3, methyl folate and B12 help increase receptor site sensitivity and ensure the breakdown of used serotonin.

Phosphatydlserine, and l-carnitine stimulate acetylcholine production. Saint John's wort may be useful, but one should make note of the herb's numerous drug interactions.

Many herbs inhibit acetylcholinesterase that breaks down this compound. Hundreds of pharmaceuticals developed, and based on the premise of inhibiting this compound, have failed Phase Three clinical trials.

Angelica seed, clubmoss (huperzine A), wild bergamot and rosemary are few natural examples. See Chapter 16.

NOTE- Ingesting in excess of 3500 mg of choline can be toxic. Raw egg yolk contains 682 mg/100 grams. Acetylcholine support on a daily use is of no concern, as repeated exposure does not cause receptor sites to become resistant. This is not true of GABA, serotonin and dopamine. Finding the right dose can take time. Start low and increase until you find improved mental acuity, and stay there. Constant stimulation of receptors makes them more responsive and sensitive, so dosage may be lowered over time.

Producing too much can result in muscle cramps or nausea in some people.

CHAPTER 5

FATS AND OILS

In Chapter One we discussed the importance of essential fatty acids, and in particular the role of Omega3/6/9.

Adding good fats to our diet, and avoiding the bad ones is an excellent start to maintaining, or improving brain health.

Avocado, coconut, flax, macadamia, olive, sesame and walnut oils, if cold pressed and organic, qualify as healthy.

Grass fed bison, beef and lamb fats are rich in CLA.

Corn, soy, peanut, cottonseed, palm oils, and fat from industrial farm raised meat and dairy, as well as trans-fats should be avoided. Palmitic acid, for example, is a saturated fat found in marbled, corn-fattened cattle.

There is growing evidence EPA (eicosapenaenoic acid) and DHA (docosahexaenoic acid) play key parts in the growth, development, maintenance, and healing of our brain.

EPA appears to be more beneficial for depression, and DHA appears better for neuro-inflammatory conditions. However, the science is still not crystal clear, suggesting a combination may be best in most cases.

The third most prevalent long chain fatty acid is DPA or docosapentaenoic acid. In most fish oils, due to manufacturing processes that concentrate DHA and EPA, this fatty acid is missing.[212]

DPA is converted in the body from EPA by an enzyme that adds two carbon units, or converted back to EPA or DHA. DPA is less actively oxidized in the body, and stored in body tissue. In fact, DPA comprises 40% of the long chain omega-3 fatty acids in mother's milk.

Higher blood levels of DPA during pregnancy are associated with a lower risk of postpartum depression.

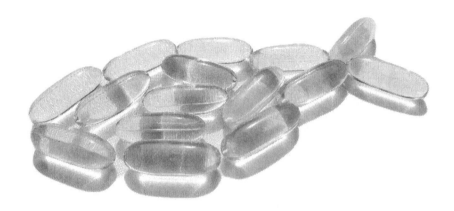

Many fish oils, derived from salmon, sardine and anchovy, are highly prone to oxidation, and subjected to heat and solvent extraction. Wild salmon oils vary in EPA/DPA/DHA ratios. Chinook oil, for example, is 17/5/12, Coho is 9/5/14, and Sockeye (my personal favorite) is 7/3/14.

Studies have found a large variation in the levels of EPA (6.5-40.9%) and DHA (8.1-26.4%) in various fish oil capsules.

Unless specified, most fish Omega-3 complex oils contain a EPA/DHA ratio of 3:2. Specific ratios may be best for certain brain health conditions.

Sardines, anchovies and other fish are abundant in L-alpha-glycerophosphorylcholine (GPC) and dimethylaminoethanol (DMAE), both precursors to acetylcholine.

Large amounts of DMAE are too stimulating to some people, creating headache, muscle tension and irritability. This supplement is to be avoided, by those suffering epilepsy, any history of convulsions, or bipolar disease.

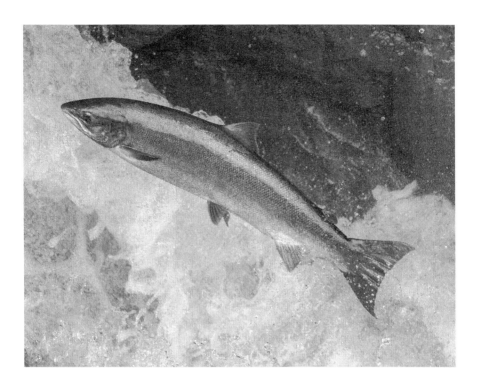

Many off-the-shelf products will not mention whether the salmon oil is from wild or farmed fish; nor its method of extraction.

Read labels carefully as some products contain egg or soy.

Green extraction, using CO_2, offers consumers a product without traces of solvent and is a move in the right direction.

Aqua™ Biome has developed a product that includes DPA.

Today, over one million tons of fish oil are produced annually, but only 5% are used to extract Omega-3 fatty acids.[213]

Algae is becoming an increasingly important, and clean source, of DHA, and the carotenoid astaxanthin. Several years ago I had the pleasure of visiting a production plant in Iceland, with its pure, clean fresh water, and geothermal electric energy. The company Algalif produces very high quality astaxanthin for the world market.

One of my favorite sources of vegetarian DHA is derived from *Schizochytrium* algae species.

See more on Micro and Macroalgae in Supplement Chapter 15.

Krill oil is rich in EPA and DHA as well as astaxanthin, but some products are solvent extracted, and the product is a bit more expensive. Ethanol extracted krill oil is available.

Some studies suggest is may be slightly better absorbed, due to its additional phospholipids. The content of astaxanthin ensures considerably less oxidative breakdown and rancidity. Sustainability is an issue facing all ocean harvests.

A small randomized, DB, PC trial of 21 people suffering mild cognitive impairment, were given a capsule containing astaxanthin and sesamin (from sesame seeds) or placebo. Significant improvement was noted in their ability to comprehend and perform complex tasks quickly and accurately after only 6 and 12 weeks.[214]

Vegetarians and vegans may choose to obtain DHA from algae source. After all, this primitive, unicellular organism is the original source of all marine oils.

Early research on algae/omega-3 was conducted in my hometown of Edmonton, at the Alberta Research Council

Over a dozen papers in the last 15 years report that alpha-linolenic acid (ALA) from nut and seed oils are not converted to DHA, but three studies do show ingestion of micro-algae increases blood erythrocyte and plasma DHA.[215]

Seeds and nuts, however, (see Chapter 15) play a key role in brain health, for numerous other reasons.

The importance of EPA and DHA to brain health is beyond question. How to efficiently deliver them, where needed, is the larger issue.

One study found combining quercitin, which helps quell allergic response, with DHA, may help increase its protective effect.[216]

Another possibility is to add EPA and/or DHA to a phospholipid complex known as lysophosphatidylcholine (LPS). This phospholipid is formed, in the degradation of phosphatidyl-choline, and combined with herbs such as milk thistle seed to ensure better absorption and liver support.

Recent studies on glymphatic tissue in the brain, lead to a lot more questions than answers. Obviously, the movement of lymphatic fluid moves nutrients and toxins in both directions, suggesting a newer model of the blood-brain barrier (BBB) is required.

The transport and absorption of these fatty acids may be significantly increased, by combining with LPS. One mouse study found the percentage of DHA recovered in lymph phospholipids was five times greater with LPC-DHA, compared to free DHA. And when micellized (water soluble), DHA increased by two fold.[217]

One study found LPS-EPA enriches both EPA and DHA in the brain, albeit a mouse study.[218]

Most DHA supplements do not increase our brain DHA, as they are hydrolyzed to free DHA and absorbed as triacylglyercol.

The transporter at the BBB is specific for phospholipids forms.

The apoliprotein E (APOE) 4 allele is the strongest risk factor for genetic forms of Alzheimer's disease. DHA is transported across the outer membrane leaflet of the blood-brain barrier, but LPC-DHA is transported across the inner membrane. APOE4 carriers may have impaired brain transport of DHA but not LPC-DPA.[219]

In clinical practice I found micellized vitamins, particularly A and E, were incredibly effective at improving absorption levels.

Let us now look at some brain health issues, and the latest medical findings on which EPA/DHA oil ratio, may be best for various conditions.

Anxiety

In anxious, nervous individuals that self medicate with nicotine or drugs, it may be best to add a high ratio DHA fish or algae oil product to the diet.

Depression

On the other hand, for individuals with depression, low energy, poor appetite, insomnia and loss of hope, EPA rich fish oil would be more applicable.[220] In a meta-analysis of 241 DB, PC randomized trials, 28 met the inclusion criteria; suggesting EPA may be more important for supplementation in cases of depression.

Anxiety/Depression

Where the moods swing between the two, a EPA/DHA ratio of 3/2 is more advised. This is a common fish oil ratio. Just ensure it is free of heavy metals, and produced under low heat.

There is scientific evidence children with either ADHD or Autism Spectrum Disorder have low omega-3 levels; the latter group more so.[221]

For ADD and ADHD I suggest a product called Equazen. It is an Omega-3/6 fatty acid product with a 9/3/1 ratio of EPA/DHA/GLA. Clinical trials found the supplement showed similar benefit in ADHD children over a 12-month period to methylphenidate.[222]

Of ten clinical trials, reviewing the benefits of Omega-3 for ADHD, only the two involving with Equazen were statistically significant.[223]

A randomized, DB, PC study[224] in Australia of 132 children, not taking stimulants (ie. Ritalin) aged 7-12 years for 30 weeks found significant cognitive improvement.

Children and adults with ADD, without hyperactivity, may find a good ratio EPA/DHA fish oil works just as well. Both oppositional and less hyperactive/impulsive children with ADHD improved teacher-rated behavior after a 15-week supplementation of EPA.[225]

Autism Spectrum Disorder (ASD) children often exhibit irritability and hyperactivity. One randomized, DB, PC trial of 111 children found vitamin D and DHA reduced irritability, and vitamin D (2000 IU/day) by itself reduced hyperactivity.[226]

A small study of autism symptoms in pre-term toddlers found DHA and GLA supplementation showed clinically significant improvements.[227]

DHA in pre-natal supplements resulted in lower diastolic and systolic blood pressure in five-year old children, compared to mothers who did not take DHA.

DHA supplementation is found in superior infant formulas.

Alzheimer's and Parkinson's disease patients may benefit from a good source of EPA/DHA.

The exact ratio for AD is unclear at the moment. It is also unknown whether EPA, as a DHA precursor, acts directly on brain health, or via DHA.[228] My suggestion for now is to consider a good quality EPA/DHA oil with close to equal ratios.

Bipolar disorder and the potential benefit of omega-3 supplementation is difficult to access. One meta-analyses found significant benefit in the depression side of equation, but no significant effect for mania.[229] DMAE should be avoided.

Many people complain about the burping and unpleasant experience of trying to digestive omega-3 fish oils. It can be a problem for many people, including Laurie, my amazing wife and life partner for the past thirty years. One solution is to take an enzyme rich in lipase at the same time, along with food.

Under supplements we will discuss the various lipo- and phospholipid products that improve digestion, and fats and oils bio-availability to the brain.

NOTE- Patients with pyroluria do not tolerate Omega-3 oils that well. See zinc under Supplements for more information.

Fish oils affect platelet function, and potential bleeding, and should be discontinued for three to five days before surgery.

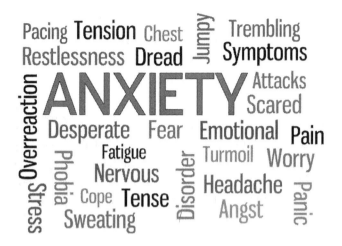

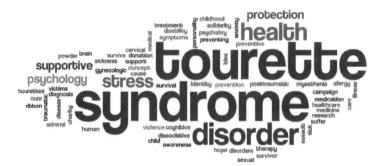

CHAPTER 6

ANXIETY, POST TRAUMATIC STRESS DISORDER (PTSD), AND TOURETTE SYNDROME

ANXIETY

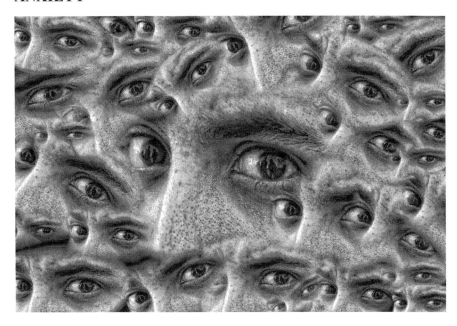

"Our age of anxiety is, in great part, the result of trying to do today's job with yesterday's tools and yesterday's concepts."

MARSHALL McLUHAN

Anxiety is a broad term that involves multiple factors, including lifestyle, diet, and a variety of psychological factors.

Physiologically, anxiety involves the basal ganglia tissue surrounding our limbic system.

This area of the brain is concerned with behaviors associated with survival, including food, reproduction and fight or flight responses. Two basic forms are panic anxiety and social anxiety, according to Jeffrey Kahn. He suggests the former developed from a primeval instinct to stay close to the tribe, and not stray too far from home and family. Social anxiety developed to keep people in line in their tribal hierarchy, to know their place.[230]

Both anxiety and depression rates are very high in young adults and teenagers. Almost 50% of university students report their anxiety so severe they can hardly function.[231]

And there is a direct link between anxiety, depression and the misuse of drugs. Low dopamine levels may be a common link.

Our limbic system responds well to nutrition, and supplements including herbs and aromatherapy. The hypothalamus is involved in limbic system activity, and is directly influenced by olfaction.

Acupuncture can calm the limbic system in a manner different than anti-depressant drugs.[232] Acupuncture may be useful for opiate-type addictions in patients that do not respond to pharmaceutical anti-depressants.

When stressed, such as being chased by a bear, the sympathetic nervous system is activated. Our modern lifestyle leans in this direction, with numerous stressors in everyday life.

Our sympathetic and parasympathetic nerves run parallel to each other. The former are quite thin and reactive, the latter are wider and thicker and are supposed to be dominant most of the time. The sympathetic nervous system is wired for emergencies and life threatening situations, but has become the dominant state of modern life. The thin wires burn out, creating inflammation that leads to exhaustion and depletion.

It was widely believed our brain controls the response to stress, but new findings suggest it is our microbiota-gut-brain axis. The gut sends messages to the hypothalamus, which talks to the pituitary and then to different glands, such as the thyroid and adrenals, which then respond.

Correcting gut health, including leaky gut and healthy bacteria is essential to finding nervous system balance. See Chapter Two.

Studies have found complaining rewires our brain for anxiety and depression.

And hence, the additional benefit of meditation, yoga and other mindful practices, which instill patience, and gratitude.

Anxious patients who self-medicate, are nervous, and anticipate worst-case scenarios, may benefit from GABA or GABA related herbal supplements, vitamin B complex, magnesium and a higher ratio of DHA in their Omega-3 combination.

In Canada, from 8-11% of women suffer generalized anxiety disorder (GAD) during pregnancy, which influences their unborn child.

A study of 26 expectant mothers in their last trimester gave one group 480 mg of choline, and other group 930 mg (double the recommended amount). The researchers measured cortisol levels in blood from the mothers and babies just after birth. The larger amount did not alter mothers' stress hormones, but did significantly lower those of the baby.[233]

Egg yolks are a rich source of choline, but supplements can sometimes be useful.

Folate supplementation as part of a multivitamin will help prevent spina bifida, in fetus of expectant mothers, as does high choline intake.[234]

Lavender essential oil, in small amounts, is relaxing and calmative, either diffused into the air, or added to baths after the hot water is poured. It helps to add a few drops to either milk, or Epsom salts (magnesium sulfate) to help emulsify and spread the fragrant scent. See Chapter 20.

Magnesium supplementation may be beneficial, particularly if nerve and muscle excitation is present. Deficiency is a widespread concern, with some estimates suggesting up to 90% of North Americans are lacking this important mineral. See Chapter 15.

Forest bathing, the art of walking mindfully in nature, can help relieve tension, anxiety, depression and fatigue. A study involving 128 volunteers (averaging 60 years old) had their mood states tested, and exhibited significantly lower anxiety levels.[235]

Mixed anxiety and depression can take a number of forms. It is important for the practitioner to distinguish the variation, as stimulating the incorrect neurotransmitter may exaggerate the issue.

For the mixed anxiety and depression individual, there is often a deficiency of both GABA and dopamine. Therefore, supplementation with GABA and dopamine supporting herbs, B6, magnesium, SAMe and a good ratio EPA/DHA fish oil would be useful.

For anxiety-depressive states with worry, ODD (oppositional defiance disorder) and over-focus on problems, a better approach would be an emphasis on 5-HTP, saffron and possibly Saint John's wort, with L-tryptophan supplements during a complex carbohydrate-rich evening meal.

Anxiety-depression associated with outbursts of temper, mood swings, irritability; as well as memory and learning problems responds better to GABA, magnesium, B6, huperzine A, acety-1-carnitine, and *Ginkgo biloba*.

And finally, anxiety-depression associated with a lack of focus, low energy, sadness, and weepiness, may do better with L-theanine or green tea, *Rhodiola rosea*, and/or L-tyrosine in the morning on empty stomach.

POST TRAUMATIC STRESS DISORDER (PTSD)

Post Traumatic Stress Disorder involves upsetting and recurring thoughts or dream-state of dramatic events. These may be incidents of abuse (including sexual), accidents, war, and trauma. Individuals can be fearful, startle easily, and have constant anxiety around possible future events. Children and grandchildren of alcoholics or drug-abusers can suffer this hyper-vigilant state.

Many people suffering PTSD turn to cannabis for temporary relief. "One preliminary study on veterans with posttraumatic stress disorder (PTSD), researchers tested cannabis (including THC) as a treatment. Results showed the use was significantly associated with higher PTSD symptom severity, as well as higher levels of violent behavior and alcohol and drug use."[236]

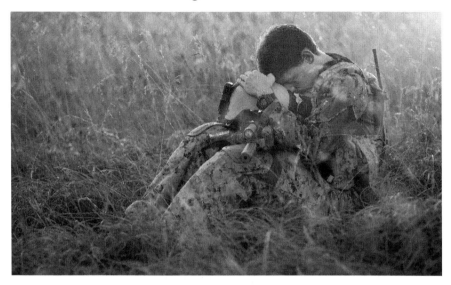

Dr. Susan Sisley recently completed research on the use of cannabis by 76 PTSD war veterans. She was fired from her position at the University of Arizona when the FDA approved her trial, so they moved it to the *Scottsdale Research Institute*. With a 2.15 million dollar contribution from the *Colorado Department of Public Health and Environment*, the study was recently completed. Results of the trial will be released in a medical journal sometime in 2019.

Cannabinoids (CBDs) cross the blood brain barrier and bind to our own endogenous cannabinoid neurotransmitter system. These are anandamide, from the Sanskrit wordk ananda, meaning bliss, and 2-AG.

These are not stored in synaptic vesicles, but produced within neurons and released to flow backward across the synapse to find their receptors CB1 and CB2. There are more CB1 receptors for cannabis in the human brain than any other known neurotransmitter.

Anandamide inhibits the release of glutamate and acetylcholine within the cortex and hippocampus, impairing the ability to form new memories.

These receptors greatly increase the release of dopamine. Munchies, a well-known side effect of cannabis ingestion, are a consequence of stimulation on this receptor in the hypothalamus.

Stimulating cannabinoid receptors may protect against consequences of stroke, chronic pain and neuro-inflammation, and some aspects of age-related memory loss.

Cannabis may protect the aging brain by preventing the damaging effects of glutamate, reducing brain inflammation, and restoring neurogenesis. A puff or dropper may be enough, according to recent research. See Chapter 16.

Supplementation with GABA or herbs such as valerian root, damiana, Canby's lovage, or ashwagandha may be helpful, as well as magnesium, vitamin B6 and Omega3 oils.

Robuvit is a red oak wood extract that exhibits benefit in the reduction of PTSD symptoms.[237]

Saint John's wort, on the other hand, should be avoided.

Both lavender and roman chamomile essential oils are calming and soothing.

Phase Two clinical trials into the benefits of MDMA (3,4-methylenedioxymethamphetamine) for PSTD have been completed. Twenty-eight people with chronic PTSD were randomized in a double blind comparison of either 100-125 mg or 40 mg (low dose) of MDMA for one year. The larger dose group, along with psychotherapy had the largest reduction in PTSD symptoms.[238] A review of the contemporary papers on potential uses, include anxiety associated with autism, and alcoholism is noted.

MDMA (3,4-Methylenedioxymethamphetamine), also known as ecstasy, assisted psychotherapy for the treatment of PTSD shows great promise. A recent publication based on six phase two randomized controlled trials, suggest another treatment option.[239]

There are ongoing Phase Three clinical trials in the United States, Canada and Israel, with results scheduled for 2021.

Brazilian Jiu Jitsu training, and Transcendental Medication (TM) show benefit in treating PTSD. A five-month training program in the former, found clinical improvements, decreased major depression and generalized anxiety, and less alcohol use.[240]

TM helped relieve symptoms, in a one-month study of 46 veterans. The median PTSD score declined from 52.5 to 22.5, a decrease of 30 points.[241]

Psilocin, from Psilocyin mushrooms, has shown great benefit in stilling the mind. A number of studies have found benefit in treating nicotine and alcohol addictions, as well as PTSD, depression and anxiety. See Chapter 17 Medicinal Mushrooms.

Eye movement desensitization and reprocessing (EMDR) may help some individuals suffering PTSD.[242]

TOURETTE SYNDROME

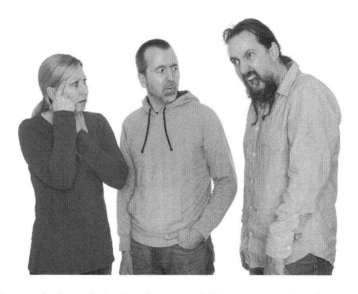

Another variation of the Anxiety Model is Tourette Syndrome (TS). Or to be more precise, it is a combination of two opposing brain related issues; attention deficit hyperactivity disorder (ADHD), and obsessive-compulsive disorder (OCD). Both are covered in greater detail in their own section.

TS disorder involves motor and vocal tics; the former involving head or limb jerking, facial and eye tics, and the latter with involuntary noises including barking, coughing, and swearing.

It runs in families genetically related to abnormalities in the dopamine group of genes.

It is estimated that 60% of people with TS have ADHD, and 50% suffer OCD. See Chapter 12.

People with ADHD have difficulty paying attention, and those with OCD pay too much attention to their own negative thoughts and behaviors.[243]

Dopamine and serotonin play a balancing act, and too much of one makes the other less effective. Raising dopamine in ADHD patients helps them focus and be motivated. Too much, and symptoms of too little serotonin, such as obsessive, moody and inflexible behaviors, appear. If tryptophan is given to ADHD patients, serotonin increases and symptoms worsen, but the patient won't care if they are worse, and will exhibit lower motivation.[244]

Care is required in choosing supplementation for TS patients.

L-theanine from green tea may be helpful, along with magnesium, scullcap, kava kava, passion flower, lemon balm and/or hops. Excitatory foods such as caffeinated beverages, and sugars should be eliminated from diet.

Useful therapies may include music, self-hypnosis, acupuncture, and cannabis.[245,246]

Other complementary and alternative medicines (CAM) considered useful are meditation (prayer), vitamins and supplements, massage, hypnosis, homeopathy, chiropractic manipulation, and EEG biofeedback. In a questionnaire of 100 TS patients or parents, 64 had used at least one CAM therapy, with 56% reporting they found some improvement.[247]

Nicotine patches or gum may be a useful adjunct.[248]

CHAPTER 7

DEPRESSION, SEASONAL AFFECTIVE DISORDER, AND POSTPARTUM DEPRESSION

DEPRESSION

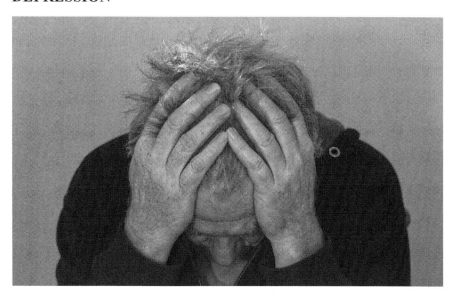

"Depression is the inability to construct a future."

ROLLO MAY

Depression at some point, will affect over 50 million Americans, and 300 million people worldwide. The World Health Organization projects that by 2030 the amount of worldwide disability and life lost to depression will be greater than cancer, stroke, heart disease, accidents and war.

Depression is being diagnosed in people at a younger and younger age. The age group of 18-29 year olds are more likely to suffer depression than those sixty or older.

Depression rates vary a great deal around the world, from a reported 2% of the population in Japan and Korea, to 7% in the USA, 11% in New Zealand and 16% in France.

In turn, depressive thoughts increase our risk of heart disease, cancer, dementia, Alzheimer's disease and diabetes.

More than twenty studies, conducted over the past decade, show the prevalence rate of diabetics with depression is three to four times greater than the general population. Instead of depression being a diabetic complication, it is now considered the reverse. That is, depression may be a cause or trigger for diabetes. A major study at Johns Hopkins tracked over eleven thousand non-diabetic adults for six years and found depressive symptoms predicted incidents of Type-2 diabetes.[249]

Symptoms include agitation, loss of appetite, sleep disturbance, confusion, feelings of hopelessness, sadness, crying, loss of self-worth, low energy, and suicidal thoughts. All of these symptoms are painful enough, but the reaction from friends and family is also problematic, leading many sufferers to avoid treatment.

Depression can be difficult to diagnose as Parkinson's disease, Alzheimer's disease, dementia, thyroid dysfunction, diabetes and stroke all exhibit similar symptoms.

One study found 67% of patients with celiac disease were also depressed, and 73% suffering high levels of anxiety.[250]

Many of the medications recommended for depression can exacerbate or mask the true cause of depression associated with brain health.

Nearly all depressed patients are told they have a chemical imbalance, as if they were deficient of a particular drug.

In fact, many of the touted benefits of anti-depressant medications "fall below accepted criteria for clinical significance."[251] Under an appeal to the Freedom of Information Act, a group of researchers obtained access to unpublished studies on anti-depressants that *Big*

Pharma tried to bury. The data found anti-depressants outperformed placebo in only 20 of 46 trials.

Irving Kirsch (2010) conducted an exhaustive study of antidepressant medications in clinical trials and found inert placebo pills are about 82% as effective.

Major medical journals, with the most pharmaceutical advertising, are associated with publishing fewer articles on dietary supplements. Articles suggesting supplements were unsafe was found in 4% of journals with the fewest ads, and 67% with the most pharmads.[252] Are you surprised?

Twenty-seven million Americans take antidepressants (as of 2014), and yet, two-thirds find no relief. One of the largest-ever multi-site treatment studies of the effectiveness of drug therapy for serious clinical depression, found 72% of the 2876 patients still had residual symptoms after fourteen weeks.[253]

One Australian study found women who sit more than seven hours a day have a 47% greater risk of depression than those sitting less than four hours.

Depression doubles the risk of cognitive impairment in women, and quadruples the risk, in men. In fact, late-life depression may be a precursor to Alzheimer's disease, with one-third of patients with mild cognitive impairment also reporting depression.

One study found just 16 of 211 elderly women with six or more depressive symptoms were being treated, in any manner.[254]

In fact, the differences between depression and dementia are subtle but distinct.

Depression is more likely with a prior family history, physical symptoms, sad or negative feelings, excess worry or anxiety, feeling life is not worth living, lonely or bored, crying for no apparent reason, difficulty with daily chores, low energy and suicidal thoughts, that come on more quickly than dementia. The single theme most consistent with depression is loss.

Dementia is related to difficulty doing familiar tasks, problems with words and language, disoriented in time and place, decreased judgment, memory loss, forgets where things are placed, problems with abstract thinking, changes in personality, loss of initiative. Suicidal thoughts are less common.[255]

And in the elderly, the two may co-exist, increasing the difficulty of adequate treatment. A sense of community, or belonging is so important, as many people feel isolated, lonely and forgotten.

Each year, in the United States, over forty-seven thousand suicides are directly, or indirectly related to depression.

Various lifestyle changes can often relieve symptoms associated with depression. Exercise such as walking, stretching, gardening, biking or swimming can be helpful. Connection with family and friends, a companion animal, music, tai chi, dance, drumming and journaling all make a difference.

One study found group drumming helped anxiety, depression social resilience and improved inflammatory immune response.[256]

Good nutrition and proper supplementation is a cornerstone to lifting depressive states.

Thyroid function plays a key role in the production of serotonin, dopamine and GABA. In the brain scans of people suffering low thyroid function, over 80% showed impaired memory.[257]

Low thyroid function is associated with depression, low sex drive, weight gain, elevated cholesterol, dry skin, menstrual issues and hypertension. One-third of depressions are directly related to low or high thyroid levels. The tens of millions of Americans with thyroid issues may be the result of increased hormone-disrupting, synthetic chemicals in our air, water (chlorine and fluoride) and food.[258] Exposure to EMFs plays a role in thyroid dysfunction.

A long-term study found people eating fast foods and baked goods were 51% more likely to suffer depression.

Constant stress is a factor that influences dietary choices, by people reaching for foods that increase dopamine, to reduce their anxiety and depression. Breathing and exercise are useful in depression. Nature deficit disorder, articulated by Richard Louv, is a big factor in modern society. We are part of nature, and watching nature on television or the internet does not help us reconnect with our core being.

High fat diets help protect against the damaging effects of chronic stress, likely through the hypothalamic-pituitary-adrenal-axis or HPAA.

However, this impulse can become obsessive, leading to reduced dopamine reward, increasing anxiety and depression leading to overeating, and obesity.

I have personally reduced excess weight by using intermittent fasting, waiting at least 12-14 hours between meals. This is not difficult for most people.

Fasting helps change our microbiome, by increasing the levels of *Akkermansia*, a microbe that encourages more mucus secretion in the gut. This is turn improves insulin sensitivity for type 2 diabetics, and increases Lacto species growth.[259]

Essential fatty acids, particularly omega-3s, are a cornerstone of healthy brain function. A 3:2 or higher ratio of EPA:DHA is a good choice for most people. See chapter 5.

DMAE (dimethylaminoethanol) derived from sardines increases acetylcholine levels, associated with elevated moods and protection of memory.

There is a direct correlation between low cholesterol and depression, including suicide risk. Low levels of omega-3s are associated with depression, and low cholesterol is associated with low serotonin receptors in brain cells.[260] One quarter of our cholesterol is found in the nervous system. Low serotonin levels in our spinal fluid is associated with aggression, and low cholesterol levels.

A cholesterol level lower than 159 is associated with a 21% increase in premature births.[261]

Folate levels are directly related to depression severity. Methylation is a problem for up to 40% of the population, and avoidance of synthetic folic acid is recommended. It is important to read food labels carefully, as folic acid is sprinkled in numerous fast food products.

A daily B-complex, including B6 and B12, with methyl-folate is important, as B vitamins have been linked to depression and bipolar disorders in a number of studies.

A study conducted over 40 years ago, estimated fully one-third of adults are low in folates.[262]

Of course, one of the difficulties in assessing studies on depression, is that patient groups are not allowed to have concurrent diseases.

Vitamin D, derived from sheep's lanolin, or mushrooms (for vegans) is important, as our ability to produce sufficient amounts for optimal brain health, declines with age. In the right climate, of course, fifteen minutes of sun exposure to bare arms and legs is sufficient for most people.

Magnesium theronate is recommended for supplementation, as patients recovering from depression, show their magnesium levels rise.[263] Many forms of magnesium are available, but many do little more than relieve constipation.

There are four neurotransmitters relevant to depression. See Chapter 4 for more information on each of the following.

Low dopamine levels can affect sleep, appetite, mood and sexual appetite.

The depression associated with low dopamine is very different from that caused by low serotonin. These individuals enjoy life, but their mood is low and they have a hard time getting motivated. Dopamine can excite the brain to new ideas, or help give focus in attention span for concentration. Learning disorders and ADHD are associated with, but not limited to, poor dopamine activity. At the same time, high dopamine is associated with psychosis and schizophrenia, with many anti-psychotic drugs classed as dopamine blockers.

Acetylcholine helps protect neuron synapses and plays a key role in short and long-term memory, as well as mood elevation.

Noradrenaline levels can affect mood. When released in excess due to short-term stress, it can have a positive effect.

Of course, some people suffer from low levels of both dopamine and serotonin.

Low serotonin levels are associated with depression and repressed anger. Increased production of serotonin helps relieve tension and create more positive moods. Unlike low dopamine people who feel worthless and hopeless in their depression, serotonin types suffer depression and anger, or OCD and anxiety disorders.

Sugar temporarily stimulates serotonin, but the rise and fall of insulin and blood sugar levels, creates a vicious cycle of needing more.

Tryptophan rich foods, or L-tryptophan supplementation helps increase brain serotonin, which elevates mood.

The herbal product 5-HTP is more easily converted into the neurotransmitter, serotonin.

Other supplements of note are cacao (chocolate), and resveratrol, which help increase hippocampal serotonin and noradrenaline.

SAMe is a major anti-oxidant and contributes to the formation of serotonin. SAMe may be more helpful in cases of depression involving males, but worth a trial in either sex.[264]

SEASONAL AFFECTIVE DISORDER (SAD)

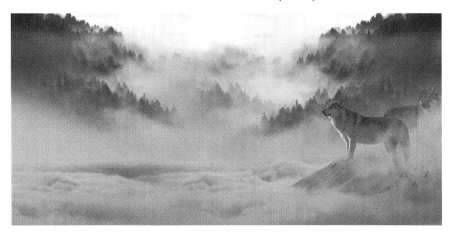

Low light levels in winter can affect feelings of depression, the desire to hibernate, and load up on carbohydrates.

Vitamin D deficiency can exacerbate the feelings of exhaustion and fatigue associated with poor sleep, and general imbalance of circadian rhythms.

Negative ions, more plentiful in nature than urban environments, show benefit in a small group of patients with SAD.[265]

Light boxes can be helpful, and act like the sunlight our pineal gland is craving. A combination of negative ions and bright lights may be very helpful.

If there is inappropriate melatonin production there may be depression and fatigue. Fifteen to thirty minutes of light exposure in the morning can help increase serotonin production.

For insomnia, use the extra light in late afternoon or early evening at least two hours before bed. Natural light around noon for an hour or so is very helpful for those affected.

Blue light, associated with smart phones and computers can worsen insomnia and symptoms of SAD.

POST PARTUM DEPRESSION (PPD)

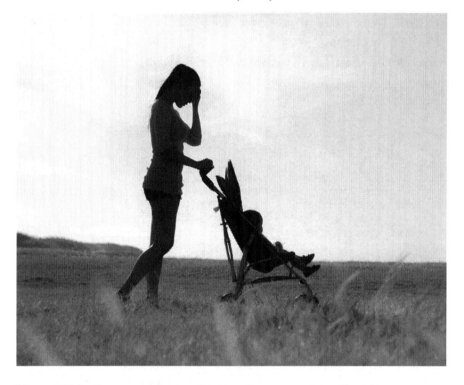

Up to 13% of new mothers will experience anxiety disorders, and this may be exacerbated by childhood trauma, intolerance of uncertainty, obsessive-compulsive disorder and depression.

Over 400,000 American women annually suffer from PPD.

Screening by pediatricians has improved, but other than cognitive and behavioral therapy, very little is offered by the biomedical model. Prescriptions for anti-depressant medications such as SSRIs, or a referral to psychiatrists are the top two options.[266]

There is a 40% increase in monamine oxidase (MAO-A) levels during PPD. Tryptophan and tyrosine supplements do not affect their concentration in breast milk. Blueberry juice and blueberry extract were included in this small (41) double-blind study, showing the benefit of supplementation.[267]

Postpartum home care shows reduced PPD, and the value of midwives and doulas in improving positive outcomes.

Studies have found late onset postpartum depression (PPD) in new mothers, may lead to delayed language development during infancy and early childhood.[268]

Omega-3, vitamin D and dietary advice show imprecise outcomes in a meta-analysis of randomized controlled trials.[269]

However, a systematic review of over 88,000 PPD patients found 22 studies, suggest protective effects from vitamins, fish oils, calcium, vitamin D, zinc and possibly selenium.[270]

Dietary supplementation of EPA and DHA during pregnancy or postpartum reduce some of the symptoms associated with depression.[271]

Remember that these important oils are required for fetal brain development, and will be depleted from an expectant mother during pregnancy.

One study found low levels of omega 3 and higher levels of omega 6 oils in early pregnancy were associated with a greater risk of PPD.[272]

Folate supplementation during pregnancy decreased the risk of PPD in one study of Chinese women.[273]

Body movement exercises and acupuncture showed benefit in a meta-analysis involving 2779 women suffering anxiety, depression and personality disorders during pregnancy.[274]

Magnesium sulfate and zinc sulfate supplements did not reduce PPD and anxiety in a triple-blind, randomized, placebo-controlled study.[275] The choice of poorly absorbed, sulfate bound minerals may have been a factor in the poor outcome.

Vitamin D (2000 IU daily) during late pregnancy was effective in decreasing PPD in a randomized, controlled trial of 169 women.[276]

Lower postpartum ferritin levels can cause depression. Supplementation with iron showed a 42.8% improvement in PPD in a randomized, PC, DB trial of 70 mothers.[277]

Saffron would be worth a trial for its anti-depressive benefit. See Chapter 16.

The benefits of placentophagy (consuming placenta) are uncertain. The freezing of tissue is probably useful in the event of immune disorders which may occur later in life.

If at all possible, breastfeeding is highly encouraged. Maternal infections with hepatitis B and C are no contraindication to giving mother's milk. Breastfeeding is correlated with slightly enhanced cognitive development in several studies.

The first three to five days of breast milk is actually colostrum, containing antibodies that modulate genes, and growth factors and hormones that close the permeability of the gut lining. This also works in supplement form for adults. One quarter of solids in colostrum are antibodies (IgG, IgE, IgA, IgD), which help colonize the microbiome. It helps repair the microvilli worn down in celiac patients.

Lavender scent, for four weeks, helped prevent stress, anxiety and depression after childbirth.[278]

No associations have been found between *Toxoplasma gondii*, associated with cats, and postpartum blues.[279]

In March 2019, the FDA approved the synthetic hormone brexanalone for treating PPD. A full course of injections costs about $34,000, and comes with significant side effects.

CHAPTER 8

AUTISM SPECTRUM DISORDER

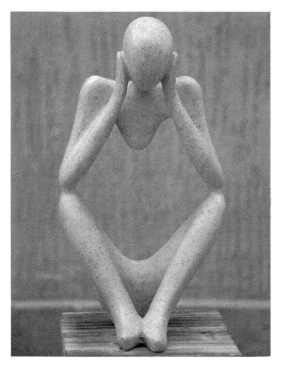

"Mild autism can give you a genius like Einstein."

TEMPLE GRANDIN

"I see people with Asperger's syndrome as a bright thread in the rich tapestry of life."

TONY ATTWOOD

The United Nations estimates that up to seventy million people fall on the autism spectrum, with over three million individuals in the U.S. alone.

Just fifty years ago, one in five thousand children were born with, or developed, the disorder by age three. In 2018 this became one in 59 (and one in every 37 boys).

At one time, Asperger's syndrome and autistic disorder were considered sub-sets of the condition, but in 2013 the umbrella of autism spectrum disorder (ASD) was put in place.

Each individual will exhibit their own unique, distinct gifts, with large number of ASD people excelling in math, music or arts.

One interesting finding shows siblings sharing the same biological parents and diagnosed with autism, don't always share the same autism-linked genes.[280] This suggests that although links to over 100 genes have been correlated to autism, environmental factors may play a larger role. In fact, only 15% of genetic autism is directly related to changes in genes.

Temple Grandin is a well-known professor with autism. In her book *The Autistic Brain: Thinking Across the Spectrum*, she does not dismiss, entirely, the connection between ASD and vaccination. She personally thinks the issue will not be settled until a study is run that separates children starting out developing normally, and those that regress around 18 months, associated with vaccination.[281]

Genetic changes can, however, happen spontaneously, due to random deleting, doubling or reversing a gene.

The DRD4 gene codes for a receptor that regulates the level of dopamine in the brain, and some people possess a variant called DRD4-7R (seven repeat allele). These individuals are less sensitive to dopamine, the neurotransmitter responsible for emotional response. This allele has been linked with anxiety, depression, epilepsy, dyslexia, ADHD, migraines, OCD as well as ASD.

If the father has the 7R variant, the children will be more likely to exhibit OCD and tic-like behavior, while a mother with 7R variant may have a child exhibiting social anxiety disorder and oppositional defiant disorder (ODD).[282]

It is likely that a genetic change, along with an environmental influence, produce symptoms associated with ASD.

Genes may increase the risk, but inflammation of the gut and brain may exert a greater influence. Toxins are a factor, as children born today have an average of two hundred toxic chemicals in their umbilical cord blood.

Differences in biochemistry include lower DNA methylation, affecting gene expression, decreased ratio of SAM (methyl donor) to SAH (methylation by-product), and increased markers for oxidative stress.

One study found 23% of mothers of autistic children had antibodies that targeted brain cells, while still in the womb.[283]

Mothers with obesity are 50% more likely to bear children with autism. A study of obese mice found more than half of their pups had a tendency toward autistic behavior, avoiding other mice and attracted to inanimate objects.

Peri-natal exposure to mercury from dental amalgams is significantly associated with increased risk of ASD and ADHD. Exposure to EMFs may increase release of mercury vapor and decrease levels of dopamine, serotonin, noreprenephrine and acetylcholine neurotransmitters in the brain.[284]

The researchers then looked at the microbiome and found a lack of *L. reuteri*, and when this bacterium was added to their diet, the anti-social behavior disappeared.

The ASD brain functions differently, and something occurred neurologically. Some individuals choose to think of the disorder as a personality trait, but I believe most parents would appreciate knowing if a treatment would be helpful.

Diagnosis of ASD is reliable in children as young as 14 months based on a recent study by Karen Pierce in *JAMA Pediatrics*.

Both adults and children with ASD are perceived as lacking empathy, due to problems with communication and socializing. Research shows they may be aware of other's feelings, but have difficult interpreting or understanding them.[285]

One thing we do know is that children with autism have distinct patterns of unhealthy gut flora. This is discussed in an earlier chapter, but it is well documented that gastrointestinal conditions are commonly associated with the spectrum.

Certain subsets of children with ASD, and ADHD suffer inflammatory bowel disease, Crohn's disease, celiac and ulcerative colitis.

One study found 87% of autistic children possess antibodies against gluten, egg, and dairy, compared to 1% of children without autism.[286]

Children with ASD exhibit immune deficiency, with low to normal antibodies, low numbers of white blood cells (including imbalanced T1 and T2), and poorly functioning natural killer cells, and/or increased levels of inflammatory cytokines. They have low secretory IgA in their gut lining and respiratory systems, making them susceptible to low-grade or sub-clinical viral infections.

One subset of children with autism react negatively to strep infections, causing the antibodies to inappropriately effect the basal ganglia of brain, and increasing obsessive-compulsive disorder.[287]

Fever has been found to improve function and behavior, and reduce "autistic" symptoms in some children. Although poorly understood, this phenomenon may relate to the pattern of acute and chronic inflammation discussed in Chapter 3.

In one study, 92% of ASD children suffered intestinal distress and 85% had chronic constipation.[288] The CDC estimates that children with autism are 3.5 times more likely to experience diarrhea and constipation than their peers.

Leaky gut is involved, with higher levels of lipo-polysaccharides, which are pro-inflammatory, finding their way into the bloodstream.

There is a great deal of controversy over dietary restrictions, and improvement of symptoms, associated with ASD patients.

One systematic review of six randomized controlled trials involving 214 participants, found no evidence that a gluten and casein-free diet was beneficial for symptom relief.[289]

On the other hand, one other randomized controlled trial of 67 children and adults with ASD found a group given supplements along with dietary restriction of soy, gluten and casein, for 12 months, showed significant benefit.[290]

Clostridial species, including the most well known *C. difficile*, appears to play a detrimental role. Antibiotics are implicated in allowing this bacterium to dominant gut flora, sometimes with deadly consequences. Clostridia species and their toxins increase sensitivity to light and noise, and affect muscle tonus. Hence, we commonly find in ASD, the walking on tiptoes, and odd stretching of arms and legs.

Different bacteria produce different forms of short chain fatty acids. Clostridial species produce propionic acid (PPA), which is toxic to the brain. It increases leaky gut weakness, where it can then slip into the bloodstream, creating inflammation. It alters the brain's mitochondrial function, and depletes the brain of anti-oxidants, omega-3s and various neurotransmitters.

One interesting study found mice, engineered to exhibit autism-like symptoms, had 46 times more PPA in their blood. When fed *Bifidobacterium fraglis*, the leaky gut in "autistic" mice sealed up, reducing levels of the destructive molecule significantly.[291]

The only problem is *B. fragilis* is considered a human pathogen.

Lactobacillus reuteri however, (see Chapter 2) increases levels of oxytocin, the "cuddle" hormone and neurotransmitter that influences people to be more social. Oxytocin reduces repetitive action in those with ASD, and improves the recognition of emotion in children with the condition.[292]

A study in Finland took 75 babies and gave half *L. rhamnosus* and other half placebo for their first six months of life. At age 13, 17% of the kids receiving the placebo exhibited ADHD or Asperger's. Those who received the healthy bacterium had no evidence of either.[293]

Other gut bacteria may be problematic. One metabolite 4EPS, on fimbria, is found in levels some 50 times higher than in non-autistic populations.

Tryptophan may be deficient in ASD. A study of 236 patients found supplementation of B vitamins and magnesium influenced the utilization and metabolic homeostasis of this precursor to serotonin and melatonin.[294]

Taurine helps ease constipation in children with ASD, due to an increased production of bile salts. It improves magnesium function and has a calming effect by activating GABA receptors. See Supplements Chapter 15.

From 40 to 80 percent of autistic people suffer from anxiety and depression, approximately twice to four times the general population. And 50 to 80 percent suffer from gut dysbiosis.

One study from Italy found not only do ASD people suffer GI tract issues, but their close relatives do as well.[295]

Sleep is critical in ASD, as brain inflammation and waste products cannot be cleared via glial cells and glymphatic tissue into the cerebral spinal fluid. When glial cells are overwhelmed, glutamate is released in large quantities, leading to hypersensitivity and a noisy brain. See glymphatic in Chapter 3.

Fortunately, glial cells regenerate, when nutrients and cofactor supplements decrease the oxidative stress and a more balanced glutamate/GABA balance is restored.

Seventy-three percent of ASD children suffer hypoperfusion, meaning they don't get enough oxygen to their brain.

When oxygen flow is restricted in the thalamus, the children show repetitive behavior patterns. When restricted in the right temporal lobe, obsessive behavior occurs. When the left temporal lobe is affected, impaired social interaction and communication has been noted.[296]

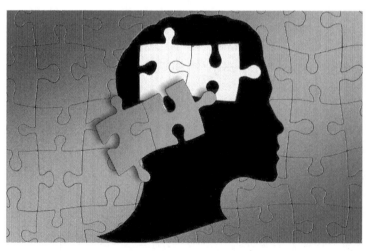

Children with autism have a higher incidence of seizure activity (up to 35%) than other developing children (1-2%). Taurine has been found helpful in preventing and treating epilepsy.

Autism is associated with abnormally high levels of dopamine activity in the brain.[297]

Another issue in ASD children concerns the auditory cortex processing the human voice. It may be poorly connected to the brain's subcorticol reward center, triggering a dopamine response that encourages motivation. This suggests an inability to experience speech as pleasurable.[298]

When a non-autistic child hears his or her mother's voice, oxytocin is released in the brain, inducing warm and tender feelings and trust. This does not happen in ASD.[299]

This creates a disastrous impediment to bonding with parents or others.

Cannabidiol (CBD) may be useful in ASD. While the jury is still out, CBD appears to modulate brain excitatory glutamate and inhibitory GABA level in brain regions linked to ASD. In a study of 34 men (17 neurotypicals/17 ASD) CBD increased GABA in the former, but decreased it in latter group. Therefore, CBD modulates glutamate-GABA system, but prefrontal-GABA systems respond differently in ASD. More research is needed.[300]

DHA and GLA supplementation have been found to decrease irritability associated with ASD. In an animal study of autism-like features, GLA showed more protection of neuronal degeneration and loss, than ALA, derived from flaxseed oil and other vegetable sources.[301]

The supplement N-acetylcysteine (NAC) shows benefit for symptoms of irritability.[302] See Chapter 15.

One case study of a nine-year-old boy with ASD followed the progress in reducing severity of symptoms with supplements of DMG (dimethylglycine), B6 and magnesium. After five months the symptoms improved by 47-53%.[303]

A good vitamin B complex with folinic acid is essential. Nearly all prepared foods contain synthetic folic acid, which without proper amounts of vitamin B12, can cause methylation problems. Cerebral folate deficiency, in the spinal fluid, can result in a number of developmental problems including autism.

Methylation is a significant issue in children with autism.[304]

Coenzyme Q10 supplementation helps relieve oxidative stress and improves relevant biomarkers in ADS.[305]

Studies in Ireland suggest zinc and vitamin A levels were within normal range in the ASD children tested.[306]

There is some preliminary evidence that prenatal vitamin D deficiency and autism are linked.[307]

Cruciferous vegetables and their derivatives, especially sulforaphane, appear to help treat and prevent neurological disorders including ASD, AD, PD and schizophrenia.

Carnosine appears to help sleep disorders in autistic children (see Chapter 15), as does melatonin.

Saccharomyces boulardii (see Chapter 2), probiotics, L-glutamine, omega fatty acids, vitamin A and zinc can help improve secretory IgA in mucus membranes.

Bee pollen appears to ameliorate acute and sub-acute brain disruption induced by propionic acid.[308] Caution is advised, as people may react to individual flower pollens.

Valproic acid, taken during pregnancy, may be associated with increased incidence of ASD, but is based on a mouse study.[309] Valproic acid is a prescription drug used to treat epilepsy, bipolar disorder and prevent migraine headaches.

CranioSacral therapy may be useful in treating ASD, based on a survey of over 400 therapists and parents.[310] The benefit to the glympathic system may be involved, and would be worthy of clinical trials involving other brain health conditions.

Music therapy improved language and communication, as well as cognitive and motor skills in 40 autistic subjects aged two to forty-nine.[311]

CHAPTER 9

ALZHEIMER'S DISEASE, AND SENILE DEMENTIA

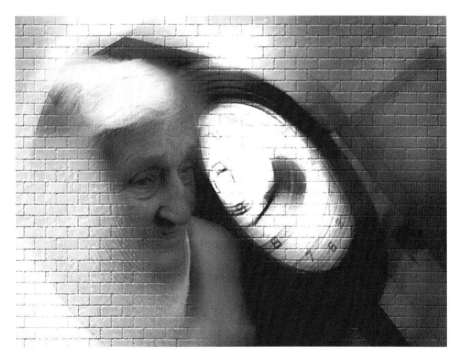

"Alzheimer's is the death of imagination."

DEVDUTT PATTANAIK

Alois Alzheimer was not the first person to identify plaques (beta-amyloid) and tangles (tau) in brain tissue. But he was the first to associate the spots with cognitive decline. When first reported in 1906, his findings were largely dismissed.

Between 1910 and 1930 only 14 articles on Alzheimer's were published in two major neurological journals. This was probably due to the assumption of the day that senile dementia was a normal part of aging.

Alzheimer's disease cannot be truly diagnosed without an after-life brain autopsy, showing the brain shrinkage, deterioration of neurons, and increased plaques and tangles.

Today, however, suspected Alzheimer's disease (AD) numbers are growing at a frightening rate. Worldwide, an estimated 48 million people suffered various forms of dementia as of 2015.

In 2017, an estimated 5.5 million Americans over 65 years old, were living with AD. It is presently considered the sixth leading cause of death.

The human hippocampus produces about 700 neuron cells per day. By age 70, our hippocampus diminishes in volume by one percent each year. This is not caused by dying neurons, but by disappearing synapses. In the cerebral cortex we lose one neuron every second, or 85,000 per day. And still, this only amounts to less than 10% of our total brain cells lost between twenty and ninety years of age.

By age 85, nearly 50% of people will be diagnosed with AD or another form of dementia; 70 % of them women. Women do live longer than men, but this figure could also relate to estrogen decline at menopause.

Psychosis is often present in Alzheimer's dementia, with the progressive reduction in frontal-lobe consciousness, rational thought and memory.[312]

Children with Down syndrome have an extra chromosome (21) that contains genes affecting AD. These individuals will often exhibit AD type dementia in middle age, with the characteristic plaques and tangles developing much earlier in life.

About 25% of the population (about 75 million Americans) is born with a single copy of ApoE4 (apolipoprotein), giving them a AD risk of about 30%. About seven million carry two copies of ApoE4 increasing their risk to nearly 50%.

Most people carry two copies of ApoE3 giving a 9% genetic risk of AD.

Apo E4 binds to 1700 different genes involving inflammation and cardiovascular disease, but in Alzheimer's it shuts down the gene that makes SirT1, linked to longevity; and is associated with activation of nuclear factor kappa B (NF_kB), that promotes inflammation.

In 2017, the FDA approved ten DNA tests from 23andMe, including one for late-onset AD, evaluating your ApoE genetics.

Years ago I took a DNA test for AD, as my mother, and her mother, developed the cognitive dysfunction. I did not test positive for ApoE4.

Dr. Bredesen has written an important book, *The End of Alzheimer's*, with a protocol for preventing and reversing cognitive decline. It is highly recommended. His understanding of AD and recommendations resulted in nine of ten patients showing significant improvement within three to six months.

He suggests the attempt to block the breakdown of acetylcholine affects neither the cause, nor progression of AD. The brain reacts to any inhibition of the enzyme cholinesterase by simply producing more.

According to Dr. Bredesen, there are three basic subtypes of AD. Type one is inflammatory (hot) and occurs more often in those who carry one or two ApoE4 alleles.

Type two is atrophic (cold) and involves one or two ApoE4 alleles, but there is little evidence of inflammation. In this case, hormone and endocrine levels are sub-optimal, vitamin D is reduced, there is insulin resistance, and homocysteine levels may be elevated. He notes type one and two can occur together, especially if glucose and insulin levels are high.

AD is sometimes referred to as Type 3 diabetes with good reason.

Insulin signaling is important for neuron health, and high levels reduce survival levels. After insulin does it job, an enzyme IDE (insulin-degrading enzyme) removes it. But IDE also degrades amyloid-beta, and if it is too occupied with insulin breakdown, the growth of plaques increases.

Type three is toxic (vile) and more common in the ApoE3 allele, where AD does not typically run in a family. This type typically shows low zinc levels, or a high copper to zinc ratio. Other heavy metals, or mycotoxins may be involved.

Beta amyloid may well be protecting our brain from various pathogens crossing the blood brain barrier (BBB), including viruses, bacteria and fungi, heavy metals, allergy-related food protein, BPA and associated toxins, EMFs and various nutrient deficiencies.

Acetylcholine loss was found in brain samples post-mortem in 1978, just over forty years ago. Four years earlier, two researchers at Northwestern University, Chicago gave student volunteers scopolamine, and in memory tests they performed as poorly as elderly patients.

Scopolamine is derived from *Scopolia tangutica*, an Asian herb that induces "twilight sleep." It is widely used, even today, in mouse and rat studies. From 1978-1982, researchers trialed AD patients with choline supplements, up to fifty times the average human intake, but to no avail.

The crisis is epidemic, with a shortage of workers and facilities to house and care for AD patients bound to become a serious problem.

Memory loss is common in the elderly, but it is never too late to improve the loss of some 200,000 brain cells every day.

Speech and finding the right words, or the ability to read and write become more difficult. Judgment and reason begin to suffer. Daily tasks become difficult.

My own mother began to leave on stove burners and water taps. As it progressed she began to use swear words that were out of character for someone who grew up beside a Baptist parsonage.

Beta amyloid plaques and tau tangles are two issues associated with AD. The word amyloid is misplaced as it means "starch". These clumped, sticky protein molecules are found outside neurons, but begin their life inside. Tau is a protein that forms inside the neurons, helping create microtubules that are flexible, but help maintain their shape.

This led to scientists debating which is more important, leading to the intellectual challenge between tau and beta amyloid (BA) believers. The *Tau*ists versus *BA*ptists! My mother, who had a dry sense of humor, would have been mildly amused.

She did not drink tea or coffee. Perhaps she should have. Tea (green or black) containing caffeine, exhibits anti-cholinesterase activity, and modulates different targets on the cholinergic pathway. It has a dual effect on our nicotinic receptors, behaving as both an agonist, and ion channel blocker.[313] Caffeine releases acetylcholine, and increases serotonin in the hippocampus, but chronic consumption reduces the excitability of acetylcholine in cerebral cortex. It exhibits a net dis-inhibitory effect on GABA transmission.

There is increasing awareness of the brain-gut microbiota axis.

A number of theories abound, but systemic gut inflammation has been found to impair blood-brain barrier protection, and promote bacterial amyloids.[314]

In fact, there are similarities to amyloid protein in our brain, and anti-microbial peptides in our gut. These gut peptides form ribbons and threads around pathogens to immobilize them for pickup by macrophages and other immune warriors.

Beta amyloids help reinforce our neuron synapses, and assist in growth of neurons, as well as protect glial cells from free radical damage.

When pathogens, whether bacteria, viruses, protein peptide particles, LPS or heavy metals, cross a leaky blood brain barrier, the glial cells respond with highly inflammatory cytokines.

Beta amyloids contain antibodies as a result of this collateral damage, and prevent the regeneration of new cells.

The herpes simplex virus type 1 (HSV1) has been implicated in the progression of AD, in over 120 publications.[315]

This suggests common cold sores need to be treated more seriously, as the development of senile dementia, AD, schizophrenia and fibromyalgia are likely related to immune suppression, peripheral infection and inflammation associated with HSV-1. Herpes virus types 6 and 7 are implicated with antiviral activity of beta amyloid, and may play a role in epilepsy.[316]

In other words, the beta amyloid plaque is trying to protect you after the herpes virus crosses the BBB.

Tau protein helps stabilize microtubules, and provides transport of nutrients into, and removal, of waste products from brain cells.

It could be that rather than causing dementia, beta-amyloid and tau are trying to save the brain from bacterial invasion. As Scott Anderson writes in the *Psychobiotic Revolution*, "They are, it seems, the firemen—not the arsonists."

This suggests an entirely novel approach to the disease and its treatment.

Prevention or dissolving beta-amyloid plaques and tau protein tangles is the present biomedical approach to this disease.

Tau (tubulin-associated unit) discovered in 1986 by three separate groups of researchers, is a sealant for microtubules that stretch along the axons to create neuron transport. Too much tau and the microtubules become rigid, while too little and they fall apart. Flexibility is needed in the fetal brain to connect and create new synapses, through the addition of phosphates.

Tau becomes tangled and hyper-phosphorylated (too much phosphorus) causing the microtubules to fall apart. When the neurons die the misshapen coils are called "ghost tangles", or "tombstone tangles."

Animals phosphorylate their brain tau when entering hibernation; an odd, and still unexplained phenomena.

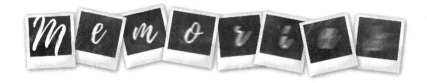

Over 200 clinical drug trials have failed to cure AD and other forms of dementia.[317] That is, all medications studied for AD in the past few years have failed Phase III trials.

Immunotherapy is a recent possible pathway, but results to date, have not been promising.

The anti-depressant drug citalopram reduced levels of beta amyloid and growth of plaque in mice, and reduced levels of beta amyloid in human cerebrospinal fluid by nearly 40%. This is an SSRI drug similar to Prozac.[318]

Maybe the attempts to eliminate amyloid and tau are not the answer.

Research has found amyloid is an anti-microbial peptide helping trap bacteria such as *Salmonella enterica*, fungi such as *Candida albicans*, or viruses like *Herpes simplex*, which lives in trigeminal ganglion cells, and migrate from this nerve to the brain.

Protista parasites such as *Toxoplasma gondii*, associated with cats, may be implicated.[319] See Chapter 13.

The mouth bacteria *Porphyromonas gingivalis* turns up quite often in Alzheimer's brains, as does the Lyme disease spirochete, *Borrelia burgdorferi*, which chronically activates our innate immune system and creates inflammation.

It may be Alzheimer deposits are our protective mechanism against various infectious, inflammatory or environmental assaults.

Microbes can access the brain through the nose, sinuses, our vagus nerve via the gut, and even the eyes.

Molds and their mycotoxins create a chronic inflammatory response syndrome by the innate immune system, and the adaptive system does not recognize and destroy them. It is estimated at least one-half million patients in the United States suffer from AD created by mycotoxin exposure. The latter may be more prevalent in high humidity climates with poorly functioning air conditioners.

Parkinson's disease, Lewy body dementia and Huntington's disease all involve protein tangles. More research into the gut connection may lead us to better approaches.

Certain genetic factors may play a role, but lifestyle, diet and supplementation can have a huge impact on our quality of life. Early treatment is important, as reversal of symptoms is only possible with nutritional intervention.

A specific type of dementia similar to AD, may be caused by TDP-43 protein deposits. This late onset condition in people over 80 years of age is called limbic-predominant age-related TDP-43 encephalopathy, or LATE. It appears to affect mainly the medial temporal lobe, according to article by lead author Peter Nelson published in *Brain* 2019 April 30.

Studies have found thousands of immature neurons in our human dentate gyrus up to the ninth decade of life. These neurons exhibit variable degrees of maturity along stages of hippocampus neurogenesis, but these neurons progressively decline as AD advances.[320]

In a Japanese study, low serum calcium levels convert mild cognitive impairment to early AD.[321] Because the body requires stable blood serum calcium, it may be that a severe magnesium, vitamin D or K deficiency is involved.

The ketogenic diet will be discussed here, in brief, as there are many excellent books discussing this effective, nutritional approach. It is not suggested for everyone, but is an important tool for those willing to move through the difficult first few weeks. It can be modified, with less strict guidelines as improvements in brain health become apparent.

Several factors in AD prevent glucose from getting to the brain, beyond simply insulin deficiency and resistance.

Two glucose transporters are involved. GLUT-1 carries glucose across the membranes of cells that make up the blood brain barrier, and GLUT-3 carries glucose across cell membranes to neurons. AD patients are deficient in pyruvate dehydrogenase, the enzyme converting glucose via a number of steps to ATP. Therefore, ketones can provide up to two-thirds of the brain's energy needs and help address these problems.[322]

But the dietary changes do require discipline.

An easier alternative would be ketone ester, which has received GRAS status from the FDA. A study of 54 healthy adults showed no significant side effects in one toxicity test.[323]

Mice models of AD were fed ketone esters and exhibited decreased plaque and tangles in brain, and reduced anxiety. Increased ketone levels with restricted carbohydrate intake helps lower blood glucose levels.

Numerous products hit the market in spring of 2018; marketed as athletic-boosting or weight loss supplements.

I personally enjoy a tablespoon of MCT from organic coconut oil in my morning coffee.

Other supplements of importance include a B-complex with folate, vitamins C, D and E; selenium, NAC, various medicinal herbs, phosphatydlserine, and good ratio EPA/DHA.

Phosphatydlserine increases acetylcholine levels and may interact with cholinesterase inhibitors if taken concurrently.

Vitamin E levels are reduced in the spinal fluid of AD patients.

Vitamin E has been shown to delay functional decline in mild to moderate AD patients, especially when taken with an acetylcholinesterase inhibitor.

Fatty acids are important but differentiation between genetic APOE genotypes may influence the proper supplementation.

AD patients should be aware vitamin E may interact with memantine, and reduce its effects.

In one study, genetic Apo E4 individuals taking polyunsaturated fats (PUFAs) showed greater levels of cerebral glutamate. The non-carriers showed benefit from PUFA intake on memory performance in 122 middle aged adults.[324] Although preliminary, this suggests great care in choosing which oils are introduced into a diet and used for supplementation, particularly for those exhibiting a genetic pre-disposition to AD.

One DB study of 485 people over 55 years old, with age-related cognitive decline was conducted over six months. The trial involved one group taking 900 mg algal DHA daily, and the control group given a placebo. The DHA group showed almost double the reduction of errors and showed memory performance and skills of someone three years younger.[325]

Vitamin C decreases beta-amyloid plaque, inhibits acetylcholinesterase activity, and prevents endothelial dysfunction regulated by nitric oxide.[326]

NAC, or N-aceytl-cysteine helps generate the important antioxidant glutathione, which is highly unstable. Glutathione is significantly depleted in the hippocampus region in mild cognitive and AD patients.[327]

Probiotic and selenium supplementation significantly reduced C-reactive protein, increased glutathione and lowered insulin levels in a randomized, DB, controlled clinical trial of 79 AD patients.

The probiotics in this particular study were *Lactobacillus acidophilus*, *Bifidobacterium bifidum* and *B. longum*.[328]

Selenium may be useful, but copper and iron concentrations are often elevated in AD blood tests.[329]

Cognitive stimulation programs improve self-reported quality of life for some patients.[330]

Research at Stanford and the Max Planck Institute suggest no convincing evidence of their efficacy, in reducing or reversing cognitive decline.

However, enriching the environment with music, intellectual and cultural richness, and creating a sense of community can help improve brain plasticity, as well as preserve and improve memory.[331]

Acupressure and shiatsu may be useful adjuvant therapies for depression associated with AD.[332]

Various herbs may be helpful (see Chapter 16), including schisandra berry, clubmoss, turmeric (curcumin) and others.

Ginkgo biloba prevents the amyloid-beta plaquing of cortical neurons, and targets the same NMDA receptors like memantine.[333]

Saint John's wort may worsen dementia in some AD patients.

AD and PD affect a sense of smell, making essential oils of limited use. In AD, the patient's left nostril is much less sensitive to odor than the right; reflecting the severity of disease in early stages is much greater on the left hemisphere.

CAUTION- Drug interactions with anti-AD drugs can create serious implications, especially for seniors taking a number of prescription or OTC medications.[334]

CHAPTER 10

PARKINSON'S DISEASE, LEWY BODY DEMENTIA, AMYOTROPHIC LATERAL SCLEROSIS (ALS), AND HUNTINGTON'S DISEASE

James Parkinson was born in 1755 and lived through an exciting time in science and technology. His contemporaries were the composer Mozart, the chemists Joseph Priestly and Humphry Davy, the poet William Wordsworth, the painter William Turner, and Edward Jenner, who discovered the smallpox vaccine.

At age sixteen he began a seven-year apprenticeship in his father's apothecary. The shop was filled with herbs, spices and minerals used to prepare medications. Later, he learned blood-letting, cupping and finally surgery.

He suffered badly from gout throughout much of his life.

James published *An Essay on the Shaking Palsy* over two hundred years ago. The disease he described in his work, was named in his honor, by Jean-Martin Charcot sixty years later. World Parkinson's Day is held each year on his birthday, April 11.

Parkinson's disease (PD) presents as a wide spectrum of conditions. Most of the public and many health practitioners focus on the tremor, the rigidity and balance problems.

Worldwide, 7-10 million people suffer from PD, with 60,000 Americans diagnosed each year. It affects about 1% of people, and typically afflicts those aged 40-70 years old.

It is treated in biomedicine by Levodopa (L-dopa), introduced in 1968. Carbidopa was later added to reduce nausea symptoms, and prevent its rapid breakdown in the liver, lungs and kidneys.

Dopamine-rich herbs such as edible faba bean and supplements derived from velvet bean, exhibit clinical benefit in treating PD, from a more holistic perspective.

MAO-B inhibitors block the enzymes responsible for the rapid breakdown of dopamine, suggesting synergistic formulas.

See Medicinal Herbs Chapter 16.

Lewy bodies accumulate in the *substantia nigra*, from damaged proteins called synuclein. They are named after Frederic Lewy, a colleague of Alois Alzheimer. Also working in the same laboratory were Hans Gerhard Creutzfeldt and Alfons Maria Jacob of Cruetzfeldt-Jacob (mad cow) disease fame.

Another protein ubiquitin, appears in Lewy bodies, in some forms of PD, associated with the inability to eliminate these damaged neurons. The Lewy body may be the cell's attempt to encapsulate worn out protein that proteasome, the cell's recycling system, can no longer accomplish.

In some ways, this is reminiscent of the beta-amyloid plaques and tau tangles present in AD.

Mitochondrial dysfunction in the neurons play a role. Coenzyme Q10 (ubiquinone) shows some promise in slowing down the progression of PD.

Lewy body disease (LBD) initially appears similar to PD but may be determined by the first onset of symptoms. PD involves dementia along with movement problems, whereas LBD is cognitive decline without involuntary muscle movements. Robin Williams suffered from the latter, progressive disease.

The issues of dementia, depression, delusional thoughts, and compulsive behavior are part of this difficult disease.

Some symptoms are predictable side-effects due to prescription drugs, but the anxiety, depression, apathy and fatigue are very real, and can apply to anyone suffering poor brain health.

There are myths associated with the Parkinson's personality, such as mental rigidity, an unwillingness to take risks, and obsessive and introspective behavior. This probably stems from psychologists of the 1940s suggesting PD patient's rigidity in muscles was related to repressed emotions, or observing that conflict produced agitation.

The tremors, stiffness and rigidity are related to degeneration of dopamine-rich cells in the pigmented substantia nigra. Many of the remaining neurons contain Lewy bodies. It is unknown why some people develop LBD in a small area of the brain (PD), and others exhibit broader distribution.

Dopamine levels can fall by up to 70% without appearing to cause problems, but at 80% levels, Parkinsonian symptoms begin to appear.

Monoamine oxidase B levels are elevated in PD. The disease appears to move from the gut to brain via the vagus nerve.

A study in Denmark, before the bacterium *Helicobacter pylori* was identified with ulcers, led fifteen thousand people to have their vagus nerve partially or completely severed. In those patients, the rate of PD was halved, suggesting vagus nerve involvement.[335]

Pesticide and/or lead exposure increases the risk of developing neurodegenerative disorders such as PD and ALS by at least 50%. Occupational exposure to EMFs increases the risk for ALS and AD by 10%.[336]

Metals such as manganese and aluminum increase the tendency of synuclein to form protein clumps, at least during *in vitro* studies.

One recent study strongly suggests exposing the brain to EMFs can decrease the number of synaptic vesicles and dopaminergic neurons in our striatum.[337]

Some authors believe PD is the result of iron deposition in striatum and substantia nigra regions of the brain. Studies refuting this claim find no significant association between iron serum levels and PD.[338] But this is a measure of blood serum levels, not deposition in the neurons, where excess iron promotes Parkin and alpha-synuclein aggregation.[339]

A study of 35 male PD patients and 35 controls, found evidence that motor dysfunction in PD correlates with alterations in brain iron.[340]

Many neurodegenerative disorders including PD, AD and Huntington's disease involve dysregulation of iron metabolism.[341]

Iron is involved in mitochondrial respiration, myelin synthesis, neurotransmitter synthesis, and metabolism. Iron is a potent source of oxidative damage from free radicals. Just picture an unpainted iron fence rusting over time due to oxidation.

In 1950, a 12% alcohol-based iron tonic, Geritol was introduced to the market, and through early television ads appealed to older viewers. It was advertised as containing, "twice the iron in a pound of calf's liver." A daily dose contained 50-100 mg of ferric ammonium citrate (FAC).

Ironically, FAC has been recently found to inhibit the influenza A, HIV, Zika viruses, as well as Enterovirus 71.[342]

Daily multi-vitamin and mineral formulations contain iron, often in forms that cannot be easily assimilated. While menstruating, women have the capacity to remove excess iron. Men do not.

Men are more likely to develop iron accumulation, compared to women, with significantly lower iron levels in five vital brain regions.[343]

Scientists from the University of Washington did a critical review of eleven studies, and concluded that the use of anti-inflammatory drugs is associated with slightly lower probability of developing PD. This suggests brain inflammation also plays a role.

A large number of PD patients suffer years of constipation, suggesting bacteria in the microbiome are out of balance.

An unhealthy gut allows iron-loving bacteria to flourish. Removing the iron, however, is another matter.

The microbiome of PD patients shows reduced levels of *Prevotella* species, and elevated levels of *Enterobacteria*.[344]

On the other hand, high levels of *Prevotella* species are found in the gut microbiome of patients suffering major depression disorder.[345]

In one study, a kefir containing six billion CFUs of *Lactobacillus casei* Shirota for six weeks improved stool consistency, and improved the quality of life, potentially slowing the progression of PD.[346]

PD patients can suffer depression. Dopamine, of course, is involved in the brain's reward system. *The Molecule of More*[347] is a recently published book on this exciting neurotransmitter.

Drugs such as cocaine and methamphetamine increase dopamine stimulation in the brain. This will all be discussed in a later chapter on addictions.

Individuals who drink coffee or smoke tobacco are less likely to develop PD. This suggests there is something in coffee or cigarettes that slow or prevent PD from developing, or the process causing PD reduces the likelihood they will smoke or drink. We know dopamine is involved in addictive behavior but to think coffee or tobacco contain substances that prevent the disease may be far-fetched.[348]

There are very few studies on dementia in PD, and yet those few show a greater reduction of acetylcholine in the brain, than Alzheimer's disease. However, any chemical that blocks acetylcholine helps PD motor skills, and doing the opposite may worsen the motor aspects, particularly the tremor.

A study of over 500 PD patients with dementia involved rivastigmine. The results were disappointing, showing that out of every 100 PD patients only 5 benefit more than placebo.[349]

Compulsive behavior is linked to anxiety. One side effect of PD patients taking dopamine agonist drugs is increased gambling, shopping, eating and sexual addiction. These impulse control disorders occur in about 10-15% of PD patients taking these drugs. From 15-25% of PD patients taking L-dopa will suffer delusional psychoses and hallucinations.

The problem with lowering levels of the drugs is it worsens other symptoms.

As mentioned above, James Parkinson suffered gout.

This condition is caused with uric acid buildup, and is associated with a higher risk of PD in 65-75 year old patients.[350]

Natural approaches include diet modification, methyl folate supplementation for prevention of uric acid kidney stones, cherry juice, and tamarack needle tea. Removing high purine foods from the diet will help.

Some authors suggest eating a low protein diet, and others suggest moving your protein meal to the evening. Maybe.

Black currant fruit and juice may be especially useful for PD.

In this condition, an increase in insulin-like factor-1 (IGF-1) is found in the cerebrospinal fluid, but its function is impaired, and thought to contribute to progression of the disease. Black currant consumption is associated with a lower risk of PD, due to its ability to alter the IGF-1 pathway.[351]

A related study found PD patients taking blackcurrant supplementation reported better emotional quality of life.[352]

Black currant, blueberry and lutein supplementation help maintain eye health. Blurred vision, poor night vision, and depth perception, are common in PD. Visual problems, accompanied by cognitive dysfunction can contribute to hallucinations.

Other issues revolve around dopamine dysregulation syndrome, in which PD patients desire more and more L-dopa, causing psychotic episodes, hallucinations and paranoid delusions.

Sleep disorders are common with PD including daytime sleepiness, insomnia (either falling asleep, staying asleep), abnormal or vivid dreaming, or an overactive bladder.

REM (rapid eye movement) sleep produces about 80% of dream states. And during sleep, the muscle tone is reduced, and one is effectively paralyzed except for breathing.

A large percentage of PD patients, whether on medications or not, experience dreams during which they are not paralyzed, and act them out. They generally dream of being attacked and fighting back. This symptom affects men more than women.

Patients will talk, yell, laugh, cry and even sing in sleep.[353] They are more likely to suffer sleep apnea. The use of a CPAP machine can greatly improve oxygen availability to the brain.

In one interesting DB study, a PET scan showed the amount of dopamine in the brain increased with ingesting L-Dopa. When patients taking the placebo, experienced improvement in their movement, the researchers also found increased levels of dopamine, similar to those actually receiving the drug.

This suggests the importance of positive mental attitude. Patients suffering tremors become worse with anxiety, stress and over-excitement.

Meditation and exercise may be useful. Nearly half of PD patients suffer anxiety for several years before diagnosis. Feelings or premonitions that something bad is going to happen are often present. The English flower essence Aspen is specific for individuals suffering from fear of the unknown.

It is problematic to instruct PD patients their loss of dopamine prevents movement. This exacerbates muscle weakness.

"Telling PD patients they have a movement disorder and leaving it at that is a self-fulfilling prophecy," writes Dr. Doidge.[354] The issue is to motivate and initiate movement.

Studies show a moderate amount of daily treadmill running, if initiated on the day dopamine is depleted, protects the basal ganglia dopamine from deteriorating.[355]

Exercise helps produce brain-derived neurotrophic factor (BDNF), and glial-derived neurotrophic factor, forming new connections between brain cells. Modalities such as Constraint-Induced Therapy, invented by Dr. Edward Taub may be helpful.

Learned non-use plays a major role in PD and by using Taub's technique, patients have achieved staggering improvement.[356]

Coconut nut oil or MCT, mentioned under Fats and Oils, may be useful in PD. Dr. Mary Newport writes, "Two men with Parkinson's disease have reported similar success while taking nine or more tablespoons per day of coconut oil. For each the improvements were gradual but ultimately profound."[357]

Supplements that may help PD symptoms include faba bean, velvet bean, *Rhodiola rosea*, green tea, *Ginkgo biloba*, turmeric (curcumin), ashwagandha, milk thistle, red wine, and magnesium.[358] Reduced progression of the disease was noted from fish oil and coenzyme Q10 supplementation, and faster progression of the disease was noted with iron supplementation.[359]

Coenzyme Q10 and creatine produce additive neuroprotection in cases of PD and HD.[360]

The addition of a MAO_B inhibitor selective to dopamine increases the amount of available dopamine for release, and protects the neurons by reducing their oxidative stress. Kaempferol, derived from *Ginkgo biloba* inhibits MAO, and protects against NMDA neuronal toxicity.[361]

Specific herbal MAO_B inhibitors include scullcap, licorice root, turmeric, damiana and green tea. All of these may be useful adjuncts with faba bean supplementation, to ensure optimal dopamine release.[362]

Damiana (*Turnera diffusa*) contains the compound, acacetin 7-methyl, which selectively inhibits MAO_B.[363]

Vitamin E supplementation may be of potential use in PD.[364]

Chocolate is rich in beta-phenylethylamine (PEA), a precursor to dopamine. It crosses the blood-brain barrier, and stimulates and modulates the release of dopamine, and improves learning and attention span. It influences endorphins, which promotes feelings of pleasure.

Green tea extracts and their polyphenol EGCG bind to iron, and cross the blood-brain barrier. This allows it to capture and isolate iron from the brain regions affected in Alzheimer's, Parkinson's, and Huntington's diseases.[365]

Baicalein, in Scullcap species, demonstrates neuroprotective properties to domaminergic neurons implicated in the development of PD. The herb protects neurons from decreased blood flow to the brain, and protects from beta-amyloid associated with AD.[366]

Curcumin, derived from turmeric root has been found to chelate both iron and copper.[367]

The brain has a high priority to receive and retain selenium even when the body is deficient. However, selenoprotein dysfunction in PD reduces its ability to lower levels of oxidative stress.[368]

Other useful supplements include nicotinamide adenine dinucleotide (NADH), L-5-methytetrahydrofolate (L-5-MTHF), and dimercaptosuccinic acid (DMSA). See Supplements Chapter 15.

The homeopathic *Argentum nitricum* 6X may help ataxia, or trembling. Massage, including aromatherapy may help to relax stiff muscles. Aquatic therapy does not appear to have any advantage over land-based rehab on freezing gait.

Amanita muscaria (*Agaricus muscaria*) in homeopathic form can be beneficial in reducing the tremor associated with PD. See Medicinal Mushrooms chapter for more information on how I used this product successfully in clinical practice.

A review of 21 studies suggests Tai Chi and Qigong benefit motor function, depression and quality of life in patients with PD.[369] Dance classes are beneficial. Five randomized controlled trials involving 159 PD patients found significant improvement in motor symptoms.[370]

Essential oils may help (see Chapter 20) but impaired sniffing and loss of smell are common in PD. In fact, impaired olfactory deficit is one early sign of the disease. Loss of smell affects our sense of taste and results in decreased appetite.

Kava Kava and iron supplements are contraindicated in PD.

Acupuncture may be useful. A systematic review and meta-analysis of 42 studies involving 2625 participants found significant improvement.[371]

Bee venom therapy may be useful for PD, AD, ASD and ALS below.[372]

One interesting study by Korean researchers discovered that stimulating a specific acupuncture spot on mice associated with Parkinson's disease, it changed the expression level of 799 genes.[373]

LEWY BODY DEMENTIA

Lewy body dementia is named after Dr. Frederick Lewy, the neurologist who discovered alpha-synuclein proteins, while working in Dr. Alois Alzheimer's laboratory.

Today, this form of dementia affects over 1.3 million Americans.

One difference between LBD and AD is that memory loss is sudden and then re-appears the next day, whereas in the latter condition it is often slow and gradual.

Loss of balance is similar to PD, with visual hallucinations often present. Patients exhibit disturbed REM sleep, often physically acting out the events in their dreams.

Survival rate is lower than AD due to increased falls and injury.

Care in diagnosis is important, as medications such as anti-psychotics, anti-spasmodics, anti-depressants, or treating them as PD patients can make their symptoms worse.

A proper diagnosis is imperative.

Anti-psychotics may increase severe neuroleptic sensitivity, worsen cognition, increase irreversible parkinsonism, or induce symptoms resembling neuroleptic malignant syndrome.[374]

Lewy bodies start to aggregate in our second brain (gut), and live inside nerve cells with help from a protein called alpha-synuclein.

The true cause is unknown, but it is best treated with natural supplementation. See Alzheimer' disease (Chapter 9).

AMYOTROPHIC LATERAL SCLEROSIS

Amyotrophic lateral sclerosis (ALS), or Lou Gehrig's disease, named for the famous baseball icon, is a degenerative disorder with loss of motor neurons, and some overlap with fronto-temporal dementia (FTLD).

Neuro-inflammation involves activated microglia. Much of the laboratory work has focused on chromosome 9 and drugs that may help reduce this debilitating disease.

The only drug approved on the market for symptom relief has a plethora of side-effects and is aimed at neuron/glutamate interactions.

ALS is very likely related to both neuro-degeneration and auto-immunity response.

Most brain issues waste away from underuse, rather than over use, as long as brain exercises are slow with rests between and ideally before the disease has progressed.

An animal study suggests ALS patients may be the exception, as female mice with the human ALS gene that were raised in enriched environments, got worse faster, than those in a "normal" environment. The application to humans is not clear.

Coconut oil may be helpful. Dr. Newport writes, "A man with ALS (also known as Lou Gehrig's disease) has had success in bringing about improvement, and then stabilization, in his condition for more than four years from taking nine tablespoons of coconut oil a day, and also by massaging the oil over his muscles. His response is quite remarkable considering that this disease is relentless in its progression and most people die within three to five years of diagnosis."[375]

In fact, Stephen Hawking was told upon his diagnosis, as a young man, that he would only live two or three more years, and passed away last year at age 76. There was nothing wrong with his intellectual capacity.

Berberine is an alkaloid found in several medicinal plants including goldenseal, goldthread and Oregon grape root. It may be useful in ALS, albeit based on preliminary *in vitro* studies. Natural compounds helpful for relieving symptoms of ALS were reviewed, in a recent paper by Nabavi et al.[376]

Curcumin (Turmeric) has been found useful in slowing down disease progression in a DB three-month study.[377] See Medicinal Herbs.

HUNTINGTON'S DISEASE

Huntington's Disease (HD) is caused by a genetic mutation of the protein, huntingtin. It is estimated about 30,000 Americans have been diagnosed, and another 150,00 are at risk due to its inherited genetic aspect. Children of parents with this mutation have a 50/50 possibility of developing HD. Woody Guthrie, the beloved folk singer/activist suffered this cruel form of dementia.

Early indications include twitching, clumsiness, restlessness, and changes in handwriting, driving, etc. The condition advances over one or two decades and is progressive. Mouth and throat muscles become impaired, making speech and swallowing difficult.

Children of HD parents are advised to test early, as healthy dietary choices and supplementation may help stave off, or delay, this debilitating condition.

Various prescription drugs have been trialed but all have known side effects.

Creatine has been found useful in HD. Good EPA fish oils, vitamin E, CoQ10 and its synthetic cousin Idebenone can be helpful. See Supplements Chapter 15.

Trehalose, a unique sugar derived from mushrooms and conifer sap, has been found useful in HD. This disaccharide is an mTOR-independent autophagy activator, meaning it helps clear the mutant huntingtin and A30P and A53T mutants of alpha-synuclein associated with HD and PD.[378]

Thymoquinone, from Black Cumin (*Nigella sativa*) and Wild Bergamot (*Monarda fistulosa*), encapsulated as lipid nanoparticles, show significant benefit in an animal study of induced Huntington's disease.[379]

One journal paper of interest to natural practitioners looked at a number of herbal compounds with possible benefit for Parkinson's and Huntington's diseases.[380]

Another review looked at 37 natural products that may prove therapeutic benefit for PD.[381]

Dancing with Elephants by author Jarem Sawatsky is a beautiful, heart-warming, and inspiring story of one man's journey with ALS. He has a website www.jaremsawatsky.com.

CHAPTER 11

EPILEPSY

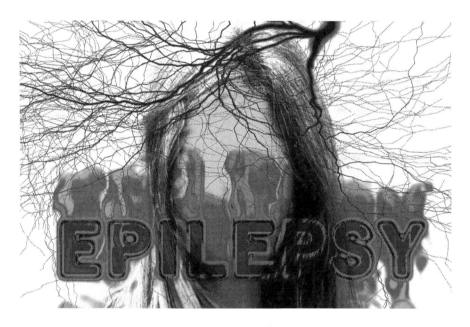

Re-examine all you have been told at school or church or in any book, dismiss whatever insults your own soul. WALT WHITMAN

Epilepsy comes in many forms. In fact, there are many conditions that appear like epileptic seizures, but are not. Some examples include jitteriness, benign myoclonus, benign paroxysmal torticollis, shuddering attacks, startle disease, paroxysmal vertigo, tics, pseudoseizures, anxiety states, dystonia, migraine, narcolepsy, head bobbing and night terrors, to name a few.

There can be many factors involved in epileptic seizure including fever, kidney or liver disease, electrolyte imbalance, hypoglycemia, low levels of calcium, abnormalities associated with hormones or metabolism, drugs or withdrawal, trauma, brain tumors, strokes and toxins.[382]

A small number of seizures are related to brain trauma, including accidents, infections or stroke. And environmental toxins can definitely play a role.

Medical science has yet to find answers for this electrical storm in the brain, but the condition is common in children and adults with cognitive disability.

However, about 70% of children suffering a single seizure episode will never have another. When put on medications, they will never be the same, with regards to mental and physical health. From 30-40% of epileptic patients eventually develop resistance to their drugs.

The sodium valproate and carbamazepine drugs have a plethora of side effects, with the warning, "avoid sudden withdrawal."

Iron supplements given to nursing home residents taking carbamazepine, decreased the efficacy of the drug by one-third.[383]

In some cases of seizure activity that does not respond to epileptic drugs, a predominance of pro-inflammatory IL-17 production is found. In these cases, a reset of immune modulation, using medicinal mushrooms may be helpful.

Reishi (*Ganoderma lucidum*) mycelium, for example, inhibited convulsions in kainic-induced seizures in lab animals.[384]

Phenytoin depletes folate and thiamine in the body, two B vitamins that alone can cause seizures, when deficient. Vitamin B6 levels are depleted after seizure, and B6 injections have reversed the condition.

B6 is activated by zinc, which is often deficient in diets and in the body tissue of those suffering epilepsy.

Essential fatty acids (Omega-3), amino acids (taurine), B complex, magnesium and selenium are recommended supplements.

Omega-3 fatty acids reduced seizure frequency and duration in a triple-blind randomized clinical trial of 50 patients for six weeks. The EPA/DHA ratio was 3:2 (180 mg/120mg) twice daily.[385]

A DB, PC randomized trial of 99 patients with drug-resistant epilepsy involved EPA, DHA and placebo. There was no difference in the reduction of seizures between EPA and DHA, but significant improvement was observed in both treatment groups.[386]

Diet can make a difference. In ancient Greece, Hippocrates called it the secret disease, and treated epilepsy with fasting.

But one can only fast for so long.

When I was eight-years old, I was put on a regime of shots to treat allergies for dust and feathers. Really! This continued for years as I suffered from hay fever, and asthma well into my teen years.

When 23 years old, I found myself on a hippy commune in northern Alberta. I had read some ill-informed books on fasting and decided to do a 30 day water fast. This is not a recommendation!

I did well after the first four days and by day ten I was feeling good. I continued another week and one day after plowing a field, I returned to my log cabin. As I took off my white t-shirt, I experienced the memory of a small, eight-year old boy sitting alone on a wooden chair, in a long, green hallway of the doctor's office, waiting for his allergy shot.

I turned the shirt around, and two distinct yellow-orange spots adjacent to my kidneys popped out at me. I smelled them, and they gave off a distinct phenolic smell.

But, as mentioned, you can only fast for so long!

The Mayo clinic developed the ketogenic diet in 1920s. It worked well, especially for children, with 95% of patients having seizure control and 60% becoming seizure free.

In 1938 anti-convulsant drugs were discovered, and the diet was ignored, except at Johns Hopkins, where the present day classic ketogenic diet was developed.

This consists of a 4:1 ratio of fat (dairy, eggs and meat) to carbs and protein. It has problems associated with acidosis, kidney stones, constipation and bone fractures. A meta-analysis of 19 studies found that half of patients reduced seizures by half, and one-third reduced seizure episodes by 90%.

One easier variation is the MCT diet, based on medium-chain triglycerides, mainly from coconut oil. It works better at creating ketones, allowing more protein and carbohydrates in the diet. However, it has some side effects including diarrhea, cramps and vomiting in a small number of people.

A modified Atkins Diet allows a 1:1 ketogenic ratio and better suits some people. Another diet, a low glycemic index treatment allows more carbohydrates in the diet, as long as they are low-glycemic.

In all cases, it is not the level of ketones that correlates with anti-convulsant effects.[387]

However, a modified ketogenic diet reduced seizure frequency, severity and improved quality of life (QOL) in a three-month study of 55 adults with refractory epilepsy. Sixty percent reported more than 50% improvements in frequency, 76% improvement in severity, and 87% in QOL.[388]

Modified ketogenic diet improved all perimeters above, including those whose seizures persisted despite surgery and vagal nerve stimulation.[389]

Ketogenic and modified Atkins diets appear to reduce seizures by a significant percent in Lennox-Gastaut syndrome, a condition belonging to the epileptic encephalopathy grouping.

This was studied on 61 patients with 20 placed on a ketogenic diet for 16 months. Fifteen remained on the diet, with three patients seizure-free, three with a 75-99% decrease, two with a 50-74% decrease, and the remaining 7 children less than 50% reduction in seizures.[390]

The modified Atkins diet was tested on 25 children with the syndrome. After three months two were seizure-free, and ten of the twenty-five had more than 50% reduction in seizure frequency. At six months, of 11 children on diet, three were seizure-free and 8 had more than 50% reduction.[391]

In many children, epilepsy seizures are the result of a damaged microbiome and leaky gut, and the resulting nutritional deficiencies. Folate, B6, B1 and manganese deficiencies are implicated.

Vitamin B6 (pyridoxal-5'-phosphate) deficiency plays a key role in B6-responsive epilepsy, even at an early age. Early diagnosis and life long treatment can help alleviate this condition.[392]

Pyridoxine-dependent epilepsy is often found in the first year of life, and is a rare autosomal recessive condition caused by antiquitin deficiency. A diet low in lysine, and high in arginine, along with pyridoxine can help ameliorate the cognitive impairment in this genetic condition.[393]

It should be noted that this lysine/arginine ratio is conducive to cold sore (*Herpes simplex* 1) outbreaks. Lysine helps prevent viral replication.

In clinical practice, I found a high fat diet along with L-taurine supplementation and a 1:1 ratio of passionflower and scullcap tincture worked well, especially in children with a relatively healthy microbiome. This is increasingly rare due to the overuse of antibiotics in young children.

Passionflower contains chrysin that protects neurons and suppresses neuro-inflammation, showing benefit in epilepsy and depression.[394]

Mistletoe (*Viscum album*) extracts may be useful. See Chapter 16.

Probiotic supplementation has been found beneficial in the treatment of drug-resistant epilepsy.[395] A four-month study of 45 patients found 29% displayed a greater than 50% reduction in the number of seizures, as well as observed, improved QOL.

Yoga may be helpful in modifying epilepsy, based on a study of randomized, controlled trials.[396]

The generic diabetic drug metformin has been found to alleviate symptoms of seizure, in a systematic review.[397] See Supplements.

CHAPTER 12

ATTENTION DEFICIT DISORDER, ATTENTION DEFICIT HYPERACTIVITY DISORDER, OBSESSIVE-COMPULSIVE DISORDER, ADHD AND OCD - THE SEEMING OPPOSITES

"Habits are at first cobwebs, then cables."

SPANISH PROVERB

"The trouble with normal is it always gets worse."

BRUCE COCKBURN

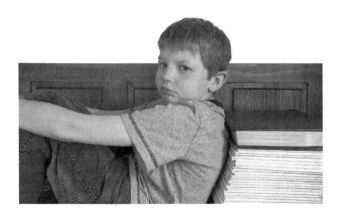

Attention Deficit Hyperactivity Disorder (ADHD) is widespread in our society, affecting from 5-10% of children and 4.7% of adults. The inattentive type was originally known as ADD, but the two variations are often found in combination.

The connotation of deficit and disorder is unfortunate as many high-profile achievers, including Sir Richard Branson have publically embraced their diagnosis.

In 2000, over six million American children were diagnosed with ADHD; and the majority given prescriptions for Ritalin, or other amphetamine medications.

About 30% of the children given stimulants suffer poor appetite, and sleep disorders.

An Icelandic epidemiological study of ADHD symptoms of nearly eleven thousand students aged 14-16, found 5.4% of them showing the criteria for ADHD, accompanied by their self-medicating with LSD, cocaine, magic mushrooms, nicotine, alcohol and amphetamines.[398]

ADHD is the most commonly diagnosed behavioral disorder in children, and the fastest growing disorder in adults.

It is three to five times more likely to be diagnosed in boys.

ADHD is believed to affect 5-10% of all school-aged children, an increase of more than 20% in the past decade. It varies widely, from state to state, with a 5.6% diagnosis rate in Nevada and a whooping 15.6% rate in North Carolina. In the United Kingdom, the rate is less than 2%, and in France less than 0.5%!

It has been suggested that Big Pharma, over-worked teachers, stressed-out parents and pop-a-pill societal conformity is a problem in search of a cure. Maybe.

A child with ADHD likely has one parent with the condition.

Diagnosis can be difficult as there is no purely objective test, so these numbers may represent an increase in awareness, or simply over-diagnosis. Practitioners must try to discern between anxiety, depression, bi-polar disorder, petit-mal or temporal lobe seizures, Asperger's syndrome, hearing or learning problems, as well as possible hypothyroidism.

In fact, stimulant prescription drugs are widely misused by 5-10% of high school students and 5-35% of college students.[399]

Adderall is strictly speaking not an amphetamine, but the chemical structure is similar. Its use, and abuse, does lead, according to various studies, to methamphetamine addiction.

Prescriptions for young women aged 26-34 rose 86% between 2008 and 2014. And rates for adults with ADHD rose 53.5% in the same period of time.

Charles Bradley first noted amphetamines calmed hyperactive children over eighty years ago.

From 25-40% of children diagnosed with ADHD show little improvement from medication, but do respond well to placebo.[400]

Symptoms include restlessness, fidgeting, constant chatter and little ability to delay immediate gratification.

ADD involves more inattention. They can, however, become easily distracted by sights and sounds, but fail to pay attention to details or follow direction.

Both ADD and ADHD diagnosis are often misapplied to children with psychological trauma, highly creative, intelligent children that are bored, or lack of play and exercise in the school setting, especially for boys that require rough housing to learn impulse control.

For an ADHD diagnosis the behavior must appear before age 7, and the inappropriate activity must interfere in home, school, or community activity. However, there is presently no single medical, physical or any test to accurately diagnose ADHD.

One study of 579 children aged 7-10 years who took ADHD drugs for over three years, showed a lower growth rate than those not on meds. Elevated levels of dopamine affect the pituitary gland, regulating growth hormones. The same study found that after three years the effectiveness of the drug was reduced, due to developing tolerance.

Many adults suffer with ADHD for much of their lives without diagnosis. They may have difficulty with daily chores, starting or finishing tasks, or being unable to focus and complete projects. They typically have lower income and higher rates of unemployment, and are impulsive, taking risks including automobile accidents.[401]

They may self-medicate or become more prone to addictions.

They are also great entrepreneurs, outside-the-box thinkers, creating new products through hyper-focus and a low boredom threshold. Both sides of this equation are true.

Tyrosine, taken on an empty stomach in the morning can improve focus, concentration and reduce procrastination. The amino acid supplement combines well with calming L-theanine.

Some known risk factors for ADD/ADHD include low birth weight, and fetal exposure to nicotine, alcohol, cocaine or lead. Fluorescent lights and early television viewing, computer screens, and video games may exacerbate the condition. Dr. John Ott published research in the 1970s relating fluorescent lighting to increased hyperactivity. This is still a problem.

Exposure to phenyalanine (either prenatal or postnatal) has been associated with ADHD.[402] The artificial sweetener Aspartame contains phenylalanine.

Diet and food sensitivities are involved due to the leaky gut/leaky brain connection. Dr. Feingold, in the 1970s, suggested elimination of colors, preservative and certain foods.

An elimination diet is often useful, even if it only removes gluten, dairy and soy. It is a good place to start.

One study of celiac children with ADHD found that after six months on a gluten-free diet, there was significant improvement in all twelve markers of the deficit.[403]

A high sugar/carbohydrate breakfast without protein increases hyperactive behavior, and a study of over 1800 three-year-olds found removing artificial colors and sodium benzoate reduced ADHD symptoms.[404] Sensitivity to the yellow dye tartrazine, produced from coal tar, may be involved. It is often marketed as FD&C yellow 5, E102 or C.I. 19140.

Avoid this toxin by reading labels, as it is found in numerous refined foods.

Artificial food colors (red and orange), and some plant-based foods contain SULT1A (sulfotransferase) inhibitors that may impact

ADHD behavior. The SULT1A enzymes protect humans from catecholamines, but some foods like grapefruit and orange juice, orange dyes (annatto) in cheese, black and green tea inhibit the enzyme. In turn, this increases plasma tyrosine and dopamine in the brain, and is related to various drugs including salicylic acid, clomiphene, danazol, various food colorants, and environmental chemicals, including bisphenol A.

Food sensitivities and intolerances must be indentified and removed from the diet. Traditional allergy testing (IgE) does not detect IgG food intolerances. The Pulse test, mentioned elsewhere, is highly specific to recognizing histamine and mast cell responses.

Early work by Dr. Wolraich in 1985, and recent work by Del-Ponte et al (2019) examined the relationship between the consumption of sugar in 2924 children 6-11 years old and incidence of ADHD. The results found no association between sucrose intake and incidence of ADHD.[405] It may be that sugar per se is not the issue, albeit excess sugar does encourage an unhealthy microbiome. It may be the additives and colors that accompany the sugar-laden product.

Quercitin, vitamin C and pantothenic acid (B5) reduce histamine response affecting brain health and inflammation.

Curcumin (turmeric), chrysin (passion flower), apigenin (chamomile) and phytoestrogens in red clover and soy inhibit this process, as does B6 (pyridoxyl-6-phosphate) in one *in vitro* study. The good news is that the SULT enzyme is dependent on reserves of sulfur-containing compounds found in the cabbage and onion family. The bad news is that many ADHD children are picky eaters, and may not like broccoli, cauliflower, cabbage, garlic and onions. Broccoli sprouts, and related concentrated supplements make life much easier for both children and parents.

We now know there is a direct correlation between the health of the microbiome and the brain. If there is a leaky gut, due to a multitude of reasons covered earlier in book, then the likelihood of a leaky brain is very possible.

The most popular theory regarding ADHD is a dopamine deficiency in the prefrontal cortex. It should be noted that people who struggle with addictions, suffer from ADD or ADHD. Ritalin is thought to alter levels of dopamine, but rat studies suggest Ritalin boosts serotonin in the brain, not dopamine. Researchers now believe there is a chemical imbalance of the two neurotransmitters.

Research at Harvard found adults with longstanding ADHD exhibit abnormally high levels of dopamine. Other studies find the dopamine D4 receptors in the prefrontal cortex do not function very well.

Food sensitivities and allergies must be addressed with strict dietary changes, including a high protein diet, free from dyes, sugars and specific allergens.

Children of ADHD parents are prone to uni-polar and bi-polar disorder, as well as traumatic brain injury later in life, in a twenty-year study of 5128 siblings over twenty years.[406]

Supplements found helpful include omega-3 with a 3:2 ratio of EPA/DHA[407], or cod liver oil, a good multivitamin with methyl folate, L-theanine, *Rhodiola rosea*, L-tyrosine (morning only), choline, magnesium[408] and phosphatydlserine.[409]

L-theanine (see Green Tea in Chapter 16) increases alpha brain waves, promoting relaxation and calmness.

Animal studies found it increases various neurotransmitters including serotonin, dopamine and GABA.

One study involved 200 mg of L-theanine given twice daily to boys with ADHD, and researchers found the sleep quality vastly improved.[410]

Iron levels should be tested, and treated if deficient. Zinc deficiency, or improper zinc/copper ratios should be addressed.[411]

A study of 14 children (aged 8-12) with ADHD involved a multi-vitamin/mineral supplement, with a four and eight week off and on regime, in a DB, PC study. Seventy-one percent showed at least a 30% decrease in ADHD symptoms, and 79% were much improved, or very much improved, at the end of five months.[412]

The same team conducted a double-blind study on 80 un-medicated ADHD adults, half given multi-vitamin/mineral supplements for eight weeks. Hyperactivity, impulsivity and inattention were statistically improved, and even depression symptoms lessened.

In utero and first year of life deficiencies, including zinc, iron, magnesium, iodine, vitamin D and DHA may play a role in the development of ADHD. Exposure to even small amounts of organopesticides by pregnant women show increased risk of birthing children with ADHD.[413]

The over-focused ADD patient may suffer low serotonin and find saffron a useful herbal supplement. 5-HTP may help boost serotonin, and a higher carbohydrate meal in evening permits better absorption of tryptophan. If sleep is an issue, tryptophan is a better choice, as 5-HTP can generate cortisol and disrupt sleep.

For a child, 25 mg of 5HTP or 250 mg of L-tryptophan, is good starting point. Do not give either one, concurrently with anti-depressants. EPA without DHA may be a better choice for this particular sub-type.

ADHD, but not ADD children may benefit from algae-based DHA. One study of 362 children (aged 7-9) with reading and behavioral difficulties were given 600 mg DHA, or placebo for six weeks. Significant improvement was observed in those children below the 20th percentile in reading ability, and exhibition of less ADHD behavioral problems.[414]

St. John's wort may be worthy of a trial, but due to its interaction with a plethora of prescription drugs, would be a secondary choice.

Learning and memory problems associated with temper tantrums, and irritability may indicate low GABA, suggesting additional B6 and magnesium threonate, as well as EPA, *Ginkgo biloba* and acetyl-L-carnitine.

If ADD and seasonal affective disorder (SAD) are present then a trial of SAMe and cod liver oil may be helpful, along with a high protein diet.

If there is sensitivity to noise and light, with hyperactivity and inattention, this may indicate low levels of both dopamine and GABA.

Zinc deficiency may be a factor. See Chapter 15 Supplements. This important mineral regulates the dopamine transporter and when children with ADHD were given zinc and methylphenidate, there was a more positive response than either the drug or placebo.[415]

Magnesium is important. One twelve-week study found zinc, magnesium and Omega-3/Omega 6 supplementation reduced symptoms in 810 children aged 5-12.[416]

Iron levels should be tested, as studies show 60-80% of children with ADHD exhibit low ferritin, with behavioral problems directly linked to lower levels. But only if levels are low should iron supplementation be considered.

Melatonin can be helpful. Long-term use is safe and effective for children, improving sleep as well as behavior and mood.[417] Start with 0.5 mg one hour before bedtime and increase as needed.

Studies have found the music of Mozart relaxing to both ADD and ADHD subjects. This is fascinating as both this musical genius and punk rock star Kurt Cobain may have suffered Tourette syndrome.[418] See Chapter Six.

Mozart composed music at age five, and wired the language of music into his brain. His work, especially with violins, is widely appreciated for its ability to connect rhythms, melodies and flow with language.

A therapy called Integrated Listening Systems, or iLs has helped over 80% of clients with ADD stop taking anti-depressants and stimulants like Ritalin. With ADHD, where distraction and impulse control create hyperactivity the rate is about 50%.

It works, in part, by stimulating the vagus system with the right kind of sound therapy, creating a calm, focused state.

Poor subcortical problems do not allow for clear auditory cortex signals, and music helps improves this sensory and learning issue.[419]

Chanting, in many parts of the world, helps energize the mind, but calm the spirit. Gregorian music has this effect, as does the music of Hildegard de Bingen. Music changes the rhythm of our brain.

I find the music of plants and mushroom, which I record with a special device, soothing and reflective.

Neurofeedback treatment is recognized by the American Academy of Pediatrics, as effective as medication, for ADD and ADHD.

People suffering these disorders have less calming, focused beta waves and more theta waves that most of us generate when we sleep. Neurofeedback therapy, and low-energy neurofeedback systems can be helpful in re-training the brain to raise beta waves, and lower theta levels when represented on a monitor.

These sound therapies may also be helpful in autism spectrum disorder (ASD) Chapter 8.

Essential oils may be helpful. Following the lead of stimulating amphetamines, it has been found that stimulating oils, such as rosemary and peppermint help bring more attention and less restlessness in ADHD.

OBSESSIVE- COMPULSIVE DISORDER (OCD)

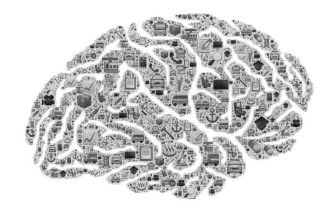

"Though a thousand times a thousand men are conquered by one in battle, the one who conquers himself is truly the master of battle."

GOTAMA BUDDHA

"Cleanliness becomes more important when godliness is unlikely."

P. J. O'ROURKE

Obsessive-Compulsive Disorder (OCD) and OC Spectrum Disorder are in some ways the opposite of ADD, in that there is too much concentration on the negative aspects of life.

Howard Hughes suffered a classic case of OCD, spending his last days in an Acapulco hotel, terrified of germs.

Obsessions are unwanted thoughts and urges that don't go away, while compulsions are the repetitive behaviors performed in a futile attempt to stop them. Over time the compulsions make the obsessions worse.

Jeffrey Kahn calls it the Clean, Arrange, Save and Behave disorder. He suggests people with OCD think they have to clean more, plan more, save more and control their behaviors.

Unlike our ancestors, today, it is all too easy to over-clean everything.

One of my favorite television series, *Monk*, featured a brilliant crime detective, whose memory recall was part of his OCD.

Studies have shown that a childhood history of ADHD is common in OCD adults who were never diagnosed, and showed up at an earlier age.[420]

One study found the lifetime prevalence of ADHD in adult OCD patients is 13.7%. These sub-type patients present some additional challenges that include an early history of rheumatic fever, and co-morbidity with Tourette syndrome. They have increased risk for academic impairment and suicide attempts.[421]

However, in one subset of children with ADHD, a syndrome known as PANDAS (Pediatric Autoimmune Neuropsychiatric Disorders Associated with Strep) occurs. This results from the production of antibodies to a *Streptococcus* infection that inappropriately reacts against brain tissue of the basal ganglia, resulting in increased OCD symptoms. A wide range of low grade or subclinical microbial infections may trigger PANS (Pediatric Acute-onset Neuropsychiatric Syndrome) with an acute or sudden onset of OCD behaviors, tics and other symptoms.

This has also been observed in cases of ASD (Chapter 8).

OCD can range from compulsive behavior with over-protective and risk avoidance fears, to body dysmorphic disorder, anorexia/bulimia, Tourette, or impulsive self-destructive behavior. Hair pulling, or TTM (trichotillomania), nail biting and compulsive skin picking are part of this disorder, as are obsessive thoughts and actions associated with sex, contamination, hoarding, religion, and superstition.

In one study of 539 adults with OCD, a substantive number suffered from compulsive sexual behavior disorder. It is more likely comorbid with other mood, obsessive-compulsive and impulse control disorders.[422]

A study[423] of 9449 university students found same sex sexuality associated with impulsive/compulsive behavior and addiction, including binge eating.

Various modalities such as acupuncture, yoga and mindful meditation do not appear to be very helpful.

Worry, and the need to find order and control dominate in OCD.

Jeffrey Schwartz has developed a four-step self-treatment method to change brain chemistry and help free those suffering obsessive-compulsive behavior. It is based on self-directed neuroplasticity, and has helped thousands of people change their brain chemistry.[424]

Glutamic acid decarboxylase (GAD) is discussed in the chapter on neurotransmitters. Antibody reactions are common and create specific symptoms. GAD is the enzyme that produces GABA and its calming effect. Elevated GAD antibodies have been linked to OCD, and "stiff man syndrome" a progressive, muscle stiffness. But not so, in Parkinson's disease.

Dysregulation of glutamate, for various reasons, may contribute to OCD spectrum disorders.

Diet is very important. A gluten-free diet, given to 29 patients with Gilles de al Tourette syndrome and OCD, for one year, led to a marked reduction in tics and OCD in children and adults.[425]

Useful therapies may include 5-HTP, as well as cognitive-behavioral therapy. Jeffrey Schwartz lists four steps for behavioral self-treatment. Relabel, reattribute, refocus and revalue. The key is helping the client recognize their obsessive thoughts are the result of OCD and brain dysfunction.

Family members can easily become enablers and create co-dependency, but this sabotages both parties; inducing guilt and self-projection.

Serotonin levels are low in people with OCD. Researchers have observed how the persistent one-track thoughts resembled those falling in love. Both groups showed 40% less serotonin, but after a year the giddy obsession of romance had normalized.

In fact, in the early stages of falling in love, the brain is flooded with dopamine, similar to an additive drug.

In some cases, however, a person with OCD and driven by poor serotonin activity, may actually find taking 5HTP makes their OCD worse.[426] Low doses may work better, and instead of causing negative plasticity in the brain, can stimulate and strengthen neurons so they function better on their own.

L-tryptophan has been found, in several studies, to be beneficial, but it should not be taken concurrently with anti-depressant medications.

Inositol, a B vitamin also found useful in anxiety and depression, may help, particularly in hair-pulling and skin picking. A small study of three women found 6 grams of inositol three times daily in juice showed improvement. Start with four grams daily and gradually increase. It may combine well with 5-HTP. Maybe.

Vitamin D supplementation reduced OCD in one reported case involving a seven-year old boy.

NAC (N-acetyl cysteine) may be helpful in TTM. A 12-week DB, PC trial of 50 patients found the NAC group showed a significant reduction in symptoms with daily doses of 1200-2400 mg daily.[427]

Thirty-four OCD outpatients (taking an SSRI) given NAC or placebo in a randomized DB, PC ten-week clinical trial, found improved resistance/control to compulsions.[428]

St. John's wort may be useful based on a small study of 12 OCD patients for one year. They were given 450 mg of 0.3% hypericin capsules twice daily. Significant change was found at week one, and continued to increase throughout trial. Forty-two percent were rated much or very much improved, 50% minimally improved, and 8% showed no change.[429]

Valerian root (*V. officinalis*) may be useful in OCD. An eight-week DB randomized trial of 31 outpatients involved a capsule of valerian root extract (765 mg/daily) or placebo. A significant improvement was found at the end of treatment.[430]

Supplementation of Milk Thistle seed extract (*Silybum marianum*) for OCD was found as effective as fluoxetine (Prozac), in an 8 week DB randomized trial of 35 adults.[431]

OCD related to cleanliness, will sometimes respond well to the English flower essence Crabapple.

One pharmaceutical, buspirone, acts on serotonin, but not on reuptake pump. It is mild, and may be helpful for OCD people who get too anxious when trying behavioral therapy.

CHAPTER 13

SCHIZOPHRENIA SPECTRUM DISORDER, BIPOLAR AND UNIPOLAR DISORDERS

"We are not ourselves. When nature, being oppressed, commands the mind To suffer with the body."

WILLIAM SHAKESPEARE

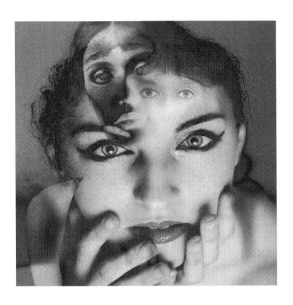

Schizophrenia spectrum disorder (SSD) is a form of psychosis associated with hallucination and delusion. A milder form is sometimes referred to as schizotypal personality disorder (STPD). The latter group use larger regions of the prefrontal cortex, have thicker connections between two sides of brain and exhibit more brain activity than the general population.

The gene, neuregulin 1, plays a key role in higher risk for both conditions. Two copies of this mutation lead to higher levels of creativity. The Nobel Prize mathematician John Nash battled schizophrenia. The 2012 film *A Beautiful Mind*, portrayed both the genius and mental issues he endured.

The most common form of hallucination is auditory, or hearing voices. Delusions are fixed beliefs, inconsistent with generally accepted views of reality. The mass delusion of religion, on the other hand, is considered normal if believed by a majority of people.

The degree to which things are important is salience. And if things are salient they trigger the desire molecule dopamine.[432]

Blocking dopamine does not make all the symptoms go away, but it can reduce instances of delusion and hallucination.

The modern medical approach is to give enough medication to block 60-80% of dopamine receptors. High doses of medication make the world a dull place, and difficulty getting out of bed.

There is increasing evidence of a correlation between schizophrenia and exposure to *Toxoplasmosis gondii*, an intracellular parasite that infects one-third of humans worldwide.

It is generally considered benign and asymptomatic, but a high level of behavioral and psychiatric disorders, including SSD may be linked to this infection[433]. The organism is transmitted by outdoor cats eating an infected prey (rats or mice), and then spread in their feces. It is now found in raw meat including pork.

In humans, acute infection with *T. gondii* can produce psychotic symptoms similar to SSD, and childhood exposure to cats is a risk factor. Some medications used to treat schizophrenia inhibit the replication of the organism in cell culture.[434]

A group in France looked at bipolar patients testing positive for *T. gondii*, and those given valproate experienced fewer lifetime depressive episodes.

Despite people with SSD having fewer children, the disorder numbers remain constant, in about 1% of people around the world.

Members of a family, with a SSD sibling, may suffer dyslexia, depression, bipolar disorder, autism, ADHD and OCD.

In fact, on average, anti-psychotic medications reduce symptoms by only 15-25%.[435] And there is evidence the long-term use of neuroleptic drugs may cause brain atrophy, as well as unpleasant side-effects.

Hyperactivity of the HPAA (hypothalamic-pituitary-adrenal axis) is common in schizophrenia spectrum disorders. This suggests a possible role for the correct adaptogenic herbal supplementation.

Caution is advised as *Rhodiola rosea*, one of my favorite adaptogens, is contraindicated in bipolar, due to possible mania. I can find no clinical study to back up this claim.

Drs. Abram Hoffer and Carl Pfeiffer treated tens of thousands of patients, showing supplementation and diet far more effective than prescription drugs.[436]

Dr. Hoffer, who passed away in 2009, found many patients suffering SSD were deficient in B3 (niacin or niacinamide). The rare condition of pellagra has many of the same symptoms.

He coined the term adrenochrome hypothesis, suggesting oxidized adrenaline, caused the LSD or mescaline-type psychosis. Large amounts of niacin appear to alleviate the symptoms. His first patient, in 1950, was a twelve-year old boy.

He coined the term *Orthomolecular Medicine*, and founded his own journal after orthodox medical journals ostracized his work and publications. Linus Pauling introduced the word orthomolecular meaning "correct molecule" in the journal *Science* in 1968.

The pineal gland may play a role in this condition, and perhaps other brain disorders. The pineal can produce N, N-dimethyl-tryptamine or DMT, the spirit molecule, based on work by Dr. Rick Strassman.[437]

DMT is abundant in plants of South America, used for entheogenic journeys. It is endogenous in the human brain. The pineal gland produces melatonin in the presence of serotonin. But this gland has the ability to convert serotonin into tryptamine, a step in DMT formation.

When tryptamine is methylated twice, it becomes DMT. But the pineal gland also produces beta-carbolines that inhibit DMT breakdown by monoamine oxidases (MAO).

Ayahuasca is an Amazonian mixture of beta-carbolines and plants with DMT, as the former prevents MAO in the gut from rapidly destroying the swallowed DMT and inhibiting the entheogenic journey.

The healthy pineal gland has a very efficient security system, the best example being the inability to stimulate daytime production of melatonin. Adrenaline and noradrenaline are neurotransmitters that activate receptors in the pineal gland and play a role in nightly production of melatonin.

Adrenaline and noradrenaline, enter the blood stream and when they approach the pineal gland, nerve cells take them up and dispose of them. This insures that stress and exercise do not stimulate daytime melatonin production.

If the pineal security system does not function properly, high levels of stress may worsen hallucinations and delusions in susceptible psychotic individuals.

Within the pineal is a small protein that protects the body from psychedelic amounts of DMT. Early studies found when schizophrenics were given pineal gland extracts, in the 1960s, their symptoms greatly improved. The anti-DMT enzymes reduced the pathological high levels, and psychotic symptoms improved.[438] Calcification of the pineal, due to fluoride, has been postulated to be involved.

Research shows methyltransferase enzymes forming DMT are more active in schizophrenia. But if the MAO system normally destroying DMT is defective, the compound will linger and produce undesired results. It is clear that MAO is less efficient in schizophrenic patients, and does not clear DMT quickly enough.

Sleep and circadian rhythm abnormalities are common in cases of SSD. In a meta-analysis of 29 studies, enlarged calcification and smaller pineal gland volume were found in schizophrenia patients than healthy controls. Melatonin supplementation leads to modest improvement of objective and subjective sleep, and metabolic adverse effects of anti-psychotics and the related tardive dyskinesia symptoms. For relief of latter symptoms see *Ginkgo biloba* in Chapter 16.

A recent study found removal of a pineal cyst in one patient relieved psychotic disorder just one month after surgery.[439]

Glutamate is the principal excitatory neurotransmitter in the brain, but this must be cleared by transporters, to avoid prolonged activity involved in both SSD, and BSD below. The excitatory amino acid transporters (EEat) play a role in this process on glial cells. Taurine (see Supplements Chapter 15) is transported by EEat2 [440], suggesting possible benefit in wakefulness and insomnia related to these disorders.

BIPOLAR SPECTRUM DISORDER

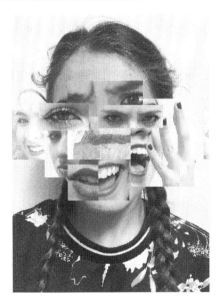

Another condition, related to excessive dopamine influence is bipolar spectrum disorder (BSD). Previously known as manic-depression, it was originally uncovered by the German psychiatrist Emil Kraeplin in the 19th century. Both bipolar and unipolar depressed patients have smaller pineal gland volume, similar to findings associated with schizophrenia.

One hypothesis suggests disruptions in circadian rhythm affect BD. Another theory suggests it derives from a pyknic (compact, cold-adapted body type) group.[441]

Vincent van Gogh, Isaac Newton and Virginia Woolf have been retrospectively diagnosed with BSD.

This is where depressive moods are abnormally low and episodes of mania are extreme due to high levels of dopamine. This is debilitating and prevents people from holding a job, or maintaining healthy relationships. The condition can be of a minor or major concern.

The upside is euphoria, energy and creativity.

It is believed to run in families and may be related to the gene responsible, chromosome 18.

In one long-term study of 700,000 students, those receiving the highest grades were three to four times more likely to develop the disorder later in life. If music and literature were exceptional talents, these individuals showed more likelihood of suffering BD, than those skilled in math, and science.

"Bipolar disorder is responsible for the loss of more disability-adjusted life years (DALYs) than all forms of cancer, or than major neurological conditions such as epilepsy and Alzheimer's disease" writes Dr. Merinkangas.[442]

Bipolar people will often self-medicate with alcohol, which normalizes the glutamate-induced elevation of intracellular sodium.[443]

The condition is not just caused by excessive dopamine, but something called the dopamine transporter. When the dopamine cell fires it releases the neurotransmitter, which binds to receptors in the brain, and the dopamine transporter sucks the dopamine back into the cell so it can start all over. It is like a re-uptake pump.

Worldwide, about 2.4% of the population suffer bipolar disorder. Research in Iceland, found people in the creative arts, such as dance, acting, music and writing are about 25% more likely to have bipolar disorder than those in noncreative jobs. I remember my first visit to that wonderful country, and the reverence shown for authors. One study at the University of Glasgow followed 1800 young people from eight to age 23. Those with a higher IQ at eight years old were predictive of a higher risk of bipolar disorder by age twenty-three.[444]

The world is full of famous, creative people with bipolar disorder. The United States is populated mainly with immigrants and their descendents, and has the highest rate of bipolar disorder (4.4%); almost twice the global average. The symptoms start earlier with about two-thirds of BD diagnosed by age 20, compared to only one-quarter in Europeans.

It is likely that an unhealthy microbiome, and the hormonal influence associated with puberty or menopause, may trigger the initial psychotic states.

This includes surgical menopause or hysterectomy. One study concluded that women suffering endometriosis, hormone therapy and hysterectomy have an increased risk of bipolar disorder.[445]

On the other hand, dopaminergic influence has led to the United States receiving 42% of all Nobel Prizes awarded between 1901 and 2013. The top three countries of origin are Canada (13%), followed by Germany and the UK (each 11%).[446]

Japan, with almost no immigration has a BSD rate of 0.7%, one of the lowest worldwide rates,[447] as well as India (0.1%).

While in clinical practice I helped numerous bipolar clients taking lithium carbonate. The list of side effects is long, but it did help reduce manic episodes in many.

However, over half of individuals prescribed lithium stop their treatment. One study found, of 873 bipolar and schizoaffective disorder patients, 54% discontinued lithium due to adverse effects including diarrhea, tremor, diabetes, elevated creatinine levels (kidney disease) and weight gain.[448]

People with BSD often suffer thyroid gland dysfunction, and lithium treatment over time creates low thyroid levels.

I wrote a herb/drug interaction booklet, with three pharmacists, back in 2001. It noted dandelion root tea was contraindicated when taking lithium, worsening the toxic effects. The book was re-printed in 2003 and subsequent years, but is now out of print.[449]

Lithia water was available in the 1990s from the Edgar Cayce group in Virginia Beach, and basically lithium-rich water from a natural source. I used this water in clinical practice due to the inability, at the time, to source natural lithium.

A company in British Columbia markets *Happy Water* from natural springs containing 0.1 ppm lithium.

An interesting study from Texas found incidences of crime, suicide and arrests for possession of opium, cocaine and its derivatives from 1981-86 were higher in counties whose drinking water contained little or no lithium, compared to those with lithium levels of 70-170 mcg/liter.[450]

Another recent study found natural lithium in drinking water may provide a protective effect on the risk of suicide in men.[451]

This is certainly a better idea than chloride and fluoride rich tap waters throughout most of North America. These chemicals, as well as bromide, used for hot tubs, are the three leading minerals that interfere with the ability of the thyroid to take up iodine for the production of thyroxin.

Lithium orotate is readily available as a supplement, is more bio-available and considered much safer than lithium carbonate. It is widely used to treat depression.

Lithium (unknown form) has been found to prevent damage associated with beta-amyloid plaque in Alzheimer', but more research is warranted. Lithium appears to work by increasing GABA receptor site sensitivity.

One test tube study suggests lithium, when added to brain cells, *in vitro*, prevented the damage of glutamate. A follow up rat study found the group taking lithium had 56% less brain cell death than controls. Lithium asparate may be useful for those who cannot tolerate lithium orotate.

Various mineral orotates, including calcium, magnesium and zinc forms are very well absorbed.

It may help in bipolar, as well as AD, PD, depression, anxiety, ALS (Lou Gehrig disease) and other mood disorders.

My advice is to work with a health practitioner in your area that is familiar with the mineral and dosage recommendations.

Low GABA levels should be addressed, as well as deficiencies of magnesium L-threonate and B6 (P5P) which may be present. A balanced EPA/DHA oil, or cod-liver oil could be a useful daily supplement. In resistant bipolar depression, higher than normal doses may be needed.

Other useful supplements are citocoline, inositol, and NAC. Citocoline (see Supplements) may be useful for cocaine and methamphetamine addiction in bipolar patients.

Know Mother root (*Anemarrhenae asphodeloides*) contains timosaponins that show anti-depressant activity by acting as a non-competitive antagonist of N-methyl-D-aspartic acid (NMDA) receptors.[452] Ginkgolide A, from *Ginkgo biloba* and Gotu Kola (*Centella asiatica*) also targets NMDA receptors. See Medicinal Herbs Chapter 16.

Essential oils may be helpful. Antidepressants work by making neurotransmitter serotonin linger in the gaps between neurons. Essential oils may work as serotonin agonists, which can push the serotonin system into overdrive, making the brain more sensitive like turning up the volume in your car radio so weaker stations can be heard.[453] Care must be taken, but good results may be obtained by intelligent selection and observation.

Essential oils antagonize NMDA receptors, suggesting rapid anti-depressant potential.[454]

Unipolar disorders (UD) are under diagnosed and patients are often lumped under the BD umbrella. The main difference is the time of onset, and the one emotional state in UD. Generally thought of as a depressive disorder, it can also be mania without the depression.

In bipolar disorder, there is often a correlation to emotional, physical and sexual abuse, and greater childhood trauma. Unipolar individuals are more likely to exhibit emotional inhibition, approval seeking, crave dependency and suffer abandonment issues.[455]

Both disorders may benefit from bright light therapy used for treating Seasonal Affective Disorder (SAD).[456]

197

Ketamine is associated with rapid, but transient anti-depressant effect in treatment resistant UD. There was no difference between lithium and placebo in continuing the response to ketamine in one double-blind randomized, controlled trial.[457]

CAUTION- SAMe, DHEA, *Rhodiola rosea* and St. John's wort are contraindicated in BD. *Gingko biloba* may reduce the side effects of Depakote.

CHAPTER 14

ADDICTIONS

"But for the unquiet heart and brain
A use in measured language lies;
The sad mechanic exercise
Like dull narcotics numbing pain."

ALFRED LORD TENNYSON

Nearly all addictions relate to issues around dopamine and its brain receptors.

Addictive narcotic and prescription drugs modify our brain's reward and motivation system. The ventral tegmentum (VT), in the midbrain is the most important region involved, containing about 400,000 neurons that release dopamine.

All addictive drugs stimulate the VT and dopamine release.

Animal studies have found cocaine, morphine, nicotine, alcohol or benzodiazepines induce long-term potentiation in the VT, that can persist for up to one week.

The density of dendritic spines in VT is increased by cocaine, and decreased by chronic use of morphine.

Users begin to feel their drug of choice is the answer to all their problems.

Twelve step problems like Alcoholics Anonymous, despite their lack of scientific validity, create a sense of community; albeit condoning addictions to coffee and nicotine.

"Many have tried Alcoholics Anonymous (AA) or twelve-step-based programs with limited success. This is not surprising," notes Lance Does in *The Sober Truth*. "Every year, our state and federal governments spend over $15 billion on substance-abuse treatment for addicts, the vast majority of which are based on a twelve-step program... There is only one problem: these programs almost always fail."[458]

Personal emotional support can make a difference. For some people, the lack of condemnation if one slips, or the guilt of letting others down, helps. But the science is underwhelming.

Drug addiction centers and holistic treatment centers offer yoga, tai chi, acupuncture, meditation, mindfulness, hypnosis and a wide range of modalities. But unless the brain gets what it desires, the rest is just window dressing.

Dopamine overtakes the rational side of the brain, and addicts feel powerless to resist. This dopaminergic compulsion of wanting takes over and is detached from anything they care for, or may be good for them.

Let us have a look at some of our society's most troublesome addictions, including those that are approved, and heavily taxed in Western society. More people, of course, are addicted to cigarettes and alcohol, than heroin. Their easy accessibility is the biggest health issue, associated with abuse.

A number of studies on the benefit of Psilocin, derived from Psilocybin mushrooms for nicotine and alcohol addiction are cited in the chapter (17) on Medicinal Mushrooms.

Essential oils may be a substitute treatment for inhalant addiction, as part of treatment program.[459] This DB, randomized controlled crossover study of 34 young males addicted to inhalation for an average of six years found benefit from the essential oil protocol.

NICOTINE

Tobacco is often smoked by cocaine users to stimulate dopamine and serotonin release. It mimics acetylcholine, is easy to obtain, legal and relatively cheap in comparison.

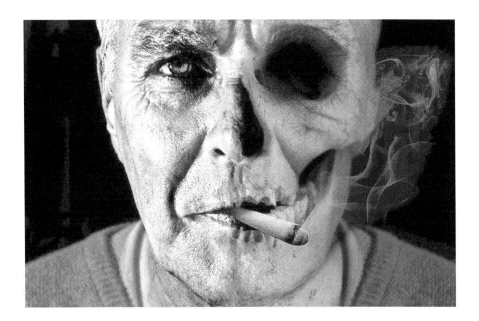

The mechanism is different as nicotine increases the firing rate of dopamine-producing ventral tegmentum neurons through action on nicotinic receptors on their surface, whereas cocaine, amphetamines and ecstacy block the dopamine transporter that normally reabsorbs the neurotransmitter after release by neurons.

Nicotine is an unusual drug in that most people don't initially enjoy the experience. It takes time. Small amounts tend to stimulate and larger amounts sedate. But the main thing it does is relieve cravings for itself. It's the perfect addiction circle.[460]

Quit smoking campaigns don't work. School programs on drugs and alcohol don't work. In fact, use of these addictive substances often goes up after the program, as student's interest is increased.

Raising taxes is controversial but the only thing that appears to work. The problem is that those who smoke tend to be less educated and poor. Nicotine appears to reduce anxiety in women more than men.

When women become pregnant, the usual steps taken to quit smoking are skipped, as the concern and empathy for the fetus becomes paramount. Olga, my beloved 89 year-old mother-in-law, smoked from age ten until a few years ago when she moved into an extended care facility. She decided to quit and that was that.

Nicotine occurs naturally in 64 species of plants around the world, but tobacco is the most well known.

Up to 90% of inhaled nicotine is absorbed, and because the lipids are soluble, it goes directly to the brain, in 2-7 seconds.

Low doses stimulate the left hemisphere, and higher doses affect the right hemisphere and are more sedative.

Brain activity is affected, with alpha and beta wave activity increased, and delta and theta waves decreased.

60% of adults diagnosed with attention deficit disorder (ADD) smoke tobacco.

The World Health Organization estimates 14% of all dementia cases, worldwide, are caused by smoking tobacco.

Individuals with serious mental illness are often the heaviest smokers.

In the United States, the health damage caused by tobacco results in almost one death every minute.

Nicotine is an agonist at nicotinic acetylcholine receptors, but with chronic use it becomes an antagonist.

It has an indirect effect on monoamine systems, and increased dopamine activity. Smokers show a 40% decrease in the level of MAO_B, and a 28% decrease in MAO_A levels, compared to non- or former smokers.

Nicotine does initially increase blood flow to brain, improving glucose utilization and supporting the dopamine reward-based activity.

But long-term use causes blood vessels to narrow, limiting oxygen and nutrients to the brain, impacting dementia and AD.[461]

One strategy that helped in my own clinical practice was medicinal herbs. Scullcap and Green Flowering Oats help calm the nervous system while undergoing nicotine withdrawal. Lobeline, a compound in *Lobelia inflata*, is almost chemically identical to nicotine. The herb is a partial agonist at receptor sites and yet is not addictive.

Other herbs that may reduce cravings and addiction are *Rhodiola rosea*[462] and St. John's wort.[463] Nicotine withdrawal reduces brain levels of serotonin, so consider tryptophan supplementation as part of an evening complex carbohydrate-based meal.

Cytisine, found in various herbs, including Scotch Broom, is a nicotinic receptor partial agonist. The compound is widely used in eastern European countries for nicotine withdrawal.

These herbs are covered in Medicinal Herbs chapter 16.

Another strategy for smoking cessation involves fresh lime juice.[464]

ALCOHOL

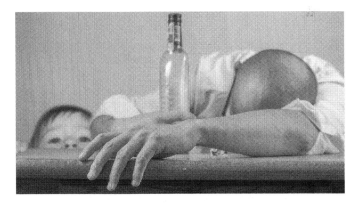

Alcohol abuse takes a great toll on modern society. And on the health of your microbiome. Prohibition did not work, and it never will. Tax revenues to various levels of government, now ensure the product will always be readily available.

Alcohol makes us feel relaxed and happy, helping form social communication, and friendships.

It helps relieve both panic and social anxiety, and is also a predictor of alcohol problems.

Various news sources suggest a daily drink of wine or beer be considered a health beverage. I am not convinced.

Don't get me wrong. I enjoy a cold, local brewpub pint as much as the next person, but the evidence is quite clear.

A study at Johns Hopkins showed daily drinkers have smaller brains.[465]

A thirty-year study of 550 men and women found moderate drinking (1-2 glasses daily) leads to atrophy of the hippocampus. It found no protective benefit from drinking one to seven small glasses of wine at week.[466]

One study found, however, after Alzheimer's disease was diagnosed, that 2-3 drinks a day slowed the progression and lowered mortality in mild cases.[467]

Several addiction psychotherapy approaches attempt to play one part of the brain against another. Unfortunately, with alcohol addiction, will power is not enough.

Alcohol abuse is connected to seven cancers, involving mouth, throat, esophagus, liver, colon, rectum and breast.[468]

And most importantly for brain health, it leads to an increase in gram-negative bacteria in the gut, and intestinal permeability by reacting with tubulin, the scaffolding inside every nerve cell. Elevated antibodies to tubulin are a biomarker of brain inflammation.

Motivational Enhancement Therapy builds up motivation by encouraging clients to talk about what they desire. Affirmations don't really work that well, unless someone believes them. It is somewhat manipulative but does help some people.

My wife Laurie uses Afformations when working with students and clients.

The concept of afformations was presented by Noah St. John, (2013) and is a way of putting new thoughts into the mind. The right afformation might nurture new thoughts to allow in new hope and possibility. Noah suggests afformations be phrased as questions. They differ from affirmations, which are presented as statements. Phrase your afformations around a goal, so it heightens the power of what you truly want or need. The supportive behavior, that follows, puts it all into action.

Most people have been taught to use affirmations, rather than afformations. I will highlight the differences between the two below.

This example is around the issue of addictions. Please feel free to create your own, so it reflects your goals.

An affirmation could be- "I am free from all desire to use substances which harm me."

The afformation might be, "How is it I so easily refrain from using all substances which harm me?"

According to Noah St. John, afformations create less resistance internally, than affirmations, as they are posed as questions and possibilities, rather than statements. He feels these questions can seep into our consciousness more easily, being less challenged by our inner judge. See Bibliography.

Cognitive Behavioral Therapy teaches clients to avoid cues that remind them of their addiction. Anything that reminds them of drinking is removed from the home. It has limited success.

Scientists have found addiction to alcohol changes how segments of DNA work, which are essential to dopamine control in the frontal cortex. A key enzyme is suppressed, interfering with the ability of neurons to transmit information.[469]

Bipolar individuals will self-medicate with alcohol due to its normalizing effect on the glutamate-induced elevation of intracellular sodium.[470]

Niacin, B3 supplementation works well for some individuals suffering alcoholic depression.

The gut peptide ghrelin circulates from the stomach to the hippocampus and enhances memory and learning. It is generally thought to be involved in appetite and adiposity, but ghrelin receptors are also present in the dopaminergic system, suggesting its use in the treatment of alcohol addiction, consumption, craving and withdrawal.[471]

Withdrawal from caffeine and tobacco increases irritability, headache, and muscle tension. These two drugs are widely used at AA meetings.

L-glutamine is particularly useful for alcohol cravings, and helps repair damaged intestinal tissue, associated with leaky gut.

An over-growth of *Candida albicans* converts sugars into alcohol (ethanol) and acetaldehyde. Pregnant women may stop drinking alcohol, but if yeast infections are an issue, fetal development may be influenced by release of the carbohydrate-fed toxins. After giving birth, breast milk will contain toxins associated with this overgrowth of yeast.

The drug Antabuse (disulfiram) is derived from a natural compound in the medicinal mushroom Inky Cap. It works as an aversion therapy by its affect on the liver enzyme acetylaldehyde dehydrogenase.

One medicinal herb helping curb desire for alcohol is Kudzu, a prolific, invasive plant of the southern United States. See Medicinal Herbs Chapter 16.

Kudzu is combined with bupleurum, gentian and tangerine peel in a product called Declinol. The combination was used in a pilot study to help reduce alcohol consumption in moderate to heavy drinkers. Bupleurum was added for its protection of liver toxicity but also benefit on regulation of endorphins, dopamine and epinephrine. Gentian and tangerine peel stimulate gut TAS2R receptors, which is synergistic with the effects of Kudzu.[472]

Another herbal combination *Relief*, containing saffron, passion flower, cocoa seed, radish and black cumin shows potential for improving alcohol withdrawal symptoms.[473]

Alcohol-free beer and wine can help the process.

COCAINE

Cocaine is derived from coca leaf (*Erythroxylum coca*), harvested in parts of South America, mainly Bolivia, Peru and Columbia.

The drug was used in the original Coca-cola over 100 years ago; a combination of cocaine and the stimulating kola nut.

Today, the Stepan Company in Maywood, New Jersey legally imports coca leaf, manufactures pure cocaine for the medical industry, and sells a cocaine-free extract to a known soft drink company.

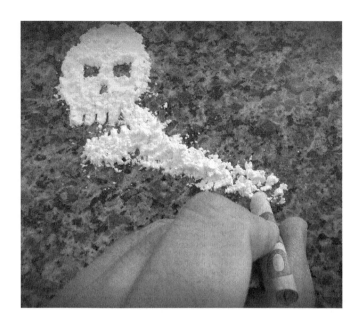

While living in Peru in the early 1980s, I used coco leaf with an alkaline ash from burned quinoa stems, to help my respiration when hiking the higher elevations of the Andes. Believe me, it is difficult to sleep at 15,000 feet when your heart is pounding and you are gasping for air.

A new bottled beverage in Peru called Kdrink is produced from coca leaves. Possession of up to two grams of cocaine or five grams of coca paste is legal for personal use in that country, as well as neighboring Bolivia and Columbia.

Addictive drugs, such as cocaine destroy our usual relationship with dopamine. They stimulate and confuse the brain, and eventually the brain think drugs are the answer to everything.

Crack cocaine has a faster onset of action than snorting the drug, producing a faster, larger dopamine rush.

As the drug blocks the dopamine transporter, it interacts with the receptor over and over again. Increased energy, goal-directed activity, self-esteem, racing thoughts and sexual drive all transpire. Cocaine intoxication is so similar to mania that health professional cannot easily tell them apart.[474]

Cocaine and Ritalin, commonly prescribed for ADHD, occupy the same receptor sites in the brain.

The South American two-plant entheogen Ayahuasca may be useful for cocaine addiction. A survey of 40 crack cocaine addicts found the herbal combination helped them reduce cocaine consumption and allowed access to a consciousness dimension that lasted well beyond the single experience.[475]

Cocaine and amphetamines inhibit or modulate the dopamine, noradrenaline and serotonin transporters; all the members of the neurotransmitter sodium symporter (NSS) family. Genetic variations of NSSs are associated with ADHD, ASD and bipolar disorder. Ibogaine (see Medicinal Herbs) is a non-competitive inhibitor of transport, but displays competitive binding towards selective serotonin reuptake inhibitors.[476]

OPIOIDS

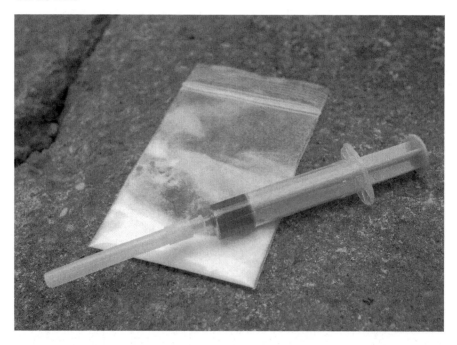

Opioids, cannabinoids and benzodiazepines increase their firing rate of dopamine indirectly, by inhibiting the activity of GABA-producing interneurons in the ventral tegmentum (VT).

Of the 89 million US adults who use prescription opioids every year, nearly four million reported misuse.[477] This is probably a low-ball figure. In 2017, more than 47,000 Americans died from opioid overdose.

Americans consume 132 pounds of wheat per person per year.

Wheat releases opiate-like molecules called exorphins that cause mental derangement if they cross the blood brain barrier (BBB).

Chocolate also stimulates opiate receptors but we don't ingest anywhere near the same amounts.

As more and more wheat products are consumed, people develop opiate receptor resistance, and more is needed to satisfy the addiction. Depression is very common in people who have damaged their opiate receptors.

Wheat contains benzodiazepines, a class of drugs used to treat anxiety and depression. Tranquilizer misuse is common among adults who misuse opioids.[478]

The type of opioid concentrated in casomorphins in cow's milk is ten times more potent to the brain, than morphine. One type bovine casomorphin-7 is associated with brain dysfunction and neurological disorders such as autism and schizophrenia. Casomorphins exaggerate the histamine release from food allergies and diminish cognitive function in ADHD and autism.

One recent study found a 1% increase in depression was associated with a 26% increase in opioid deaths.[479]

Drugs such as heroin and OxyContin act on both the dopamine and endorphin circuits, making them highly addictive.

The Sackler family that marketed OxyContin was once worth over $13 billion dollars. The approval of the drug by the FDA was based on misleading information about its addictive nature. In 2017, over 72,000 deaths were associated with heroin and prescription drugs like OxyContin.

A recent study revealed sixty-seven thousand physicians received over four hundred and thirty thousand payments totaling nearly $40 million dollars in non-research opioid marketing.[480]

Scientists have long believed that the brain could not change, and never anticipated bombarding the opioid receptors with medications could do harm. Really?

But we now know that once these receptors are saturated, the brain makes new ones.[481]

The Sackler's company, *Purdue Pharma* filed for bankruptcy in 2019 following the filing of over 2000 lawsuits alleging it contributed to the deadly opioid crisis sweeping America. In late March of the same year, they agreed to pay $270 million to the State of Oklahoma in the first, of many settlements to come.

Long-term opioid use causes the brain to become less sensitive, and more dependent, making the problem worse. Dr. Michael Moskowitz is a psychiatrist turned pain specialist, who discovered chronic pain can be unlearned.[482]

Fentanyl is a synthetic opioid that has been linked to tens of thousands of deaths in the past few years. It is often used alone, or mixed with heroin or cocaine.

Morphine, a valuable medicinal drug, and heroin are derived from the opium poppy. Spirulina (see Supplements) may be useful in treating opioid addiction.

Codeine, in cough syrups is another constituent widely used in OTC medications.

Its use in children's cough syrup was only recently reviewed by Health Canada.

Kratom (*Mitragyna speciosa*) exerts opioid and alpha-2 receptor agonistic effects and may be useful in helping addicted clients.

The alkaloids mitragynine and 7-hydroxymitragynine modulate opioid receptors, without addictiveness and overdose risk associated with opioid analgesics, such as morphine. Mild withdrawal symptoms have been noted.[483]

It is a partial agonist for mu-opioid receptors and a competitive antagonist at kappa- and delta-opioid receptors.

The alkaloids appear to exert diverse activity against adrenergic, serotonergic and dopaminergic receptors, suggesting a complex pathway of targets.

It has low respiratory depression and abuse potential, compared to opioids, due to its biased antagonist molecular structure.[484]

The herb deserves supervised clinical trials before it is dismissed as another illegal drug.

Kratom use is linked to 36 deaths, according to the FDA, that issued a public warning in November 2017. This may not be specifically true, as kratom exposure alone has not been causally associated with human fatalities.[485] It is the mixing and matching of kratom with opioids and various pharmaceuticals that have led to serious complications, including these deaths.

Ibogaine (see Medicinal Herbs) has shown benefit in opioid, cocaine and nicotine addiction. In the hands of a qualified practitioner, it has proven of significant benefit in various treatment center studies around the world.

Red clover, a medicinal herb generally associated with relief of menopausal symptoms, has an affinity for both mu and delta opiate receptors.[486]

The isoflavone pratensein significantly protects against amyloid-beta induced cognitive impairment by enhancement of synaptic plasticity and cholinergic function, albeit in a rat study.[487]

Purple Prairie Clover (*Dalea purpurea*) is native to the southern half of Alberta, where I live. The root may have application for opioid treatment, and is something I am exploring with an indigenous health center. The compound pawhuskin A is the strongest of three stilbenes with an affinity to opioid receptors.[488]

Also see the non-addictive California poppy, Green flowering Oats and Scullcap in the Medicinal Herbs Chapter 16.

SEX ADDICTION

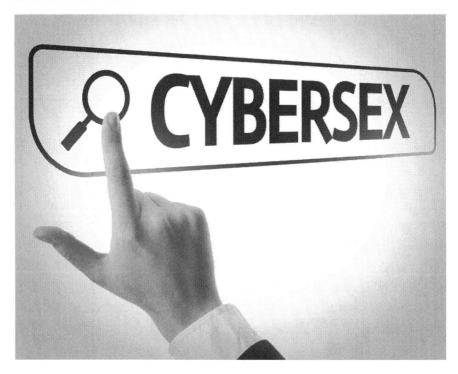

When I was a young teenager, back in the mid-1960s it was difficult to find sexually explicit material. There were magazines in drugstores, but it was not commonly available like today, where pornography sites are instantly available on the web.

The science is not clear, but porn addiction may be classified in the same category as drug addiction. Dopamine receptors light up when exposed to sexual images, and after awhile the interest in the same pictures diminishes. Chronic viewing of pornography becomes compulsive. Sex addicts need the continually new rush associated with dopamine. Elvis Presley, the famed singer, was reportedly addicted to both prescription drugs and pornography.

Parkinson's disease (PD) patients lack dopamine, and are given supplements such L-dopa to boost dopamine's effect in the brain.

About 16% of PD patients taking medication get into trouble, ranging from pathological gambling, to hypersexuality, to compulsive shopping.

GAMBLING
VIDEO GAMES
TELEVISION
SHOPPING

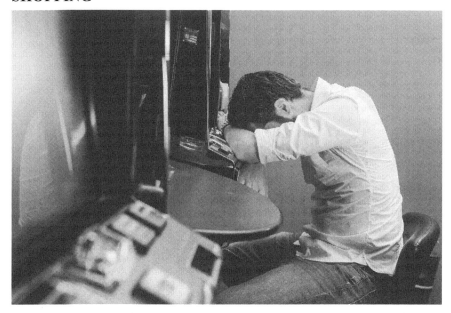

In one study, 30 healthy volunteers were given L-Dopa or placebo and invited to gamble. The former group placed larger and riskier bets. When both groups were later asked how happy they were, there was no difference. When they looked inside the brains they found the more active the dopamine cells were, the more money the volunteers expected to win.[489]

Research has found that people who had gambling addiction before starting Parkinson's medication are more likely to become worse.

Higher levels of depression and poorer motivation is found in problem gamblers, as well as higher incidents of OCD, and more frequent and extreme childhood ADD.[490]

Other mental health issues including PTSD and bipolar disorder may be linked to self-medicating as a response to the anxiety and depression.

One study of 3421 university students found gambling disorder was significantly associated with the past year use of cocaine, heroin/opiate pain medications, sedatives, alcohol and tobacco.[491]

Dopamine is the molecule of anticipation. Think of a casino floor in Las Vegas. The real money is in slot machines, which occupy 80% of floor space. People buy lottery tickets, hoping to win the big one, with odds of 14 million to one.

Video games contain unpredictable rewards. One in ten gamers aged eight to eighteen are addicted to video games, a rate five times higher than gamblers.[492]

The frontal lobe is not fully developed in adolescent brains, causing them to act impulsively.

Video games are based on surprise, and about making the future better than the present. Young people risk obesity, reduced sleep time and excessive sugary drink consumption when video gaming. Research suggests addiction to video games is a serious, emergent pediatric problem.[493]

Nicholas Kardaras, author of *Glow Kids*, suggests television, to children, is like electronic cocaine.[494] The dopamine rush grows old, and more and more is needed to fill the void, leading to anxiety, depression and aggression.

The next time you visit a casino observe the number of older people trying to shake off their low spirit and depression for points, rewards and money.

Obviously the excess of dopamine creates major problems with addictive personalities. Serotonin and dopamine tend to balance each other so herbs like saffron, or *Griffonia simplifolia* (5-HTP) may be useful. NAC or N-acetyl carnitine may be useful in helping individuals with gambling, or video game addiction.

Rhodiola rosea (see Medicinal Herbs) helps balance the hypothalamic-pituitary-adrenal axis (HPAA) and may be useful.

Anxious, tense addicts may suffer low levels of GABA, magnesium and B6 (P5P).

Moody individuals, with memory and learning difficulties, and those prone to temper tantrums may benefit from the above suggestions, as well as *Ginkgo biloba* or Clubmoss (Huperzine A).

Acetyl-l-carnitine may be useful, but this supplement is contraindicated with mania, in bi-polar disorder.

On the emotional level, a variety of flower and mushroom essences help address some of these specific issues. See Chapter 19.

CHAPTER 15

SUPPLEMENTS

Whenever you add new supplements to your personal healthcare regime, it is best to introduce only one for the first three or four days, and observe any untoward effects. Begin with one-quarter of the recommended dosage and move up every few days.

Children are often resistant to supplements, even when told they are good for them. Capsules can be opened, or tablets crushed and added to juice, smoothies, nut butters, etc.

MICROALGAE

Fresh water algae are a rich source of easily assimilated amino acids, vitamin and minerals.

There are over twenty species of Chlorella, that have thrived on the planet for billions of years. The name is derived from Greek *chloros*, meaning green.

I suggested Chlorella cracked wall tablets in my clients for various health issues. *Chlorella vulgaris* is the most popular cultivated product, rich in chlorophyll and the benefits of green leafy vegetables. It is rich in B1, B6, B12, vitamin A, K and C, and more nutrient dense per gram than kale, spinach or broccoli.

One review of DB, PC, randomized human clinical trials on 55 subjects with fibromyalgia, 33 with hypertension and 9 with ulcerative colitis was conducted at a Medical College in Virginia. The daily intake of 10 grams of *Chlorella pyrenoidosa* for two or three months reduced of blood pressure, lower serum cholesterol, and accelerated wound healing and enhanced immune functions.[495]

Chlorella vulgaris was found in a mice study to reduce the impact of stress on the HPAA, or hypothalmic-pituitary-adrenal axis.[496]

It is calming to those suffering anxiety and nervous energy.

Looked for products that are organic, processed at low temperatures and have cracked cell walls for optimal absorption.

It is a useful addition during heavy metal detoxification.

Side-effects are usually associated with the rapid detoxification due to consuming large doses.

CAUTION- Chlorella interacts with immune suppressive drugs and blood thinners such as Coumadin.

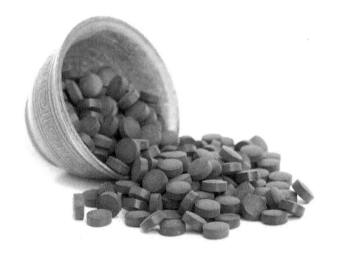

Spirulina is a close cousin, with similar uses, and more published clinical studies. It is richer, than Chlorella, in protein (up to 70%), iron, and GLA (gamma-linolenic acid). Several studies suggest its benefit in brain health.

In one mouse study, amyloid beta-protein was significantly reduced in the hippocampus and whole brain in both spirulina groups.[497]

A rat model of Parkinson's disease showed a mediation of alpha-synuclein neurotoxicity and a decrease in activated microglia when given a spirulina-enhanced diet. The increased expression of the fractalkine receptor (CX3CR) suggests a possible action.[498]

A mice study found spirulina (*S. platensis*) reduced kainic acid neuron death in CA3 hippocampal cells.[499]

Spirulina (*S. maxima*) prevents cell death caused by amyloid beta 1-42-induced neurotoxicity in PC cells, via the activation of brain-derived neurotrophic factor (BDNF) involved in neuron survival and protection.[500]

The phycocyanobilin chromophore of spirulina, a structural analogue of biliverdin, shares bilirubin's ability to inhibit NAPDH oxidase complexes. It may help prevent morphine tolerance, with possible use as adjuvant in clinical opiate therapy.[501]

I recommended Klamath Lake blue-green Algae (*Aphanizomenon flos-aquae*) for a period of time in clinical practice. One client complained of kidney pain so I completed a urinalysis; finding considerable blood in his urine. He was a fruitarian (eating only fruit) and taking massive (in my opinion) doses of blue-green algae. I urged him to stop and in three days the pain and blood resolved.

I began to question its source, as a colleague from the university studied the harmful effects of blue-green algae on prairie lakes. I stopped recommending it in the early 2000s. Since that time there have been both good and bad reports on the product.

On the one side, the microalgae is rich in phenylethylamine and appears to inhibit MAO-B activity. This suggests possibilities associated with improving mood disorders and neurodegenerative diseases.[502]

The same commercial extract Klamin® interferes with amyloid-beta aggregation, supporting formation of smaller and non-toxic structures. This suggests neuro-degenerative protection.[503]

On the other hand, cyanotoxins have been found in some spirulina and blue-green algae supplements, mainly mycrocystins. In one study 8 out of 18 products off the shelf showed the presence of cyanotoxins. This is due to the fact that in some environmental conditions, algae blooms can occur. This can lead to serious health issues.

The neurotoxin beta-N-methylamino-L-alanine (BMAA) is produced by aquatic cyanobacteria and microalgae. Bivalves contain higher levels of toxin than fish muscle, and are associated with the Amyotrophic Lateral Sclerosis-Parkinsonism-Dementia complex of neurodegenerative diseases.[504]

It may be best to stick with controlled, cultivated microalgae to avoid problems.

MACROALGAE

Fucoxanthin, derived from a marine carotenoid, might prevent beta-amyloid induced neuronal loss, suggesting possible benefit in treating AD.[505]

The brown Korean seaweed *Hizikia fusiforme* improves intestinal tight junction integrity.[506]

Seaweeds generally show promise for neuroprotection in PD. The Atlantic marine brown seaweed *Bifurcaria bifucata* shows antioxidant and neuroprotective potential in one *in vitro* Parkinson's disease model.[507] Various other seaweeds showed promise for neuroprotection, by the same research team.[508]

Homotaurine, derived from red algae, may be useful in various neurodegenerative conditions. See below.

PPQ (pyrroloquinoline quinone) is a cofactor for redox enzymes originally identified in methanol-utilizing bacteria. It has been identified, in very small amounts, in parsley, celery and few other foods.

PPQ reduces levels of C-reactive protein, indicative of inflammation, and enhanced mitochrondrial function in a human study.[509]

A group of twenty healthy subjects (50-70 years old) were given 20 mg of PPQ or placebo for 12 weeks. Concentrations of hemoglobin and oxygen saturation in the right prefrontal cortex increased in the PQQ group, suggesting enhanced cognitive function.[510]

Forty-one elderly patients were given 20 mg of PPQ or placebo for twelve weeks. The results suggest PPQ can prevent reduction of brain function in aged, especially in attention and working memory.[511]

PQQ prevents mitochondrial dysfunction by promoting biogenesis and regulating fission and fusion, suggesting neuroprotective effect in Parkinson's disease models.[512]

AMINO ACIDS and related COMPOUNDS

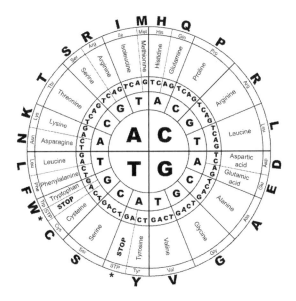

Acetyl-L-carnitine (ALC) is a different form than the amino acid L-carnitine, by having an attached acetic acid group.

This acetyl group can be donated to choline, to form acetylcholine, the valuable neurotransmitter.

ALC provides an acetyl moiety incorporated into glutamate, glutamine and GABA, or into lipids for myelination and cell growth.[513]

ALC shows positive effects on mitochondrial metabolism and in the treatment of neurodegenerative conditions. It plays neuromodulatory effects on both synapse health and transmission. It is widely distributed in the brain, blood-brain barrier, brain neurons and astrocytes. It reduces the concentration of glutamate in the synapses and improves nerve regeneration and damage repair after trauma by enhancing neurite growth.

This may help in mental cognition, including Alzheimer's (AD) and Parkinson's disease (PD) because synaptic energy states and mitochondrial dysfunction are a core factor in their pathology.[514]

Unlike L-carnitine, ALC protects the nervous system due to its faster transportation. Depression, impaired cognition and other memory-deficient states, including mild AD may be helped with supplementation.

The use of methamphetamines increases blood-brain barrier permeability. Studies suggest ALC promotes alpha tubulin deacetylation and protects against histone deacetylases.[515]

A meta-analysis of 21 DB, PC, randomized controlled clinical trials of ALC involved 1.5 to 3 grams, taken daily for three, six and twelve months. Significant improvement compared to placebo was observed.[516]

A review of 12 randomized controlled trials of 231 individuals showed significant reduction of depressive symptoms.

It helps increase dopamine production, and may possess possible application in PD (author opinion).[517] ALC reduces glutamate overflow associated with depression.[518]

ALC is a histone acetylation modulator and should be studied for benefit in various psychosis spectrum disorders.

And unlike its cousin, ALC protects cellular mitochondria by restoring levels of the phospholipid, cardiolipin.

One rich natural source is lamb, but all animal protein supplies some amounts.

It combines well with alpha lipoic acid (ALA) in the production of cellular energy, and the prevention of glycation associated with blood sugar dysregulation.

There is one recorded case of a man with bipolar disorder relapsing when taking ALC to aid weight loss. Start with 500 mg daily and increase over time.

NOTE- the D and DL forms of carnitine are not functional and can cause problems. Because of possible side effects, in rare disorders, L-carnitine should not be used without blood testing.

Valproic acid and other seizure medications lower carnitine levels.

ALPHA-LIPOIC ACID (ALA)

Alpha-lipoic acid is a water and fat-soluble supplement that helps lower blood sugar levels in type 2 diabetes.

It is a powerful anti-oxidant that helps regenerate vitamins C and E, as well as recycling coenzyme Q10 and glutathione.

An early PC study of 40 bipolar depression subjects found a combination of ALC and ALA exhibited no anti-depressant effect.[519]

Recent studies suggest, however, ALA may be a useful adjunctive treatment for schizophrenia. One study looked at the benefit in 10 patients taking 100 mg daily, with a 63.9% reduction in Brief Psychiatric Rating Scale scores.[520]

Schizophrenics treated with atypical anti-psychotic drugs often gain considerable weight. ALA supplementation, in a DB, PC, randomized trial of 22 overweight and clinically stable patients for twelve weeks, found significant weight loss.[521]

A systematic review of 32 articles found ALA effective in the prevention of Alzheimer's disease progression.[522]

A combination of carnosine and ALA shows neuro-protection in a rat model of early-stage Parkinson's disease.[523]

Thimerosal, a mercury containing preservative used in various drugs, including vaccines, has been linked to neurodevelopment disorders such as autism. A rat study found ALA prevented the adverse effects of associated behavior.[524] This suggests one possible prophylactic approach to preventing side effects of immunization. More research is needed. In clinical practice I found homeopathic Echinacea and Thuja reduced the immediate fevers, often suffered by young children after vaccination.

A review of the literature suggests that many cases of idiopathic autism are induced by early mercury exposure from thimerosal.[525] Genetic and non-genetic factors establish a predisposition of adverse effects in only some children. The issue is highly controversial.

The R form is found naturally in food and the one I prefer.

300 mg twice daily between meals appears to work well.

My good friend, brilliant nutritionist, and former student John Biggs has developed a product called Cell Fuel. It contains CoQ10, PPQ, NAC, ALC and ALA in a balanced formula.

Alpha GPC (alpha-glycerylphosphorylcholine) occurs naturally in our cells, and has been shown to improve memory in AD. It is present in breast milk in high concentration. Choline-derived supplements help produce acetylcholine. See Chapter Four under Acetylcholine for more information.

Adult dose starts at 600 mg daily.

Taurine (2-aminoethanesulfonate) is a free amino acid that hyperpolarizes brain neurons and inhibits their firing. It is abundant in the brain, retina, muscle tissue and various organs, and plays a key role in eye health, diabetes and epilepsy.

Its high concentration in the retina serves as a neuroprotectant against glutamate-induced toxicity.

It calms the excitatory and nervous system without being sedating, working as an inhibitory neurotransmitter. It is a calming amino acid that supports and activates GABA receptors.

Deficiencies result in a reduction of oxygen consumption, an elevation in blood sugar and lactate production, and a decline in ATP production. Taurine may have a role to play in congestive heart disease, acute hepatitis, and cystic fibrosis.

Although similar in molecular structure, taurine and GABA act on different receptors, but it is definitely a modulator of neuronal activity.[526]

Taurine helps boost the creation of new brain cells, a process known as neurogenesis, in both young and old.[527]

Taurine is added to the energy drink Red Bull (Taurus) to quell the jittery effect caused by mega doses of caffeine.

Caffeine is an effective adenosine receptor antagonist that binds to its receptor on acetylcholine neurons, slowing activity. The concentration of adenosine increases during the day, inhibiting acetylcholine neurons, as your brain slows down and you begin to feel drowsy.

Coffee drinking has been associated with a lower risk of Parkinson's disease in men, and lower incidence of type 2 diabetes in women.

Moderate consumption may lower the risk of developing Alzheimer's disease. In an animal study, taurine protected brain cells from toxicity associated with beta-amyloid deposits.[528]

Caffeine sets free the activity of dopamine neurons to increase euphoria and bliss. It is estimated that some 80% of all people in North America have measureable amounts of caffeine in their brains from embryo to death.

Theobromine and theophylline, from chocolate and tea also block adenosine receptors.

Chocolate contains phenethylamine, a molecule that resembles amphetamine, and a small amount of anandamide, found in cannabis.

It contains estrogen-like compounds, and findings suggest men who eat chocolate live longer.

Chocolate contains magnesium salts, useful for menopausal women, and in fact, improves magnesium cellular uptake and utilization.

Anandamide activity is synergistic with Tylenol, reducing the experience of pain.

Multiple sclerosis patients find a combination of cannabis and acetaminophen provides a measure of symptom relief.

Taurine may not work in all cases of epilepsy, as a deficiency is not the only prerequisite for seizure activity.[529]

The transport of taurine, rather than its concentration in plasma and urine, may explain why it works in some cases of epilepsy and not in others.[530] It interacts with other nutrients, biochemicals and xenobiotics, making its pathway to brain health, unclear.[531]

In autism, when there is persistent inflammation and oxidative stress, cysteine, from which taurine is derived, is used to make glutathione (see NAC).

Taurine is very safe. High doses are diuretic, but 1000 to 2000 mg supplementation is good place to start.

CAUTION- A subset of children with autism spectrum disorder have a metabolic disorder which makes them intolerant of specific amino acids including taurine. Discuss your condition with a health practitioner as blood and urine amino acid testing will determine its benefit, or not.

HOMOTAURINE

Homotaurine is derived from red algae. It is similar to taurine but contains one additional carbon.

It shows great promise in both primary and secondary prevention of AD, including reduction in hippocampal volume loss and reduction in genetic APOE e4 allele carriers.[532]

Homotaurine exhibits inflammation reduction in amnestic mild cognitive impairment. In one study of supplementation in 20 patients carrying the e4 allele or not, there was a positive improvement, and decrease in IL-18 associated with pro-inflammatory brain health.[533]

A single blinded, randomized controlled study looked at safety and efficacy in 47 Parkinson's disease patients for six months. The data showed the benefit of homotaurine for excessive daytime sleepiness, and promoting sleep/awake cycles in PD.[534]

TYROSINE

Tyrosine is a precursor, along with iodine, for the production of thyroxin, as well as L-dopa, dopamine, and noradrenaline.

These are involved in fight or flight, so supplementing can be overly stimulating and cause anxiety, insomnia and irritability.

Dopamine is rapidly depleted during stress, as the body uses the amino acid to make stress hormones. A lack of dopamine results in many of the symptoms associated with chronic stress.

Tyrosine helps manufacture melanin; our hair and skin pigment.

In times of stress it helps produce natural pain-reducing endorphins and is a precursor of Coenzyme Q10.

Although useful in some forms of depression, it may not be helpful for individuals suffering acute stress response, but more useful for chronic stress conditions.

Tyrosine is an effective enhancer of cognition, but only when neurotransmitter function is intact, and dopamine and/or norepinephrine are temporarily depleted.[535]

When brain levels are depleted, tyrosine helps to increase working memory and information processing.

Athletes, public speakers and those working in demanding information fields may benefit from tyrosine.

It can be useful in preventing PTSD, and aids stress associated with military life.[536]

One study found that with increased aging, tyrosine negatively affected proactive response slowing, and associated frontal-striatal activation; highlighting the importance of dopamine for proactive response inhibition in older adults.[537]

Tyrosine supplementation in a double-blind case showed a clear antidepressant effect.[538]

Tyrosine is contraindicated in patients with malignant melanoma, as it is a precursor to melanin. Patients with a deficiency of hepatic enzyme tyrosine aminotransferase develop neurological and developmental issues due to high levels of tyrosine. Tyrosinemia Type II patients are deficient in Omega-3 fatty acids.[539]

However, N-acetyl-L-tyrosine activates the dopamine pathways more so than simply affecting the adrenals.[540]

Due to its stimulating nature, tyrosine is best taken in morning 30 minutes before breakfast. 500 mg capsules, up to four daily.

DL-PHENYLALANINE

DL-phenylalanine (DLPA) is an amino acid precursor to tyrosine, noradrenaline and dopamine, as well as an enhancer of beta-endorphins. The D-fraction may be most useful when there is addiction to pleasure-seeking stimuli. It helps enhance the function of endorphins by functioning as an endorphinase inhibitor.[541]

CREATINE

Creatine helps increase phosphocreatine stores in the brain, which in turn requires sufficient ATP (adenosine triphosphate) to function properly. In PD, ALS, AD, PTSD and HD, as well as ischemic stroke and epilepsy, where brain function is impaired, there is a depletion of ATP. Creatine helps restore ATP and maintain cellular energy.

A study by Hersch on 64 patients with HD, or its genetic inheritance, found creatine slowed its progression, and regional brain atrophy.

A combination of creatine and cyclocreatine helps attenuate PD brain neurotoxicity.[542]

In an animal model study of ALS, creatine showed neuro-protection,[543] and possible benefit in AD.[544]

Creatine deficiency, due to inborn metabolism error, can affect epilepsy at any age.[545]

A deficiency may exacerbate autism spectrum disorder (ASD), affecting language delay, intellectual disability and movement disorders.[546]

The ratio of glutamate and glutamine/creatine may be affected in cases of PTSD, and the supplement should be studied for possible clinical intervention.[547]

Di-acetyl creatine is a highly lipophilic derivative that crosses the blood-brain barrier more readily, in the presence of AGAT and GAMT deficiency.[548]

Guanidinoacetic acid (GAA) is a dietary supplement that increases creatine in the human brain. A small eight-week oral trial on five healthy men, using brain magnetic resonance spectroscopy and clinical chemistry, suggest it may be helpful in neurodegenerative diseases.[549]

CARNOSINE

Carnosine (L-carnosine) supplementation helps sleep disorders in ASD in a randomized, controlled clinical trial.[550]

L-GLUTAMINE

L-glutamine helps form the epithelial cells on the wall of the gastrointestinal tract, by up-regulating a number of genes associated with gut healing.

Although it is the most plentiful amino acid in the body, supplementation may help irritable bowel and leaky gut syndrome. Deficiency may occur after major stress or infections, radiation and/ or chemotherapy, and immune disorders.

A guinea-pig model of ulcerative colitis found glutamine beneficial in carrageenan-induced animals.[551]

It may however, increase Candida and other yeast growth.

It is a precursor to the neurotransmitter glutamate in the brain. Caution is advised as it may aggravate an already inflamed intestine. Optimal amounts are required for a Th1 cytokine response to pathogens.[552]

Certain cancer tumors feed off L-glutamine, and individuals with kidney and liver disease, or Reye's syndrome should avoid supplementation.

Red cabbage, bone broth, spirulina and whey are rich natural sources of L-glutamine. Vitamin B12 controls glutamine storage in the body.

BETAINE

Betaine (trimethylglycine) is an amino acid found naturally in wheat, beets, spinach, amaranth and quinoa. Due to many patients issues with wheat allergies, this is no longer a viable source. Betaine is a derivative of choline, and a methyl donor, helping convert harmful homocysteine into methionine. Homocysteine levels may be elevated due to genetic factors, or alcoholism.

Betaine and folate supplementation may help prevent fetal alcohol syndrome, based on one animal study.[553]

Betaine is taken, along with folate, B6 and B12. Natural sources are preferred to supplements that may raise cholesterol levels. Betaine supplements are not recommended in cases of diabetes or heart disease.

PHOSPHOTIDYLCHOLINE

Plasma levels of phosphatidylcholine (PC) appear related to states of depression. However, supplementation for brain health lacks enough clinical evidence to make a recommendation.

It would seem sources of choline would be useful for the production of acetylcholine in the brain, but this does not appear to be the case. PC can, however, be synthesized to phosphatidylserine, in the endoplasmic reticulum.

PC is the most abundant phospholipid in the human body.

NOTE: Supplementation of dietary phosphatidylcholine may be contraindicated in diabetic patients, with cardiovascular disease (CVD). Gut microbiota may convert it to trimethlamine-N-oxide, which has been related to CVD mortality.[554]

CITOCOLINE

Choline is the natural precursor to acetylcholine. Citocoline (cytidine 5' diphosphocholine) is a form of choline found in our brain and available as a supplement. It is a precursor to the synthesis of phospholipids, and increases various neurotransmitters including acetylcholine, dopamine and noradrenaline.

It has long been used in Europe for vascular dementia and Parkinson's disease.[555]

Citicoline stimulates neurons to increase dopamine receptors, and protect them from overstimulation and death.

In one student of 58 students and teachers with cognitive, emotional, autonomic and asthenic disorders, the group taking 500 mg showed positive results after 30 days.[556]

It may be useful for some adults suffering ADHD, and teenagers with impulse control issues, and poor reaction times.[557]

Recent studies suggest it may protect brain cells from lead-induced injury.[558]

Citocoline may be useful for cocaine dependence in bipolar disorder, based on a DB, PC study of 130 outpatients.[559]

It increases neurotransmitter levels via influence on brain phospholipids, including increased ATP and phosphocreatine.

It may be helpful for methamphetamine patients, but does not appear helpful for alcoholism.

DOSE- 250 mg twice daily

PHOSPHATIDYLSERINE

Phosphatidylserine (PS) crosses our blood-brain barrier, and safely slows down, halts and reverses destruction of nerve cells. It helps cognitive function, improving short and long term memory and the ability to create new memory, and retrieve old ones. It helps focus attention and concentration, and supports locomotor functions.[560]

The brain is highly enriched with DHA and brain PS is rich in DHA content. By promoting PS synthesis, DHA can expand the pool into neuronal membranes and influence signaling and protein function. Alcohol (ethanol) decreases DHA-promoted synthesis contributing to its negative effects.[561]

PS, supplemented in both rats and AD patients, showed improved learning ability, vocabulary and picture matching scores. PS decreased cholinesterase, improved memory and improved hippocampus inflammation injury.[562]

A blend of PS and phosphatidic acid was given to two human groups; one elderly people without depression, and the other patients with AD. The first group in the DB, PC trial showed improved memory, mood and cognition; and the AD group showed stabilizing effect on daily functioning, emotional state and self-reported general condition.[563]

Adult dose is 200-300 mg daily.

A third phospholipid is phosphatidylethanolamine, also known as cephalin. This is responsible for cognition and memory. It is converted to PC with the help of methyl groups.

All three are derived from our food, but faulty liver health can wreak havoc with the availability of these important lipids. Soy-free sources of PS are derived from sunflower-based lecithin.

ALPHA GPC

The supplement alpha-glycerylphosphorylcholine (alpha GPC) is isolated from lecithin and well absorbed by the intestine for the production of acetylcholine. A study of 126 patients with senile dementia showed significant improvement, even slightly better than the group given acetyl-l-carnitine (ALC), mentioned above.[564]

Sardines, anchovies and other fish oil contain alpha GPC and dimethylaminoethanol (DMAE); which are both precursors of acetylcholine. The pigmentation of skin and brain, known as lipofuscin, or age spots, is resolved with the regular intake of DMAE.

In one study, DMAE increased improvement in hyperactive children in just ten weeks.[565]

MONOLAURIN AND CAPRYLIC ACID

These two useful compounds are derived from coconut oil. Monolaurin possesses powerful inhibition of *Candida albicans* biofilm, which is often present in patients with unhealthy microbiomes.

The yeast to hyphal transition occurs when antibiotics, corticosteroids and birth control pills upset our normal flora and create an unhealthy microbiome.

The fungi feed on sugars and release cell-wall deficient toxins into our bloodstream, affecting every part of the body including the brain. Oral candidiasis or thrush is commonly treated as a topical issue, but is really a more chronic condition that requires systematic treatment.

I spent a great deal of time in clinical practice discerning whether or not candidiasis was part of my client's health issues. It can resemble hypo or hyper-thyroidism, hypoglycemia, and various other auto-immune inflammatory diseases.

Caprylic acid is derived from coconut oil and considered a medium chain saturated fatty acid (MCFAs). It is used by the brain for energy and shows benefit for memory in Type one diabetes.[566]

Caprylic acid is an aggressive anti-fungal against *Candida albicans* biofilm. The short length of its carbon chain allows for easier penetration into the cell walls of yeast and fungus. I preferred to give my clients a capsule form called Capricin, an enteric-coated product that opened up in the intestine. This quick die-off creates a flood of toxins that can cause a Herxheimer reaction, with very unpleasant results. Taking a few charcoal tablets helps to absorb these released toxins and reduce the ill effect.

COENZYME Q10

Coenzyme Q10 (Ubiquinone) is an anti-oxidant that plays a key role in mitochondrial function, and is hence useful in neurodegenerative diseases such as Alzheimer's, Parkinson's and Huntington's.[567] It is found in nearly all cell membranes and hence it is ubiquitous, and responsible for 95% of energy produced by mitochondria in our cells. It does this by shuttling electrons into the mitochondria to generate ATP.

It may be useful in a nutritional plan for autism spectrum disorder (ASD), based on the results of a year long trial of 67 children and adults aged 3-58.[568]

An open-panel, parallel, add on, match-controlled trial of 80 migraine patients found a reduction in headache frequency, a shortening of its duration, and lessened severity.[569]

A recent systematic review of 221 participants found it may reduce the frequency of migraine attacks per month but not the severity or duration.[570]

At rates of 500 mg daily, it can improve fatigue and depression in patients with multiple sclerosis.[571]

Also present in oily fish and organ meats, the whole human body content is only about 500-1500 mg and decreases with age. It is fat-soluble so best taken in a meal with healthy fats and oils.

NOTE- One pleasant and unexpected benefit of CoQ10 is progressive disappearance of the contractures on both hands of Dupuytren's disease.[572]

Soft gel capsules containing ubiquinol appear the most bioavailable source of CoQ10 for humans. It is usually produced through a unique fermentation process of yeast strains involving beets and sugar cane.

Lipitor, Crestor and other statin drugs deplete the body of CoQ10. Beta blockers and tricyclic anti-depressant drugs deplete the body, as well, of this valuable compound.

NAC

N-acetyl cysteine (NAC) is a widely available dietary supplement and precursor of L-cysteine used in the production of glutathione. NAC has shown some pro-cognitive benefit in Alzheimer's and other progressive neurodegenerative conditions. It crosses the blood-brain barrier (BBB), but is low in bioavailability. NAC-amide has shown in preclinical studies to have higher permeability through cellular and mitochondrial membranes and increased central nervous system bioavailability.[573]

NAC helps optimize selenium uptake. Selenate is a potent inhibitor of tau hyper-phosphorylation, associated with formation of neurofibrillary tangles in AD. Other selenium compounds such as selenoprotein P appear to protect amyloid precursor protein from precipitating beta-amyloid due to excessive copper and iron deposition.[574]

Glutathione is a powerful anti-oxidant and assists the liver and other parts of the body, break down and remove toxins. In fact, it is so necessary the body uses 7% of its total energy production, on a daily basis, to ensure it has enough glutathione available. There are numerous glutathione products on the market, but it is a highly unstable compound, and is best supported in its creation by NAC supplementation.

NAC taken on a regular basis increases urinary output of copper. This is either good or bad. Excess copper is problematic to brain inflammation, and Wilson's disease, but small amounts help ensure zinc utilization. A hair analysis can be useful.

SAMe

S-Adenosyl-L-Methionine (SAMe) is a major methyl donor affecting neurotransmitters, epigenetic changes through methylation of DNA, RNA, RNA-binding proteins and histones; and promoting phospholipid methylation.

It shows great promise in pediatric and perinatal depression, major depressive disorders, and Alzheimer's disease.[575]

Two comprehensive reviews of SAMe for depression have been published in the last few years. Both papers consider it efficacious and safe, especially in major depressive disorders and drug treatment-resistant forms.[576] [577]

Catechol-O-Methyl-Transferase (COMT) is one of the main enzymes involved in the breakdown of monoamine (MAO) neurotransmitters including dopamine, norepinephrine and epinephrine. In order for this system to function there must be sufficient amounts of SAMe.

However, if an individual already has high dopamine levels, this will increase. In Parkinson's disease, for example, levels of dopamine are low.

Some individuals possess a particular form of the COMT enzyme (COMT Val[158]Met) making them more paranoid and risk-taking when exposed to high stress levels. This can result in a build up of neurotransmitters leading to anxiety, depression, bipolar disorder and schizophrenia.[578]

If SAMe helps, you may find magnesium, NAC, B complex and D vitamins, useful as well.

People with this genetic variant are more prone to problems of cognition, behavior, emotions, sleep, neurodegeneration and addictive behavior.[579] There may be increased susceptibility to cardiovascular disorders and hormone related cancers.

One example of problems with higher COMT in this genotype is lower dopaminergic signaling in the frontal cortex. The individual may react unusually to stimulants, and have difficulty with sleep-wake regulation, commonly found in Parkinson's disease (PD) and other neurological problems.

This is different than the methylation associated with folic acid/folate covered in Chapter One under B vitamins. This pathway builds up neurotransmitters, and COMT is involved in breaking them down. COMT inhibitors, MAO inhibitors, and dopamine agonists, as well as L-dopa are used in treating PD.

Green tea, quercitin, rutin and luteolin all target COMT and will contribute to worsening of symptoms.

DIM (dimethylglycine) supplements may be useful in those with high estrogen levels that further inhibit COMT and its ability to degrade neurotransmitters.

Both COMT and methylation can be tested, using a simple cheek swab, provided by natural health practitioners and some MDs.

Sunflower seeds are a rich source of SAMe and phenylalanine. The latter helps enhance the effect of opioid-like compounds in mice. SAMe increases the production of serotonin and dopamine and improves binding of neurotransmitters to receptor sites.

SAMe undergoes methylation and during its breakdown releases homocysteine that in presence of B vitamins, especially B6, B12 and methyl folate, re-methylates into methionine, or is converted to glutathione, a powerful anti-oxidant.

The seeds are rich in vitamin D, choline, lecithin and betaine, all of which help reduce homocysteine levels.

Sunflower seeds are rich in phenylalanine that enhances and extends opioid effects, helping with addiction withdrawal. It methylates monoamines, neurotransmitters and phospholipids.

The seeds contain trehalose, a unique sugar also found in medicinal mushrooms and conifer tree sap.

In Huntington's disease, a protein binds to a transcription regulator within cells and the genetic activity is disturbed and the cell's control of protein synthesis breaks down. This leads to glutamate remaining between the neurons, acting as an excitotoxin. The elongated Huntington protein causes the neurons to commit apoptosis, or programmed cell death. Trehalose reduces this polyglutamine aggregation.[580]

The seeds should be organic, unroasted, unsalted and kept refrigerated for optimal benefit.

NOTE. Long term use of SAMe may be problematic in individuals with poor methylation (see vitamins Chapter One). Proper folate (not synthetic folic acid) and riboflavin intake may help prevent the build up of homocysteine.

SAMe is contraindicated in bipolar disorder. A single case of mania was observed in a SSRI patient taking SAMe at the same time.[581]

Twenty-four individuals with AD were given a formulation containing NAC, SAMe, ALC, B12, folate and alpha tocopherol. Participants maintained their baseline cognitive performance and behavioral and psychological symptoms of dementia over twelve months.[582]

DOSE- 400 mg up to three, or four times daily. This can be reduced to 200 mg twice daily once symptoms abate.

SULFORAPHANES and other Crucifer compounds

Adding cruciferous vegetables, such as broccoli, cabbage, brussel sprouts, and particularly sulforaphane to the diet, helps prevent and treat neurological disorders including ASD, PD, AD, epilepsy and schizophrenia.[583,584]

A randomized DB study suggests sulforaphane supplements may be useful in reducing symptoms of ASD.[585]

Broccoli sprouts and its juice increase the secretion of benzene toxins by over 60%. Both sulforaphane and glucoraphanin help pull toxic chemicals from the body. Acrolein is produced when cooking oils are allowed to burn. Broccoli sprout juice increases its removal from our bodies by 23%.[586]

It has been observed that behaviors in a substantial percentage of children tend to improve with the onset of febrile illness. Broccoli sprouts, a rich source of sulforaphane, has metabolic effects that resemble a fever.[587] The induction of fever, that is not suppressed, may help chronic brain inflammation become more acute in nature, and allow for increased immune balance. See Chapter 3.

SEEDS AND NUTS

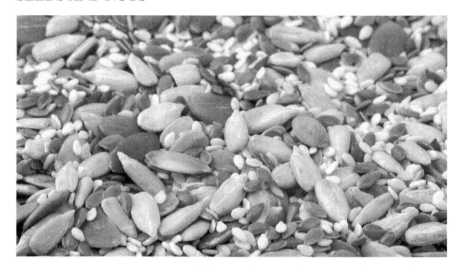

Seeds and nuts are great snack foods for better brain health. They are best raw, organic and refrigerated until eaten. Raw, unroasted nut and seed butters are a preferred source.

The exception may be roasted peanuts that contain more resveratrol than raw form.

Almonds, walnuts and hazelnuts reduce amyloid genesis, tau phosphorylation, oxidative stress and cholinergic pathways in AD prevention and management.[588]

Hazelnuts, in particular, improved memory and anxiety in rats by ameliorating neuro-inflammation and apoptosis caused by amyloid-beta tissue.[589]

Brazil nuts are rich in organic selenium, one nut ranging from 68-91 micrograms of this valuable mineral.

Cashews are only a fair source of selenium, depending upon the levels of the mineral in soil, varying from 11-288% of our recommended daily allowance. They are touted for patients with autoimmune thyroid issues, but some cautions are noted.[590]

Anacardic acid from cashew nuts showed promising neuro-protection against degenerative changes in an experimental model of Parkinson's disease.[591]

Sesame seeds are particularly beneficial in the prevention of dementia. The lignans, sesamin and sesamolin, find their way to blood serum and brain, and show potent beta-secretase inhibition that prevents the build up of beta-amyloid plaque in AD.[592]

Sesame seeds contain pinoresinol, also found in good olive oil. In a mouse study, the compound blocked acetylcholinesterase, and improved memory impairment and synaptic plasticity.[593]

Sesamol attenuated Huntington-like induced behavior in rats. Pre-treatment improved behavorial, biochemical and cellular alterations in 3-nitropropionic, acid-induced neurotoxicity. The authors of the study suggest sesamol may be effective in the management of Huntington's disease.[594]

Black sesame pigment prevents acetylcholinesterase-induced aggregation of beta-amyloid tissue, in a simulated digestion.[595]

It efficiently binds to heavy metals such as lead, cadmium and mercury, without interfering with zinc, calcium and iron uptake.[596]

Sunflower seeds are covered under SAMe above.

BERBERINE

Berberine is a powerful anti-microbial alkaloid present in several important medicinal herbs, including goldenseal, goldthread and Oregon grape root. As an isolated alkaloid, Berberine HCL or Berberine Sulfate, it helps reduce populations of unhealthy bacteria in the microbiome.

TAR DNA binding protein 43 (TDP-43) is involved in RNA metabolism. Hyper-phosphorylated and ubiquitinated TDP-43 deposits are found in the brain and spinal cord of patients with ALS and FTLD. Recent research found berberine is able to reverse the processing of insoluble TDP-43, *in vitro*.[597]

Various species of the above herbs contain tetrahydro-protoberberine and related derivatives. They show affinity at dopamine receptors and may have application in treating cocaine addiction.[598]

Berberine has shown therapeutic effect in epilepsy and Huntington's disease mouse models.[599]

METFORMIN

This low-cost, generic pharmaceutical, improving insulin sensitivity in type 2 diabetes, was originally derived from Goat's Rue (*Galega officinalis*). In the early 20th century, the compound guanidine was isolated and found to lower blood sugar in animals. The herb was traditionally used in herbal medicine as a galactagogue to increase breast milk production in new mothers.

Binding two guanidines together, chemists created a biguanide, which was less toxic. In the late 1950s the French doctor Jean Sterne clinically developed, and gave it the first trade name Glucophage, meaning "glucose eater." The FDA formally approved metformin in 1994, and it became generic in 2002.

It is relatively safe as pharmaceutical drugs go. In some patients, however, it may cause a build up of lactic acid in the muscles.

The control of blood sugar levels in type 2 diabetes is absolutely imperative for maintaining or regaining brain health. Insulin and glucose play a key role in maintaining optimal neuron health.

Diabetes and pre-diabetes now affect 50% of the entire American population.[600]

The drug may help reverse mitochondrial dysfunction in Parkinson's disease.[601]

Metformin helps ameliorate anti-psychotic induced metabolic dysfunction. This group of drugs interacts with dopamine receptors, and in turn, influences our gut microbiota. Metformin influences gut flora and activates AMP-kinase in the hypothalamus suggesting an area for further research.[602]

Twenty non-diabetic patients with mild cognitive impairment or dementia due to AD, were given metformin, or placebo, for eight weeks each, or vice versa. Metformin was associated with improved executive function, and trends suggesting improved learning, memory and attention.[603]

It helped reduce lithium-induced weight gain[604], and in a randomized controlled trial review metformin reduced weight gain in 732 patients taking anti-psychotic medication.[605]

Metformin may provide neuroprotection against methamphetamine induced anxiety, depression and cognitive impairment, albeit based on a rat study.[606]

Even mildly elevated blood sugar is problematic. In those individuals not classified as diabetic, blood glucose levels of 115 mg/dL compared to average of 100 mg/dL, were 18% more at risk of developing dementia.

Metformin prevents vitamin B 12 production and absorption. Supplementing this important vitamin is imperative for type 2 diabetics.

VITAMIN DERIVATIVES

Vitamins A to E have been covered in Chapter One.

Nicotinamide adenine dinucleotide (NADH) is the active coenzyme form of B3 (niacin or niacinamide).

It provides energy to the brain, nerves and muscles. One molecule of NADH creates three molecules of ATP.[607]

NADH is transported across the plasma membranes of astrocytes, and NAD^+ markedly decreases ischemic brain injury.[608]

Sirtuins are a class of NAD^+ dependent deacylases associated with brain aging and dysfunction.[609] They deacetylate histone and non-histone targets, and play a role in modulation of anti-oxidants and oxidative stress. Sirtuin 1 regulates cell metabolism and plays a role in forebrain neurons associated with depression.

The NAD^+ precursor nicotinamide mononucleotide (NMN) alleviated mouse models of the neurological and mitochondrial disease known as Leigh syndrome.[610] Mitochondria in neurons become less fragmented against reactive oxygen species.

Both niacinamide and NMN activate sirtuins, and hence provide neuron protection.

MINERALS

MAGNESIUM

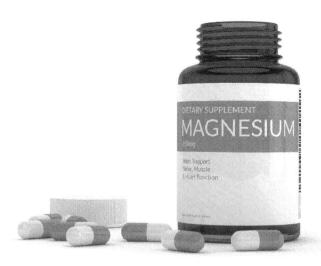

Magnesium is mentioned time and again when it comes to mineral deficiency, in our modern diet. There is also a great deal of controversy surrounding our ability to assimilate, and utilize this important mineral.

Magnesium is involved in over 600 enzymatic reactions in our body, including the manufacture of neurotransmitters, energy production and cardiovascular health.

Without adequate magnesium, we cannot convert tyrosine into dopamine, noradrenaline and adrenaline. In Canada around 40% of young people are not getting enough, and in people over 70 years old, more than 70% do not meet minimum daily requirements.

Everyone, of course, is familiar with Epsom salts (Magnesium sulfate), and their relaxing effect on muscles and nerves. Magnesium will actually absorb into the muscle tissue when cellular deficiencies are noted. Float tanks are a personal favorite relaxation, helping my mind to turn off, similar to meditation. The magnesium sulfate helps me let go of muscle tension and I twist and turn to give myself a spinal adjustment.

But eating more magnesium rich foods, or supplementing with magnesium oxide powders will not function at the blood-brain barrier.[611]

My favorite magnesium for brain health is a form called magnesium L-threonate (MgT). This combination was discovered through research, less than a decade ago, at the Massachusetts Institute of Technology.[612] They found typical magnesium compounds do not reach the brain. Studies showed raising human blood magnesium levels by 300% only changed levels by less than 19% in our cerebrospinal fluid.[613]

MgT absorbs rapidly and helps to reverse aspects of brain aging. One DB, PC human trial found benefits in adults with cognitive dysfunction, insomnia and anxiety.[614] After twelve weeks significant red blood cell concentration and urinary excretion was found in the MgT group. Visual attention, and task switching showed significant improvement. And it reversed clinical measures of brain aging.

Magnesium chloride was found effective for mild to moderate depression in a randomized, crossover six-week trial of 126 adults.[615]

Magnesium helps increase synaptic density for more efficient cognitive processing, and plasticity associated with connections from new stimuli.

Animal studies demonstrate MgT reduces fear-related memories, and may be helpful in post-traumatic stress disorder (PTSD).[616]

Magnesium phosphorica is one of the 12 cell salts, or 6X homeopathic remedies developed by Dr. Schuessler. It quickly relieves cramps and muscle tension, due to its rapid absorption.

On the other hand, phosphoric acid in sodas impairs absorption of magnesium.

Drug-induced nutrient depletion in seniors is common, with over two-thirds of seniors taking at least five pharmaceuticals at the same time. Polypharmacy, including antacids, acid blockers, antibiotics, anti-hypertensives and cardiac glycosides can severely affect blood magnesium levels. Oxalic acid and tannins in food and drink can bind to magnesium ions.

So too can healthy, high fiber foods such as chia and hemp seeds. Take supplements apart. Magnesium and B complex go well together, in a synergistic manner.

ZINC

Zinc deficiency is linked to depression, learning disabilities, autism, ADD/ADHD, cognitive dysfunction, Parkinson's, delinquent behavior and eating disorders.

It is estimated a fully two billion people worldwide are deficient in zinc. And yet, it is part of over 300 different proteins.

Stress can create great loss of zinc, due to excess excretion.

Animal protein is rich in zinc, but many grains, legumes and beans, especially soy, contain phytic acid that prevents full utilization of this valuable mineral.

A rare, genetic condition pyroluria affects zinc levels, but more commonly, a deficiency is associated with low stomach acid, chronic stress and infection, as well as eating disorders. Lack of zinc affects taste buds, making foods unpalatable.

While in clinical practice I would conduct a zinc tally test, which involves a zinc sulphate solution. This is more bio-available, along with zinc-rich foods. It is best taken aside from other supplements. Start with one teaspoon for children, two with adults.

If there is no taste, there is a zinc deficiency. If there is a slight taste but its mild, there is likely a moderate deficiency. But, a strong, offensive metallic taste indicates zinc levels are already sufficient.

Parkinson's patients suffer vision problems, as well as olfactory and taste loss, related to zinc deficiency.[617]

Zinc tablets or capsules, are poorly absorbed, by patients most deficient, and many contain excess copper to be avoided by those suffering brain health.

When zinc is deficient, the heavy, toxic minerals cadmium and mercury replace zinc at receptor sites.

The proper zinc/copper ration should be between 8:1 and 12:1 for optimal neurological health. Excess copper creates toxicity that aggravates ADD/ADHD, Parkinson's, cognitive function and is related to criminal behavior.

Zinc helps transport vitamin A to the liver, and impacts the skin and epithelial tissue of mucus membranes.

Zinc deficiency reduces insulin signaling, synthesis, storage and release, affecting diabetes and AD.

Ionic zinc is useful in severe deficiencies, including pyroluria. This little-known genetic condition affects 11% of people, who produce excess amounts of a byproduct from hemoglobin synthesis called hydroxyhemoppyrrolin-2-one. When elevated, this waste product binds to zinc and B6, leading to severe deficiencies. Elevated kryptopyrroles, found in urine, can help detect this condition. Problems associated with this condition include depression (30%), autism (50%), anxiety, ADD/ADHD (30%) Tourette syndrome, bipolar disorders, alcoholism (40%), and schizophrenia (70%).

Did I mention it affects 11% of people? Pyroluria should be more widely tested in those suffering brain health.

Supplementation of zinc, B6 and GLA (evening primrose or borage oil) and diets higher in arachidonic acid and omega-6 fatty acids can help. Omega-3 fatty acids are generally not well tolerated.[618]

Zinc attached to citrate, picolinate, chelates, gluconates and bisglycinates are best absorbed. 20-30 mg daily is recommended, unless otherwise noted. Children under ten years of age can take half dosage. It is best absorbed on an empty stomach but may cause upset or nausea. Try to take separately from B vitamins, phosphorylated supplements and iron.

HEAVY METAL DETOX

DMSA (Dimercaptosuccinic acid) is a sulphur-based, water-soluble, non-toxic compound that helps chelate and remove heavy metals from the brain. This is a major problem in cases of Parkinson's disease, epilepsy and dementia.

Cadmium, lead, mercury and arsenic poisonings of an acute nature are rare, but are generally accumulative, and chronic over time. DMSA has been used since the 1950s for helping promote urinary excretion. DMSA has considerably lower toxicity compared to other metal chelators, including calcium EDTA. If used, several intermittent courses are advised, along with professional supervision.

A 54-year old patient with early onset dementia, epilepsy and peripheral polyneuropathy was diagnosed with mercury intoxication, due to the daily use of a skin lightening cream for six years. Treatment with DMSA resulted in blood and urine mercury levels falling, and memory function improvement.[619]

CHAPTER 16

MEDICINAL HERBS

I have practiced herbal medicine for nearly fifty years. I love plant medicine and I have been witness to its healing powers.

Phytomedicines have multiple uses, but this chapter will largely be restricted to their influence on the brain neurotransmitters, serotonin, dopamine, acetylcholine and GABA.

For proper assessment and dosage, it would be best to work with a natural health practitioner, especially a trained herbalist. *The American Herbalist Guild* lists qualified herbalists, and their contact information, in different bioregions of North America. Cautions and contraindications of the herbs are noted, but individual sensitivities can occur with any substance.

As an herbalist I like to work with fresh and dried plant tinctures or standardized extracts. All doses suggested below are based on 150-pound adults. For children divide their weight into 150 and reduce the dosage to that amount. For example, a 75-pound child would take one-half the recommended dose. A hundred pound individual would start with two-thirds the suggested dosage.

All herbs have possible interactions with numerous pharmaceuticals. Avoid grapefruit juice with many of these herbs.

For those readers who prefer water infusions or decoctions, or need to avoid alcohol, there are plenty of sites on the internet to help with preparation and dosage. Capsules can also be effective if prepared from quality product.

I do not recommend home use of herbs for children under two years of age.

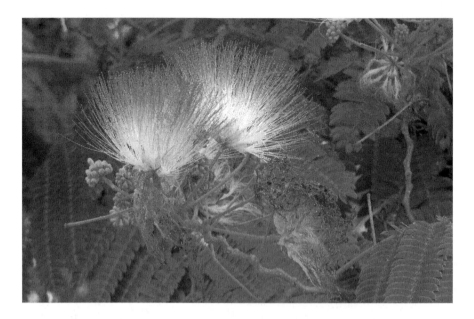

Albizia (*Albizia julibrissin*), the Tree of Happiness, is found in temperate part of the United States as well as its native bio-regions in China, Korea and Japan.

In Mandarin, the flowers are known as HUAN HUA, and the bark HE HUAN PI. In Cantonese, the flower is HAP FUN FA, the bark HAP FUN PEI. They are known as the Happiness Herb and Collective Happiness Bark, respectively.

The medicinal benefit was first recorded in the 2nd century A.D. in the book, *Shen Nong Ben Cao*, as a calmative and mood tonic, for those suffering loss of a loved one, or a similar calamity.

According to noted herbalist Michael Tierra, "the bark is thought to 'anchor' the spirit, while the flowers 'lighten' it." He writes. "As well as giving albizia to many patients suffering from acute and chronic depression and anxiety, I've also given it to those who complain of high stress, with noticed marked improvement even after a single day of use...Albizia is a good choice for probably greater than 50% of those who are presently taking a pharmaceutical drug. At a mere fraction of the price, albizia is devoid of the adverse side effects of the drugs and can be easily stopped at anytime."

Early work on mice brains with water extracts of albizia suggest the anti-anxiety effect is mediated by changes in serotonergic, especially 5-HT1A receptors.[620]

More recent lab work found a compound from flowers reduced anxiety via influence on brain neurotransmitters.[621]

David Winston writes. "I have patients who have had significant recoveries from post traumatic stress disorder, long-term unresolved grief, depression and fear."[622]

An unusual chicken study found albizia protected brain mitochondria against copper sulfate, due to anti-oxidant, or direct free radical scavenging, that prevented lipid and protein alteration.[623] Copper toxicity is problematic in some conditions of brain health, especially Wilson's disease.

Dose- up to 3-5 ml daily in divided doses of 1:5 tincture prepared from flowers and/or bark.

CAUTION- Do not use concurrently with any of MAOs, SSRIs or tricyclic anti-depressants, or during pregnancy.

Ashwagandha root (*Withania somnifera*) comes to us from the Ayurvedic system of India, where it is sometimes referred to as Indian Ginseng.

Ashwagandha is a small, evergreen member of the Solanaceae family. In Sanskrit the name means "odor of the horse", due to sweaty horse odor of fresh root. This is suggestive of the sexual potency of a stallion, and thus its use for treating infertility, and impotence.

Somnifera is derived from the Latin meaning "sleep-inducer", due to its use in relieving stress and insomnia.

The root has been used for over three millennia to help restore energy, strength, memory, and counteract stress on the mind and body. It helps to calm the mind and promote inner peace and tranquility.

A mouse trial suggests the herb may be useful in ALS (amyotrophic lateral sclerosis), associated with misfolded superoxide dismutase.

When given the extract, there was reduced glial activation and phosphorylation of nuclear factor kappa B.[624]

A randomized, double-blind, placebo-controlled trial of 66 patients with schizophrenia, showed significantly greater reductions in Positive and Negative Syndrome Scale, negative, general and total symptoms. The Perceived Stress Scale was significantly improved compared to placebo. All patients remained on anti-psychotic medication, suggesting an adjuvant benefit with minimal side effects.[625]

A randomized, placebo-controlled trial of 53 patients with bipolar disorder (BD) involved ashwagandha root extract. Those taking the herb showed significant benefit in three cognitive tasks, suggesting improvement in auditory-verbal working memory, compared to placebo.[626]

A study on epileptic rat brain showed the herb, and the active withanolide A, significantly reversed the altered muscarinic receptor expression, and reversed the oxidative stress and resultant derailment in cell signaling, in temporal lobe epilepsy.[627]

Ashwagandha was one of ten herb herbs identified in a published systematic review of GABA modulating phytomedicines. The others were kava kava, valerian, hops, chamomile, *Ginkgo biloba*, passionflower, scullcap and lemon balm.[628]

The herb combines well with blue vervain and scullcap for nervous tics, restless leg syndrome, mild Tourette syndrome and tardive dyskinesia associated with Parkinson's disease medications.

Withonone, isolated from the root, was administered to wistar rats for 21 days. Significant improvements in cognitive skill was noted, by inhibiting amyloid beta-42 and reversing the decline of acetylcholine and glutathione. Elevated levels of pro-inflammatory cytokines were attenuated. This suggests ashwagandha root, or withonone, may be useful in Alzheimer's disease due to the various mechanisms of action.[629]

A prospective, randomized, double-blind, placebo-controlled study was conducted on 50 adults. After eight weeks, the treatment group demonstrated significant improvements compared to placebo in both immediate and general memory, executive function, sustained attention and processing speed.[630]

Most of the studies have been conducted on the root, but the leaves also show differentiation of neuroblastoma and glioma cells, as well as potential for preventing and treating AD and PD.[631]

The herb lengthens the analgesic efficacy of opioids in chronic therapy.[632]

The leaf extract (which contains withanolides) restored levels of brain-derived neurotrophic factor (BDNF), and increased synaptic plasticity.[633] The leaf is widely used to adulterate root products, so manufacturers and consumers should be aware.

The root is rich in organic iron and may be useful for anemia.

DOSE- standardized extract- 250-500 mg twice daily. Tincture 1:5 2-4 ml three times daily.

CAUTION- do not use in cases of hyperthyroidism, hemochromatosis, or if there is any sensitivity to the Nightshade family. Avoid during pregnancy.

Bacopa or Brahmi (*Bacopa monniera*) is a memory enhancer from the Ayurvedic tradition of India. The plant is known by several common names including Thyme-leaved Gratiola, Bamb, Lonika, and Shvet Chamni. It has become naturalized in Florida.

Bacopa is widely used in Ayurvedic medicine for epilepsy, memory loss, anxiety, poor cognition, loss of concentration and inflammation.

The herb is used in Traditional Chinese Medicine, and known as PA CHI T'IEN.

Bacopa is used for "relaxed smartness", with a more even and consistent mood conducive to learning, and helping increase the expression of ideas and feelings. In fact, it is recommended by numerous herbalists to treat attention deficit disorder (ADD) and ADHD, combining well with green oats and holy basil.

Nine studies confirm an 11.2 to 17.9 percent improvement in cognition, and 9-12 percent faster reaction time, in subjects consuming the herb.[634]

According to scientists with the *Central Drug Research Institute* in India, bacosides help repair damaged neurons by adding muscle to kinase, the protein involved in the synthesis of new neurons. Depleted synaptic activity is thus restored, leading to increased memory capacity. Triterpenoid saponins and their bacosides are believed responsible for enhancing nerve impulse transmission. The latter aids in repairing damaged neurons and restoring synaptic activity.

One study found the herb reduces inflammatory pathways in the brain, by inhibiting the release of cytokines from microglial cells.[635]

Both bacoside A and bacopaside I protect neuroreceptors in the brain and liver, suppress lipid peroxidation and activate anti-oxidant enzymes.[636]

Bacopa may work by improving mitochondrial function and alleviating oxidative stress; suggesting its possible benefit in Parkinson's disease (PD).[637]

The herb has been found in several randomized BD, PC trials of benefit in dementia, PD and epilepsy. It inhibits acetyl-cholinesterase, reduces beta-amyloid plaquing, and improves neurotransmitter modulation of acetylcholine, 5-hydroxy-tryptamine (5-HP) and dopamine.[638]

Bacopa and Velvet Bean (*Mucuna pruriens*) were tested on Parkinsonian mice, and found to significantly decrease oxidative stress. Bacopa showed more improvement in factors influencing the substantia nigra region of brain.[639]

Twenty-four volunteers involved an acute, double-blind, placebo-controlled crossover were given either 320 mg or 620 mg of bacopa. The lower daily dose improved cognitive performance.[640]

A study of 54 elderly participants (mean of 73.5 years) involved 300 mg of the herb or placebo.

The Bacopa group showed improved cognition and reduced anxiety and depression, suggesting benefit for the elderly.[641]

The herb relieves the brain fog associated with the epileptic drug Dilantin. Animal studies suggest it reduces hepatotoxicity and neurotoxicity associated with morphine.

DOSE: Look for a product standardized to 20% bacosides A & bacopaside I. Synapsa, a standardized, concentrated product is recommended at 250 to 500 mg daily. Clinical trials show improved memory in aging brains, both healthy and those at risk for AD.[642]

For 55% bacosides, the standard dose is 300 mg daily. Tincture is 1.5-2.5 ml of 1:5 preparation 3-4 times daily.

The herb is best taken with a meal that contains healthy fats.

CAUTION- In animal studies, it stimulates T4 activity and may cause elevated thyroid hormone levels. Caution is advised if patients are taking thyroxin, or thyroid suppressing drugs. In this study the T3 levels were not stimulated, but mouse dosage was very high.

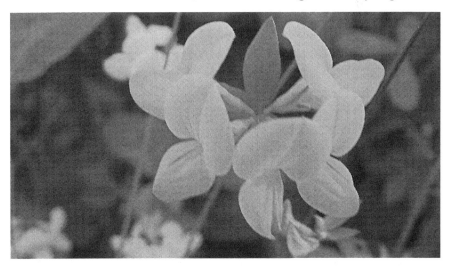

Bird's Foot Trefoil (*Lotus corniculatus*) is grown as pasture herbage, and one of the few fodder plants to contain condensed tannin (CT). One bonus of a patch of bird's foot trefoil in your pasture, is the control of internal parasites in livestock.

Lotus is from the Greek LOTOS, referring to several legumes. Corniculatus means, "with small horns", and refers to the appearance of small seedpods.

The Lotus-eaters of mythology ate fruit from a shrub that inspired happy indolence. Bird's foot refers to the slender seedpods appearance, while trefoil alludes to a similarity with red clover, also known as trefoil.

The French herbalist, Henri Leclerc first discovered, and reported the medicinal properties of this herb. He recommended using an eyewash of sweet clover, to treat an attack of pink eye in a woman suffering from insomnia and heart palpitations.

By mistake, the distraught patient made a tea of the aerial parts of bird's foot trefoil, drank it, and discovered her nervous troubles disappeared within the week!

This plant contains constituents similar in nature to those found in passionflower, but more research is required.

Further study is required, but it appears that the sedative, anti-anxiety, anti-spasmodic and tranquilizing properties may be similar. The plant is considered by some to have exhilarating properties; and useful in cases of neuro-vegetative dystonia, anguish and depression.

The plant is a central nervous system sedative, for treating tachycardia, anxiety, depression and insomnia. It appears to support the parasympathetic nervous system, helping balance the dominant sympathetic influence associated with stress and competition in our society.

The herb helps inhibit nitric oxide and interleukin 17, suggesting benefit in reducing inflammation, and inhibits both adenosine deaminase and myeloperoxidase.

Reduced adenosine deaminase activity prevents the release of excitatory amino acids. It is interesting to note a deficiency of adenosine deaminase; one factor associated with inborn errors of metabolism associated with autism.[643]

Bird's foot trefoil inhibits myeloperoxidase and its cytotoxic product hypochlorous acid associated with a number of neurodegenerative diseases including Alzheimer's disease, Parkinson's disease, ALS, MS, and epilepsy.[644]

DOSE- 1-3 ml twice daily of a 1:5 fresh aerial parts tincture.

Blueberries

Blueberry (*Vaccinium*) fruit is rich in flavonoids that possess anti-oxidant and anti-inflammatory properties.

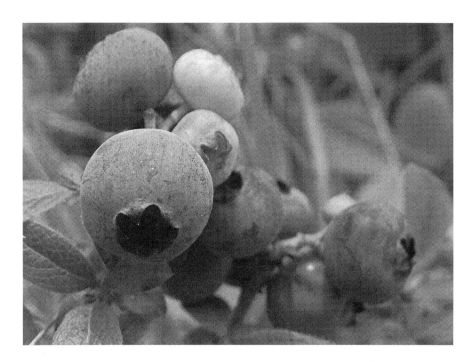

A twelve-week study of 12 adults (mean age of 67-68) who consumed 30 ml of blueberry extract or isoenergetic placebo, found significant increases in brain activity from the former. Evidence of increased working memory was noted.[645]

A randomized DB, PC trial examined older adults with mild cognitive impairment. After 16 weeks of blueberry supplementation, there was enhanced neural response in working memory.[646]

Young children can benefit from wild blueberry drink. In a study of 54 children, aged 7-10, executive function, short-term memory improved just two to six hours later.[647]

A study on blueberry extract and lithium for possible synergistic benefit in bipolar disorder, found no such effect, but both showed neuroprotection.[648]

Pterostilbene found in blueberries, may be effective in preventing or treating Alzheimer's disease. It attenuated the neuroinflammation induced by beta-amyloid by inhibiting the NLRP3/ caspase-1 inflammasome pathway.[649]

255

Bilberry (*V. myrtillus*) may enhance hyaluronic acid and glycosaminoglycan expression.[650]

DOSE- 1-2 capsules daily of 1:60 fruit extract.

Canby's Lovage (*Ligusticum canbyi*) is a close relative of Osha root (*L. porteri*).

Lovage derives from love-ache, meaning love parsley, in an early translation from the Old French to Middle English. Ligusticum is from the Greek for a related plant mentioned by Dioscorides. Perhaps, obscurely, it derives from Liguria, Italy, where a medicinal Lovage was first described.

Canbyi is named for William Canby, a 19th century businessman from Delaware, who enjoyed adding new plants to his extensive herbarium collection.

Canby's Lovage has not yet been found, to my knowledge, on the eastern side of the continental divide in Canada.

It is common west of the divide in British Columbia, Montana, and Idaho at higher elevations. At least that is where I find it.

The concentration of serotonin (5HTP) is significantly greater in the leaf than root. More melatonin is found in the root tissue of Osha than Canby's lovage, but similar amounts are found in the shoots of both.

The concentration of E-3-butylidenephthalide is higher in leaves. Z-ligustilide is found in both shoots and roots.

A number of compounds including Z-ligustilide, Z-butyliddenephthalide, senkyunolide and others exhibit affinity for serotonin (5-HT) receptors. [651]

Ferulic acid is highest in stems. An excellent identification of compounds by Christina Turi and Susan Murch was conducted in Kelowna, at the University of British Columbia, Okanagan campus.[652]

Z-ligustilide may reduce ischemia/reperfusion-induced increase in brain iron by regulating the expression of iron transport proteins.[653] This should be examined for possible PD support.

Both Z-ligustilide and senkyunolide I have a protective effect on PC 12 cells, suggestive of neuron protection.[654]

The latter compound may be useful in migraines, by adjusting the levels of MAO neurotransmitters and their turnover rate, as well as decreasing nitric oxide levels in the blood and brain.[655]

DOSE- 20-40 drops several times daily of 1:5 dried root tincture.

CAUTION- Do not ingest during pregnancy, as it may cause miscarriage.

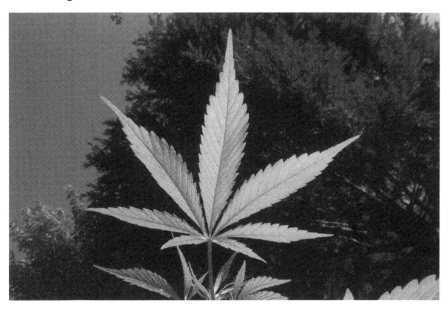

Cannabis (*C. sativa/C. indica*)

Cannabis has been used both medicinally and recreationally for thousands of years. The active compound THC is responsible for the "high" associated with smoking or ingesting the mature plant flower buds.

Cannabis use in Parkinson's and multiple sclerosis shows positive impact on mood, memory, fatigue and obesity in people suffering these conditions.[656]

For medicinal purposes, the cannabidiols (CBD) have garnered far more interest.

Cannabinoid 1 receptors and ligands have been found in our brain and immune system. CB2 receptors and ligands are mainly in the body periphery and especially in immune cells. Cannabinoids modulate a variety of immune cell functions in humans, including T helper cell development, chemotaxis and preventing tumor development. In fact, it appears the immunocannabinoid system is involved in regulating the brain-immune axis and might be exploited in future therapies for treating chronic disease and immune deficiency.[657]

Cannabinoids are common in animal nervous systems. Anandamide, our body's own neurotransmitter binds to the same receptors sites in the brain. It is responsible for pleasurable and euphoric sensations, and recently found, as well, in cocoa beans and red wine. Anandamine is from the Sanskrit ANANDA meaning, "bliss."

Drugs that boost endocannabinoid activity, and inhibit their breakdown, may be useful in epilepsy, which occurs when neurons fire excessively; or in degenerative diseases such as Alzheimer's and Parkinson's disease, where excito-toxicity or lack of neuron firing plays a causative role. Families seeking help for children suffering from up to 300 daily seizures moved to Colorado so they could legally use extracted CBD oils, showing real benefit. Severe refractory epilepsy in children is significantly reduced by cannabinoid products.[658]

Cannabidiol products for pediatric epilepsy were subjected to a systematic review, with significant reductions in frequency of monthly seizures, suggesting benefit in drug-resistant epilepsy.[659]

The FDA approved drug, Epidiolex, which is just CBD oil, shows efficacy in both Dravet and Lennon Gastaut syndrome, and reduced seizures, after 4-6 other drugs proved ineffective.

Astrocyte activity in the brain is linked to pro-inflammatory function in Alzheimer-like, multiple sclerosis-like, epileptic and schizophrenic models. CBD has been shown to decrease inflammation, suggesting neuroprotection.[660]

Dystonia is a painful condition of painful muscle rigidity, causing spasms in various neurological disorders, including Parkinson's disease and stroke. In one study, five patients experienced 20-50% improvement of their severe dystonia.

Chorea is another neurological condition characterized by rapid, jerky, involuntary movements.

Cerebral palsy, Sydenham's chorea and Huntington's disease are other examples of conditions responsive to CBD.

Various cannabinoids, terpenes and flavonoids in cannabis show benefit in the treatment of migraine, headaches and potential in assisting opioid detoxification.[661]

Cannabinoids possess noradrenergic, serotoninergic, glutamatergic, neurotransmission, neuroprotective activity; and modulate the hypothalamic-pituitary adrenal axis (HPAA).[662]

Tourette syndrome (TS) is a lifelong neurological condition from childhood with repetitive grimaces and facial tics that progresses to involuntary barks, and outbursts of foul language.

In one study of 3 TS patients, partially helped by conventional anti-psychotic drugs, there was significant improvement after smoking cannabis.

Cannabidiols enhance the passage of lipid nanocapsules across the BBB both *in vitro* and *in vivo*.[663]

CAUTION- There is scientific evidence linking schizophrenic genetics and early exposure to cannabis, which may lead to psychiatric disorders in adolescence.[664]

DOSE- Start with 2.5 mg up to 10 mg CBD oil daily and go from there. Wait four hours to see how it affects you.

Chamomile, German (*Matricaria chamomilla*) is the most well-known and used herbal beverage around the world, with some sixty million cups consumed daily.

Matricaria is from the Latin MATRIX meaning womb and CARIA, for dear. The Romans called cowrie shells MATRICULUS, meaning, little womb or little matrix. These seashells were considered charms associated with fertility, rebirth and healing. Chamomile is from the Greek CHAMAI, on the ground, and MELON, meaning apple.

Apigenin, a major constituent, binds to the benzodiazepine receptors.

A two phase, eight-week open label trial of 179 subjects looked at chamomile for the treatment of moderate to severe anxiety. Significant improvement was noted.[665]

An earlier study of 57 participants found chamomile may provide relief in anxiety and depression. Nineteen had anxiety with comorbid depression, 16 suffered anxiety with past history of depression, and 22 suffered anxiety.[666]

German chamomile inhibits glutamic acid decarboxylase, suggesting it should not be used with autistic subjects. See chapter on GABA.

On the other hand, the herb may be useful for postpartum women suffering depression and sleep problems.[667]

An unique German chamomile extract has been developed by Dr. Kevin Morin in Edmonton, Alberta, Canada. Standardized to 1.2% apigenin, and derived from the flowers, the product modulates GABA-A receptors and may be useful for generalized anxiety disorders.[668]

DOSE- Tincture- 10 to 30 drops three times daily, or 60 drops before bed. Prepare fresh flower tincture at 1:4 and 40% alcohol.

Capsules mentioned above, one to two up to twice daily.

An infused cup or three of tea works well for young children and adults. One tea bag is used for each eight ounces of hot water. Steep for 30 minutes. Allow to cool. Enjoy.

CAUTION- Herbs from the Asteraceae family may cause allergic reaction, especially if you are sensitive to ragweed pollen.

Cinnamon bark (*Cinnamomum zeylandicum*) is anti-microbial, helps lower blood sugar, blood pressure and serum cholesterol, possesses anti-oxidant, free-radical scavenging, and inhibits tau aggregation and filament formation associated with Alzheimer's disease.[669]

Cinnamon efficiently inhibits tau accumulations, amyloid-beta aggregation and toxicity in both *in vitro* and *in vivo* models. It possesses neuroprotective effects, modulates endothelial functions and may induce AD epigenetic modification.[670]

Cinnamon extract improves insulin action in the brain, as well as activity and locomotion, and lowers liver fat in a mouse model of obesity.[671]

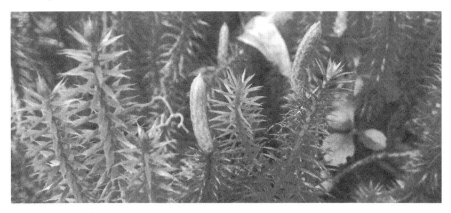

Clubmoss (*Huperzia serrata*) is known as CHIEN TSENG TA, or SHUANG YI PING in Traditional Chinese Medicine. The aerial parts contain huperzine A, which is three times more potent than phytostigmine, as an acetylcholinesterase (AChE) inhibitor.

Other names include QIAN CENG TA, meaning "thousand layered pagoda", and JIN BU HUAN, "more valuable than gold".

Huperzine A is also found in the North American *Huperzia selago* clubmoss.

In one double-blind, randomized study, huperzine A was tested in 56 patients with senile dementia and 104 patients with senile and pre-senile simple memory disorders. The injectable form showed the most significant positive effects.

A study of 50 AD patients showed significant improvement in 58%, in a multi-centre, randomized, double-blind, placebo-controlled study.

A placebo-controlled, double-blind study of 160 Alzheimer's patients found huperzine A significantly superior to either placebo, tacrine or physostigmine, a cholinesterase inhibitor, with longer lasting activity than the two drugs.

Twenty randomized, clinical trials involving 1823 participants, found huperzine A recorded significant benefit in cognitive function at 8, 12 and 16 weeks.[672]

It reduces glutamate excitotoxicity by acting as NMDA receptor antagonist.[673]

Huperzine A works on acetylcholine, only in the brain, giving it a vast advantage over cholinesterase inhibitor drugs developed for AD. It is non-toxic at up to 100 times the human therapeutic dosage, and antidotes atropine.

Alzheimer's patients are prone to seizures, with more than 20% of patients having a least one seizure, and up to 7% having recurring episodes. Many anti-epileptic drugs worsen cognitive function, whereas huperzine A exhibits anti-convulsant properties.[674]

It is not only an acetylcholinesterase (AChE) inhibitor, but protects from excitotoxicity and neuronal death via GABAergic transmission associated with anti-convulsant activity.[675]

Huperzine A, when compared to tacrine, donepezil and rivastigmine, shows better penetration of the blood brain barrier (BBB), higher oral bioavailability, and longer AChE inhibition.

Huperzine A is today, commonly produced by *Paecilomyces tenuis*, an endophytic fungus isolated from *H. serrata*.

DOSE- 50-200 mcg twice daily for AD. 50 mcg daily for cases of senile dementia.

COW ITCH
COWHAGE
VELVET BEAN (*Mucuna pruriens*)

Mucuna was a name used by Marggraf in the 1650s for a Brazilian species, derived from the Tupi word MUCUMAN. Cowhage or Cowage is derived from KAWANCH or KOANCH, two Hindustani words. The name has nothing to do with itchy cows.

The young pods are eaten as a vegetable in India and China, where they are known as T'AO HUNG KING.

In Sanskrit, the plant was known as ATMAGUPTA. It has been used to treat symptoms similar to Parkinson's disease for over 4500 years, when it was known as KAMPA VATA. James Parkinson re-described the condition, in 1817.

Mucuna pruriens seeds contain L-dopa (3, 4 dihydroxy-phenylalanine), various amines such as 5-hydroxy-tryptamine (serotonin), N, N-dimethyl-tryptamine, bufotenine, bufotenidine, a 5-oxindole-3-alkylamine derivative, DMT, DMT-N-oxide, N,N-DMT, 5-MeO-DMT, two beta carbolines, various amino acids, globulins, albumins and the alkaloids mucunadine, mucunine, prurienine, prurieninine, prurienidine, mucunadine, and mucuadinine; as well as mucuanain, a proteolytic enzyme, cytisine, tyrosine and nicotine.

Mucuna contains natural dopamine that shows a protective benefit in Parkinson's disease. In one study, the dopamine content was separated and the bean still showed effect on the disease, suggesting that more than dopamine derivatives are at work. It may well be that unidentified compounds enhance L-dopa efficacy, or other anti-Parkinson compounds, are present.

L-dopa is the naturally occurring form of the amino acid 3,4 dihydroxy-phenylalanine, a precursor to norepinephrine and epinephrine, and melanin, a pigment in the hair, skin and substantia nigra of the brain. It is classified as a natural product in Sweden.

A randomized, double-blind, controlled trial with eight Parkinson's disease patients found 30 gram preparations led to "considerably faster onset of effect", in comparison to standard L-dopa/carbidopa pharmaceuticals, concluding "this natural source of L-dopa might possess advantages over conventional L-dopa preparations in the long-term management of PD".[676]

A recent DB, randomized, controlled crossover study of eighteen patients found roasted bean powder produced similar effects as levodopa/benserazide, with more favorable tolerability. This suggested an alternative for those individuals with Parkinson's disease who cannot afford long-term prescription levodopa.[677]

Velvet bean modulates the immune system including TNF-alpha, IL-6, IL-1beta, iNOS, IL-2, and NFkappaB that plays a role in the inflammation and progression of PD.[678]

DOSE- 350 mg two to four times daily of standardized 15% capsuled product.

Elderflower (*Sambucus caerulea*) has been used in Lumbee traditional medicine and was investigated for the benefit in prevention or treatment of PD. An extract appears to suppress neurotoxicity elicited by environmental and genetic PD-related brain insults.[679]

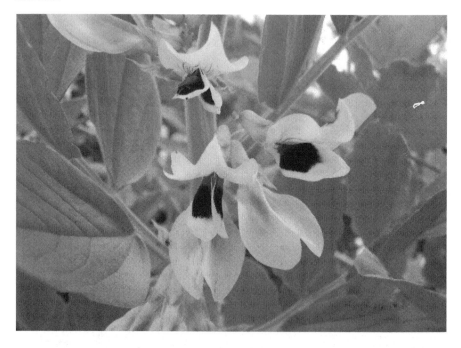

Faba Bean (*Vicia faba*) is also known as fava bean, broad bean, horse bean and Windsor bean.

Vicia is from the Latin VINCIO, to bind. Vetch is thought to be a corruption derived from the same root. Fava is an English corruption of the Latin faba meaning, "bean."

Faba beans were in cultivation for over 6,000 years before *Phaseolus* beans reached the Old World. They spread to China several thousand years later, and then were moved on to Japan and India.

Faba beans contain natural L-dopa (levo-dihydroxy phenylalanine) that penetrates the intestinal epithelial cells and is transported through the blood stream to the brain capillaries, where it is converted into dopamine.

The beans also contain Carbidopa (C-dopa), a peripheral decarboxylase inhibitor. This compound cannot cross the blood-brain barrier, but allow more L-dopa to cross into the brain. The beans should be eaten not fully mature, but when young, with a thin skin and easier to digest. Up to 90% of patients afflicted with Parkinson's disease (PD) at an early age respond quickly. Fresh leaves contain the highest L-dopa content ($22.4 \ mg/g^{-1}$).

It is easily oxidized two to three days after harvest and vanishes completely as the plant stops growing and begins to dry.

When sprouted, the L-dopa content increases ten times (10x), and is worth investigating as a potential commercial product.

The commercial product AtreMorine, has been studied in experimental models of PD.

In one study, it modulated the expression levels of tyrosine hydroxylase, glial proteins, apoptosis and endogenous dopamine and neuromelanin concentration, helping the basal ganglia recover.[680]

AtreMorine has a neuroprotective effect on dopaminergic neurons of the substantia nigra, helping improve the life quality of PD patients.[681]

While in clinical practice I worked with DopaBean, an extracted, capsule, natural health product, still available on the market.

DOSE- 15% L-dopa capsule product (Solaray) as directed.

NOTE- Favism is a hemolytic anemia disease occurring in individuals suffering from a blood enzyme deficiency, glucose-6-phosphate de-hydrogenase (G6PD), which can be fatal in infants. The deficiency occurs almost exclusively in populations living around the Mediterranean, but today affects about 400 million people worldwide, including Southeast Asia.

The condition is believed caused by the presence of faba beans, especially green pods and seeds, of two glycosidic pyrimidine derivatives, vicine and convicine, and/or their hydrolytic products (aglycones) divicine and isouramil. Some sensitive individuals will react to the pollen. Jaundice is one striking symptom that is more obvious.

The genetic coding is believed a trade off for malaria resistance, as this condition produces red blood cells that starve the malaria parasite of oxygen. Or, more accurately, G6PD deficient red blood cells contain too little of a metabolite essential for survival of the parasite.

Ironically, all known anti-malarial drugs are contraindicated for these susceptible individuals.

The gene for G6PD enzyme is carried on the X chromosome, so males are more likely to be afflicted. For a female to suffer the condition, genes on both of her X chromosomes would have to be affected.

Excessive levels of dopamine may lead to priapism, or painful, long-lasting erections.

Fig Marigold (*Sceletium tortuosum*) is native to southern Africa, but you can easily grow it in your rock garden.

The fermented plant is known as Kanna, or Channa, in its native country. The root was prized by the Hottentots as a narcotic, or cocaine-like stimulant, for more than two hundred years.

They chewed the root and kept it in their mouth for some time, until excited and intoxicated. When the Dutch arrived, they called it KAUGOED, meaning literally "chewable things."

Kolbe, an anthropologist of 260 years ago, wrote, "their animal spirits were awakened, their eyes sparkled and their faces manifested laughter and gaiety. Thousands of delightsome ideas appeared, and a pleasant jollity which enabled them to be amused by the simplest jests. By taking the substance to excess they lost consciousness and fell into a terrible delirium."

In 1914, Zwicky isolated the alkaloids mesembrine and mesembrenine. He dissolved 0.15 gram of mesembrine in hydrochloric acid, ingested it, and heard buzzing in his ears, suffered weakness of limbs, with slight trembling. It contains tortuosamine, all three interacting with the brain's dopamine and serotonin receptors. It elevates mood, decreases anxiety, stress and tension, increases energy levels and the ability to concentrate.

Laidler, in 1928, noted it was "chewed and retained in the mouth for awhile, when their spirits would rise, eyes brighten and faces take on a jovial air, and they would commence to dance."

Today, the root, leaves and bark of various ice plants are crushed, then chewed or smoked. Kaugoed (*S. tortuosum*) contains alkaloids with sedative activity. As little as five grams can create a state of stupor and lanquidity, leaving a prickly sensation on the tongue. Higher doses can produce a headache. It is used in South Africa as a narcotic to relieve pain, and as a party drug similar to use of *Cannabis sativa*.

It may be Africa's oldest natural mood enhancer and anti-depressant. It is stronger, and works more quickly than St. John's wort.

Recent studies suggest it may be a phosphodiesterase inhibitor (PDE-4). These inhibitors augment intracellular secondary messenger signaling in our brain cells, and prevent the breakdown of the key intracellular messenger, cyclic AMP.

AMP is involved in modulating multiple molecular processes involved in cognitive function, mood and inflammation.

The treatment of Alzheimer's disease involves an influence on the PDE-4-cAMP-CREB cascade.

A nutraceutical extract of the plant is available as Zembrin.

Simon Chiu presented findings on the benefit of Zembrin for twenty healthy adults in a double-blind, placebo-controlled, crossover clinical study. Twenty-five milligrams or placebo were given once a day for three weeks, then a three-week washout and a further switch with herb or placebo.

Compared to placebo, Zembrin at 25 mg per day selectively and significantly improved two key cognitive function domains, compromised by stress. Cognitive flexibility and executive function were improved, quality of sleep improved, and the change in Hamilton Depression score also improved, albeit none of the 25 were previously assessed as depressed patients.

This suggests a benefit for enhancing cognition during stress, improving cognitive decline in the elderly, and treating neuro-degenerative disorders and mood-related conditions.[682]

A study of sixteen students, receiving 25 mg of Zembrin or placebo two hours prior to MRI scan revealed interesting results. During perceptual load task, amygdala reactivity to facial fear was significantly reduced, compared to placebo. Emotion matching task showed activation of the midbrain, hypothalamus, amygdala and prefrontal cortex. There was a significant decrease in functional connectivity between the amygdala and hypothalamus with Zembrin, compared to placebo. This suggests reduction of anxiety-related effects.[683]

The herb works by inhibiting serotonin 5-hydroxytryptamine reuptake transporters and selectively inhibiting phosphodiesterase-4 in the CNS.

Work by Coetzee et al[684] found the herbal extract down-regulated serotonin transport in a manner similar to citalopram. Vesicular monoamine transporter-2 was significantly up-regulated.

Sceletium exerts significant cytoprotective effect in the presence of endotoxins, suggesting immune modulation. It up-regulated IL-10 and increased mitochondrial viability, and reduced cytokine inflammation, without hindering adequate immune response in acute situations.[685]

Recent lab studies looked at attenuation of AMPA mediated transmission, suggesting the two alkaloids (mesembrenol and mesembranol) may be useful leads for the treatment of epilepsy.[686]

DOSE- Zembrin- 2:1 extract as directed.

Ginger (*Zingiber officinalis*) rhizome is a well-known culinary and medicinal herb. Zingiber is derived from the Arabic *zinschebil*, meaning root of *Zindschi*, or India. It is a close relative of turmeric.

Although generally thought of for its gastrointestinal, anti-emetic and anti-inflammatory properties, it has some benefits in brain health. Ginger root helps reduce anxiety, possibly due to its antagonist activity on 5-HT (serotonin) receptors.

Another possibility is the inhibition of arachidonic acid metabolites, which act on GABAergic receptors. Ginger helps reduce hypercortisol levels, found in 50% of patients with major depression, via an anti-thromboxane effect.[687]

DOSE- Add fresh daily to various foods. Large amount may interfere with blood thinners. Maybe. 500 mg powder capsules can be taken several times daily with food.

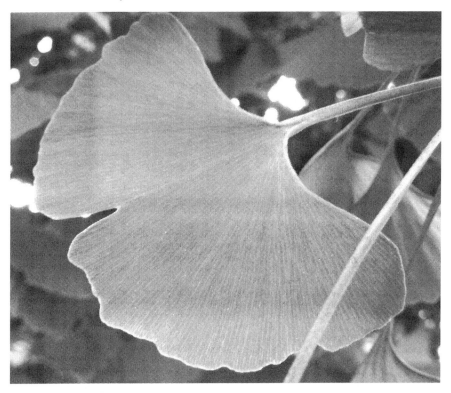

Ginkgo (*Ginkgo biloba*)

Ginkgo is one of our oldest living trees, dating back over 225 million years. It is nearly extinct in the wild, but is now widely cultivated. It is revered for its longevity, as suggested by the Chinese colloquial name KUNG SUN SHU meaning, grandfather and grandson tree. Other names include Ancestor tree, Buddha's Fingernail Tree and Eyes of the Cosmic Spirit Tree. In ancient China, it was known as I-cho (duck's foot tree).

The oldest known specimen, the Li Jiawan Grand Ginkgo King, is found near Guiyang, the capital of Guizhou province. It is three thousand years old, 30 meters tall and measures 15.6 meters in girth at breast height. In China and Korea, the plant is revered by Buddhists and planted as a temple tree. In Japan, followers of Shinto do the same.

Ginkgo is derived from the Japanese, from the Chinese ideogram pronounced Yin-Kuo meaning, "silver apricot".

The Chinese emperor Shen Nung in his famous text *Pen T'sao Ching* wrote about the use of ginkgo for memory loss.

It was mentioned briefly in TCM during the Ming dynasty in 1436 AD, but really did not become a well-known medicinal until the latter half of 20th century. The name Maidenhair is related to the similarity of ginkgo leaf to that of the fern. In fact, many scientists believe it may be the first tree to evolve. At least four different species of Ginkgo shared the planet, with dinosaurs, making it a true living fossil.

Today, over 50 million ginkgo trees are in cultivation yielding 4000 tons of dried leaves annually in the United States and France. In the latter country, prescriptions for the herb make up 4% of all drugstore requests.

The active ingredients in the leaf are ginkgolides and the sesquiterpene bilobalide usually standardized to 24/6. Look for this number on the bottle label.

The ginkgolides, particularly ginkgolide B inhibit platelet activating factor (PAF) and 3'5'-cyclic GMP phosphodiesterase, which relax the endothelium. The flavonoid fraction particularly quercitin, increases serotonin release and uptake, inhibits age-related reduction of muscarinergic cholinoceptors and alpha-adrenoceptors, and stimulates choline uptake in the hippocampus. Hundreds of studies have been conducted and a few of the more recent ones are cited here.

Eighteen studies involving 1672 patients support the use of ginkgo to treat dementia due to cardiovascular insufficiency.

A systematic review and met-analysis looked at nine trials with 2372 patients, and found ginkgo more effective than placebo, for senile dementia and possible Alzheimer's disease.

In a 24-week clinical trial of 410 outpatients with mild to moderate dementia, ginkgo helped alleviate behavioral and neuropsychiatric symptoms, and improved the well being of caregivers as well.[688]

A combination of ginkgo and bacopa showed improvement of memory and attention in adult mice.[689]

Ginkgo biloba may be useful in mild to moderate cognitive impairment, particularly when patients do not benefit from acetycholinesterase inhibitors or NMDA antagonists.[690]

A review of four DB, PC randomized trials involving 1628 patients for at least 22 weeks, confirmed ginkgo's benefit in behavioral and psychological symptoms of dementia. It also reduced caregiver distress caused by their symptoms.[691]

A retrospective analysis compared the herb with donepezil for 12 months in 189 Alzheimer's patients eighty years or older. Similar effects on cognition were noted for both, but ginkgo showed more favorable safety.[692]

The herb is approved in Germany for the treatment of cerebral insufficiency (senile dementia), tinnitus, vertigo and intermittent claudication, or poor circulation to the lower legs. In fact, ginkgo is a peripheral circulatory stimulant, allowing increased blood flow to the extremities of the body including the brain, hands, feet and genital organs.

One study found increased alpha brain wave, and decreased theta wave activity.

Many years ago I developed a line of herbal supplements for the company femMed. The product Libido was created to enhance sexual desire and included ginkgo to increase blood flow to the genital region by relaxing smooth muscle via nitric oxide influence.

A study of 68 women given ginkgo for eight weeks, along with sex therapy, found enhanced orgasm function compared with placebo.[693] The herb has been shown to potentiate papaverine in men suffering erectile dysfunction, and improved blood flow to clitoral arteries. It shows benefit in anti-depressant drug-induced sexual dysfunction. This includes SSRIs, MAOIs and tricyclic medications.[694]

Ritalin and Adderall are often used as stimulants for ADHD, but some children do not respond or tolerate them very well. A DB, PC, parallel trial for six weeks compared *Ginkgo biloba* or placebo, along with methylphenidate. The herb was an effective complementary treatment, with the drug, according to both teacher and parent rating scores.[695]

Ginkgo biloba may have a role to play in Parkinson's disease (PD). Amentoflavone, a main bioactive compound shows activity at the benzodiazepine site of the gamma-aminobutryic acid-A (GABA-A) receptor as a negative allosteric modulator.[696]

Tardive dyskinesia (TD) is a side effect of L-dopa, as well as anti-depressants such as Prozac, Paxil and Zoloft, anti-seizure drugs, and schizophrenia medications. Adjunctive *Ginkgo biloba* (240 mg daily) appears to be effective and improved TD in 299 schizophrenia patients, in a randomized controlled trial.[697]

DOSE- 60 mg capsules (24/6) up to four times daily. Start slow and take early in the day due to its stimulating effect.

CAUTION- Fifteen published case reports describe the use of ginkgo and a bleeding event. Most involved serious medical conditions including 8 cases of intracranial bleeding. Thirteen of the 15 cases identified other risk factors for bleeding. Only six cases reported that when ginkgo was stopped, bleeding did not recur.[698]

A one-year DB, PC randomized study of 309 patients taking Coumadin or aspirin, along with the herb, reported one stroke and one subdural hematoma, both in the placebo group. Overall, ginkgo was safe and improved cognitive performance over placebo.[699]

A randomized DB PC crossover study of outpatients on stable long-term warfarin found no change with the addition of *Ginkgo biloba* or CoQ10.[700]

However, it may be best to avoid any blood thinners, anti-platelets including aspirin and concurrent use of *Ginkgo biloba*. Also discontinue use of the herb for two weeks before surgery.

Recently, the daily dose of 81 mg aspirin, recommended to tens of millions of people, has been challenged and no longer suggested for those individuals without a previous history of stroke or heart attack.

In an analysis of 147 cases of herb-drug interactions, 27.45% involved hemorrhagic complications when *Ginkgo biloba* was taken with SSRI and SNRI anti-depressants.[701]

The literature cites a number of positive herb-drug interactions. Combined with trimipramine in eight patients with major depression for four weeks, sleep patterns improved. When ginkgo supplementation was stopped, the effect was reversed.

When taken with haloperidol for schizophrenia, it increased effectiveness of the drug and reduced the extrapyramidal side effect. Immune function also improved.

NOTE: A tea or tincture of the leaves is ineffective, as up to sixty pounds of leaves are used to produce one pound of extract with precise ratios. Use a standardized extract.

Goldenseal (*Hydrastis canadensis*)
Goldthread (*Coptis species*)
Oregon Graperoot (*Berberis* species)

All three of these herbs offer a multitude of health benefits. The roots contain berberine, which is helpful in various neurodegenerative conditions, including inhibition of acetylcholinesterase. Berberine may be useful in epilepsy and Huntington's disease. See Supplements.

Goldenseal is much mis-used in the health food industry, as it is not a great antibiotic, but is remarkable for reducing inflammation and helping repair damage to mucus membranes, including the gastrointestinal tract. Taken over time, it does negatively influence the production of B vitamins, so supplementation is necessary.

Palmitine and berberine in Goldthread rhizomes inhibit acetylcholinesterase, synergistically.[702]

Oregon Graperoot is rich in berberine, and has the added advantage of assisting liver health and supporting low thyroid function. It is contraindicated in glaucoma.

DOSE- see Supplements

Gotu Kola/Brahmi (*Centella asiatica*)

Gotu Kola is derived from the Sinhala name for the plant. Brahmi relates to the development of Brahman, the Supreme Reality, helping to strengthen nervous function, and promote longevity, intelligence and memory.

Gotu Kola is a slender, creeping perennial with long stems that root at the nodes.

It is eaten as a green vegetable throughout India and south-east Asia.

Apparently, it is relished as food by elephants, in Sri Lanka. And we all know elephants have good memories!

Gotu Kola is well-known for its ability to improve memory. A number of human studies on children and the elderly suggests more attention be paid to this remarkable herb for the treatment of senile dementia and Alzheimer's disease.

In a group of mentally-challenged children given either 500 mg of dried whole plant powder in capsules or placebo, intelligence quotient tests were repeated after three months. Those taking the herb showed significant improvement in memory, concentration, attention, vocabulary, social cooperation and adjustment.

A study of 20-month old CB6F mice given gotu kola in drinking water for two week showed improved performance by increasing synaptic density, anti-oxidant activity, and improved mitochondrial proteins.[703] Later work suggested it improves mitochondrial function in the absence of amyloid-beta, suggesting use in conditions other than AD, where neuronal dysfunction occurs.

A randomized, double-blind, placebo-controlled study of 28 senior citizens found 750 mg of herb taken once daily for two months enhanced working memory, and improved self-rated mood.[704]

The exact mode of action has not been determined but neuro-protection may be related to enzyme inhibition, prevention of amyloid plaque formation leading to Alzheimer's disease, prevention of dopamine neurotoxicity in Parkinson's disease and decreased oxidative stress.[705]

Asiatic acid 1 may enhance cognition and memory by its influence on GABA-A receptors.[706]

Aluminum toxicity is controversial, but may be one of many factors in senile dementia and onset of Alzheimer's disease.

A rat model of AD was exposed to aluminum chloride for 42 days. The triterpene asiatic acid mitigated induced AD associated pathologies.[707]

Pesticide exposure is linked to Parkinson's disease and related synapse dysfunction. Asiaticoside significantly improved working memory and motor coordination in rotenone-poisoned rats.[708]

Gotu kola improves vascular cognitive impairment after stroke, and is more effective than folic acid in the improvement of memory.[709]

It prevents neuronal degeneration, particularly from beta amyloid exposure, and shows positive neuroprotection on post-stroke cognitive impairment, and Parkinson's disease.[710]

Valproic acid (VPA) is commonly prescribed for epilepsy and bipolar disorder. However, due to reduced histone deacetylase, this causes impairment of spatial working memory. Gotu kola, as concurrent treatment, helps prevent the spatial memory and neurogenesis impairments caused by VPA.[711]

Its bioavailability is enhanced when taken with phospholipids.

DOSE- 2-4 300 mg capsules standardized to 8% triterpene glycosides daily with food. Tincture- 1-2 ml, three times daily.

CAUTION- Concurrent use with barbiturates or benzodiazepines is not advised due to GABAnergic activity. It should not be used during pregnancy and caution is advised when patients are actively treating high cholesterol or blood sugar conditions. The herb may aggravate pruritis. It may increase effects of other sedatives and barbiturates.

Green Tea

Green tea (*Camellia sinensis*) is a healthy beverage addition for brain health. The dried leaf is, of course, rich in anti-oxidants, helping protect cellular integrity and preventing free radical damage.

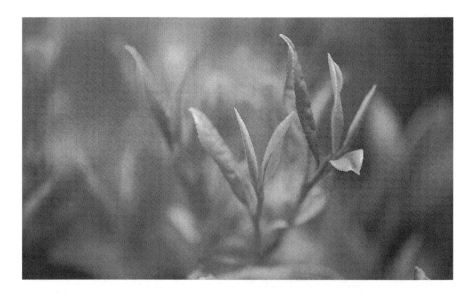

Epigallocatechin-3-gallate (EGCG) is abundant in green tea, along with other catechins, and shows anti-inflammatory benefits. It modulates genes to heal intestinal permeability, and protect from damaging pharmaceuticals that reduce TNF production.

Green tea extracts and the polyphenol EGCG bind to iron, and cross the blood-brain barrier. This allows it to capture and isolate iron from the brain regions, affected in Alzheimer's, Parkinson's, and Huntington's disease.[712]

Studies on mice show prevention of age-related cognitive dysfunction, and brain neuron proliferation.[713] It ameliorates high fat, high-fructose induced learning and memory loss.

Green tea increases our microbiome content of *Bifidobacterium*, and reduces harmful colonies of *Clostridium difficile*, *C. perfringens* and *Streptococcus pyogenes* in the gut.[714]

Taken daily, green tea may improve depression, lower the risk of cognitive decline, particularly in females, and those with genetic risk of Alzheimer's.[715]

Green tea reduces the formation of beta-amyloid plaque in AD and alpha-synuclein fibrals in PD.[716]

A meta-analysis of 48,000 participants found consuming three cups of tea daily decreased cognitive disorders by 36%.[717]

Both green and black tea contain the non-protein amino acid L-theanine, which shows benefit in generalized anxiety (GAD), depression, panic disorders, obsessive-compulsive disorder (OCD), AD and possibly schizophrenia and bipolar disorder. White tea contains L-theanine and GABA.

L-theanine (N-ethyl-L-glutamine) elicits selective changes in alpha wave activity with improved attention during execution of mental tasks.[718] Start with 200 to 400 mg on an empty stomach.

Twenty patients with major depressive disorder were given L-theanine along with their current meds for 8 weeks in an open-label study. The Hamilton Depression Rating Scale showed improvement, as did anxiety-trait scores.[719]

A ten-week, DB, PC study involving 46 participants with GAD found improved sleep satisfaction over placebo. This study of clients taking anti-depressants did not find any benefit for GAD.[720]

GABA and L-theanine may be synergistic for sleep quality and duration, improving REM and non-REM, but based on an animal trial.[721]

A recent mouse study found L-theanine ameliorates the impairment of memory and hippocampal long-term potentiation, probably through dopamine D1/5 receptor-PKA pathway activation. This suggests more study in preventing and treating AD.[722]

L-theanine has a very similar structure to GABA, and easily crosses the blood-brain barrier, helping raise brain levels.

It has positive effects on serotonin and dopamine levels, with small doses mildly stimulating, and larger doses calming.

DOSE- Two green tea capsules twice daily standardized to 95% polyphenols. One product on the market, Green T-Max, contains the catechin equivalent of up to 12 cups of green tea in one capsule.

L-theanine- 250 mg capsule- one daily.

CAUTION- Only drink organic green tea, and L-theanine derived from the same sources. Unfortunately, many tea plantations use pesticides. Mice studies suggest green tea does not improve cognition in Down syndrome, and shows some detrimental skeletal effects. More study is needed.

Griffonia simplicifolia

Griffonia simplicifolia is a climbing shrub from West Africa that produces black pods with seeds, which are harvested for their content of 5-hydroxytryptophan (5HTP), the precursor of serotonin.

When tryptophan became unavailable, the herbal supplement was used as a replacement. See Chapter 4 for more on tryptophan.

One rat study found the seed powder relieved anxiety.[723]

One advantage of 5-HTP over L-tryptophan is the intestinal absorption of the former does not require a transport molecule, and is not reduced by the presence of other amino acids. It cannot be shunted into niacin or protein production. About 70% of 5-HTP as an oral dose ends up in the blood, and crosses the blood-brain barrier (BBB). It increases dopamine and norepinephrine levels in brain. Since the early 1970s at least 15 studies have evaluated 5-HTP for treatment of depression.[724]

A DB, multi-center study of 36 patients with depression, compared an SSRI (selective serotonin reuptake inhibitor) with 5-HTP. Both groups should significant reduction in depression beginning in week two, and after six weeks both showed 50% improvement in patient's symptoms.[725]

The product helps address issues around depression, persistent nightmares, migraines and other headaches, and mood disorders.[726]

DOSE- 100-200 mg capsules (sustained release) as directed. Some individuals experience nausea, vomiting or diarrhea.

Hibiscus, or Red Sorrel (*Hibiscus sabdariffa*) flower and calyx make a pleasant herbal tea. I remember its popularity back in 1972 when combined with peppermint, lemongrass and sweet orange in Red Zinger herbal tea, produced by Celestial Seasonings. It was the hippie herbal drink of choice.

The herb is a potent antioxidant that protects against serum/glucose deprivation induced PC12 cell injury. This suggests benefit in neurodegenerative disorders.[727]

It protects against ethanol-induced deficits in the Purkinje cells of the cerebellum, in an animal study, suggesting benefit reducing brain damage associated with alcohol addiction.[728]

Purkinje cells release the neurotransmitter GABA.

The herb inhibits acetylcholinesterase, butyrylcholinesterase and monoamine oxidase (MAO), suggesting benefit in Alzheimer's and Parkinson's disease.[729]

A seed extract promotes the growth of sulfated glycosaminoglycans, suggesting benefit in gut tissue repair.[730]

DOSE- Drink as infused tea. Hibiscus may lower blood pressure and blood sugar levels. It is contraindicated for concurrent use with the anti-malaria drug chloroquine.

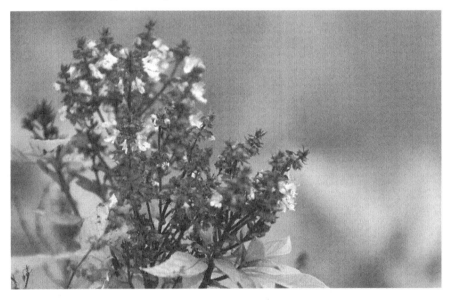

Holy Basil

Holy Basil or Tulsi (*Ocimum sanctum*) has been used for thousands of years in Ayurvedic medicine. Tulsi means "the incomparable one." Some herbalists classify it as an adaptogen, but Donald Yance suggests it is a secondary adaptogen, and I agree. It modulates stress response, inhibits cortisol release[731], increases adaptive energy and elevates the spirit.

The herb shows promise on generalized anxiety disorder (GAD), based on a small trial of 35 young people (average 38 years) for sixty days. The herb (500 mg capsules twice daily) significantly attenuated GAD as well as stress and depression.[732]

Lab studies suggest it may be helpful in reducing symptoms of Parkinson's disease.[733]

A rat model found the herbal tincture enhanced cognition by increasing choline acetyl transferase activity.[734]

A week-long rat study found a tincture prevents noise-induced changes in the brain, including reduction of acetylcholine and an increase activity of acetylcholinesterase.[735] Autism spectrum disorder is aggravated by loud noises and bright lights, suggesting holy basil tea may be worthy of a try.

Noted herbalist David Winston wrote. "In my clinical practice I use holy basil to enhance cerebral circulation and memory. It is used in ayurvedic medicine to relieve 'mental fog' caused by chronic cannabis smoking…I also use holy basil as an antidepressant for 'stagnant depression.' The term *stagnant depression* is one that I coined, and it describes a specific type of situational depression. In this case, some type of traumatic event occurred in a person's life, and because he is unable to move on, his life comes to revolve around the trauma."[736]

Sounds a lot like PTSD to me!

A systematic review of 24 studies, involving 1111 subjects found tulsi improved cognitive flexibility, attention, and working memory by day fifteen, and decreased anxiety, stress and depression.[737]

DOSE- capsules 500 mg twice daily. Tincture 20-40 drops three times daily produced at 1:5 ratio in 40% alcohol. Infused tea as often as desired.

Hops (*Humulus lupulus*)

Hop strobiles are the small green cones found on this climbing vine. Although an important medicinal herb, it is best known for its addition to beer. Hops and Cannabis are the two most well-known members of the Cannabaceae family. They are so closely related that tops of one can be successfully grafted onto the roots of the other.

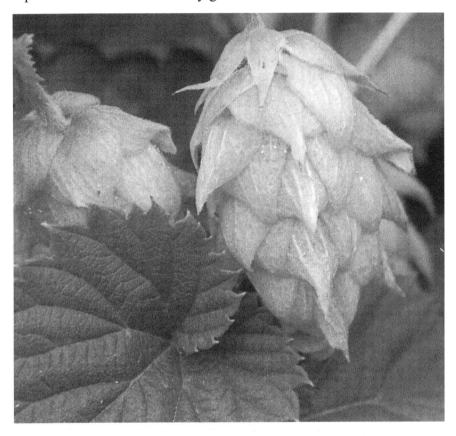

Humulus is derived from the Old German HUMELA or perennial climber, and may be from the Old Slavic CHUMELI. Hops were known as HYMELE, to the Saxons.

This may stem from the Greek HUMUS, the ground (humility) because it runs along the ground if not supported, or more likely "soil" in allusion to the ground hugging habit of the vine. The Latin HUMUS means fresh, damp earth, and HUMUDUS, wet or humidity, as the plant prefers moist soil.

Lupulus is a small WOLF and refers to its old name of wolf among willow, from its habit of climbing over Salix species. This is derived from ancient Rome where hop was known as *Lupulus salictarius*.

Hop derives from the Anglo Saxon HOPPAN "to climb"; originally from the Dutch HOPPE and, in turn, from the Old High German HOPFO, which means a plant, "which gropes or fumbles around." In Russia, the word HMEL describes both hops and a drunk.

In the 9th century, an Arabian physician claimed hops induced sleep. Hops act like melatonin, whereas valerian is more adenosine-like in action, helping the body get ready for sleep.[738]

This is no great surprise, as beer contain high levels of melatonin. Higher alcohol content yields higher melatonin content.

Cannabidiol, also found in cannabis, is a dopamine transporter, 5HT and cannabinoid receptor, and both GABA and norepinephrine transporter.

Hop resins influence GABA-A receptors, but have no influence on benzodiazipine receptors.

As a budding herbalist, I read repeatedly in a number of books, suggesting hops was contraindicated for clients with depression.

A recent randomized, DB, PC, cross-over pilot study of 36 participants with mild depression, anxiety and stress were studied for two 4-week intervention periods. Daily supplementation significantly improved all symptoms in the Depression Anxiety Stress Scale-21.[739]

DOSE- 300 mg capsules- one to two capsules twice daily. Tincture is 1.5-2.5 ml of 1:5 ratio up to four times daily.

NOTE- Both hops and German chamomile are significant inhibitors of GAD, or glutamic acid decarboxylase. See GABA under chapter on neurotransmitters. This suggests hops would not be an appropriate herbal supplementation in autism spectrum disorder (ASD).

However, for ADHD with hyperactivity, lack of attention and impulsive behavior, it works well.

Iboga (*Tabernanthe iboga*) is a shrub native to west-central Africa. It was traditionally used in ceremony to communicate spiritually with ancestors.

In African cultures a journey with the herb is believed associated with the person's soul leaving their body, and traveling to the spirit world. Rainbow-like auras and feelings of levitation and time perception are common. This is due, in part to its monoamine and indole action on 5-HT$_2$ receptors.

Ibogaine is being used very successfully in treatment centers for opioid addiction.

One study of 30 subjects with DSM-IV Opioid Dependence found that after one month, 50% reported no further opioid use.[740]

A research study in New Zealand, where ibogaine is legal by prescription, involved 14 participants. It found a single ibogaine treatment reduced opioid withdrawal symptoms and achieved opioid cessation or reduced use over the next twelve months.[741]

Ibogaine is illegal in United States, but not explicitly so in Canada and UK. Various countries including Mexico, Brazil, and Costa Rica embrace ibogaine treatment centers.

Ibogaine blocks the uptake of dopamine and serotonin, and both ibogaine and noribogaine bind to the cocaine site of the serotonin transporter. It prevents cocaine-induced increases in serotonin levels in the brain, and reduces release of dopamine induced by nicotine, cocaine and morphine.[742]

DOSE- under qualified supervision

Kava-kava (*Piper methysticum*)

Kava Kava is a Polynesian plant that shows great benefit in treating anxiety. It was traditionally used as a ceremonial water- soluble beverage in Hawaii, Tahiti, Fiji and other South Pacific islands. It is called the Root of Happiness. Methysticum translates as "intoxicating."

There is a noticeable bitter taste and numbing of the mouth upon ingestion.

The herb was approved in 1990, by German Commission E, for the treatment of anxiety, stress, and nervous restlessness. At the same time, the Commission contraindicated kava for treating endogenous depression.

In the 1990s I worked part-time as the herbal consultant to a well known nutritional bar company. One bar I helped develop, Calm, contained kava kava and poppy seeds. It did not make it to market, thank goodness, as soon after its projected release to the market, the herb was banned in North America. The poppy seeds also left a residual opiate-like compound in urine samples. Oops!

Kava-kava (kava) shows efficacy in the treatment of non-psychotic anxiety, following pre-treatment with benzodiazepines.[743]

A three-week placebo-controlled trial of 60 adults with generalized anxiety and depression (GAD) were given 250 mg of kavalactones per day, resulting in significant benefit.[744]

Other work has found kava to possess non-addictive and non-hypnotic anxiety relief. Kavalactones are considered the markers of action on GABA-A receptors, with kavain identified as a major contributor. In studies, it was found kavain does not work via classical benzodiazepine binding sites.[745]

Kavalactone displacement of the $GABA_A$ agonist muscimol is higher in the hippocampus and amygdala.[746]

A systematic review and analysis of randomized clinical trials suggests kava was more effective than placebo in three of seven trials involving short-term treatment.[747]

Dose- Capsules 70- 210 mg of kavalactones daily for anxiety and stress. Tincture (3% kavalactones) 40 drops 2-3 times daily.

CAUTION- Kava had a growing supplement market until it was withdrawn from markets due to an acetone or ethanol extract causing liver toxicity in German patients taking four or more pharmaceutical drugs concurrently.

Due to its activity on liver, it is not advised to combine other pharmaceuticals with this herb. It is contraindicated in pregnancy and breast-feeding; and avoid driving if taken in excess.

Consumers should be aware that two varieties of Kava are in the market. Historically, Tudei kava was used for medicine and special ceremony, but never for daily consumption. Noble kava was used for everyday drinking. As demand for the herb grew, farmers planted varieties giving quicker growth, higher yields and higher levels of kavalactones. Tudei effects last several days, but include lethargy and nausea, and the roots contain a chalcone, flavokawain B, proven toxic to liver cells. This cultivar contains up to twenty times the amount of this compound, and if improperly extracted (acetone?) may be even higher. Some unscrupulous companies even include the stems and leaves of Tudei. Fiji and other countries have made exportation of this cultivar illegal.

Dried roots of Noble and Tudei are indistinguishable from one another. Lateral roots contain the highest kavalactone levels but are more hot and spicy than stump. Kava lactones dissolve more easily in alcohol than water. Insist on Noble cultivar preparations.

The herb may increase effects of certain MAO inhibitors.

DOSE- 200-250 mg capsules one to two times daily.

Kratom (*Mitragyna speciosa*)

Kratom is a medicinal plant indigenous to South-East Asia. Traditionally, the leaves were chewed for energy, similar to coca use in the Andes. It is legal to possess and use in Thailand.

It possesses analgesic activity, and has been used to overcome opioid withdrawal, possessing agonist affinity on the receptors, including mu and kappa. One constituent, 7-hydroxymitragynine is 13 times more potent than morphine, but less addictive.

Mitragynine has analgesic effects that could replace codeine.

It is still highly controversial, with a least one case of naloxone reversal from recreational use. Effects kick in after ten minutes and can last two hours or longer.

Kratom and other opioid-related plant medicines will be discussed in more detail in the chapter on addictions. It appears to be less addictive and have milder withdrawal symptoms than opioid drugs. It may be useful for replacing methadone in the treatment of heroin addiction.

Note- Cases of neonatal abstinence syndrome have been noted in a term baby whose mother was drinking kratom tea. Liver injuries have been noted. Interactions with other opioids can result in deadly consequences. As of May 2018, there were no recorded human fatalities due to Kratom alone.[748]

DOSE- under professional supervision

Kudzu (*Pueraria montana*)

Kudzu is an invasive plant throughout the southeastern United States, and has now crept up to southern Ontario. It was introduced from Asia, at the Philadelphia Centennial Exposition in 1876 as an ornamental and forage crop.

A single dose of kudzu extract, from root, reduced alcohol consumption in a binge-drinking paradigm of 20 men in a PC, DB experiment.[749]

A randomized PC,DB study of 17 men over two months who reported drinking 27 drinks per week, found kudzu extract reduced the number of drink by 34-57%, reduced the number of heavy drinking days, and increased the percent of days abstinent.[750]

It does not appear to disturb sleep/wake cycles in moderate alcohol drinkers, and may be a useful adjunct therapy.

DOSE- 600 mg capsules. Take two capsules three times daily.

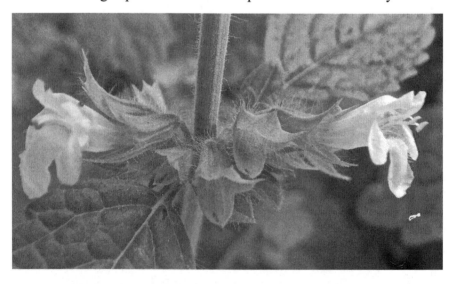

Lemon Balm (*Melissa officinalis*)

Melissa, or Lemon Balm, has been cultivated in the Mediterranean region for over two millennium.

Avicenna, the ancient herbalist, mentions use of the plant "to make the heart merry." This led to the name "heart's delight".

It has a relationship with bees, and was known to the Greeks as MELISOPHYLLON, meaning "bee leaf". The Romans carried on the tradition and called it APIASTRUM derived from *Apias* for bee. Balm is short for balsam, a description given to many aromatic herbs. Melissa was the daughter of Melisseus and Amalthea, and the sister of Adastrea and Ida in Greek mythology. She was turned into a bee by the gods and helped her sisters care for the infant Zeus by providing honey for him.

Various laboratory studies confirm its activity on nicotinic, muscarinic, and acetylcholine receptors. The herb inhibits MAO-A and acetylcholinesterase.

A DB, PC, randomized trial of forty-two Alzheimer's patients was conducted over four months. Lemon balm extract produced significantly better outcome on cognitive function than placebo, and had a positive effect on agitation in patients.[751]

A pilot trial on stressed volunteers found an herbal extract reduced anxiety by 18%, ameliorated anxiety-associated symptoms by 15% and reduced insomnia by 42%. Fully 95% (19 out of 20) of volunteers responded favorably to the herb.[752]

Twenty healthy, young volunteers were given various doses of the herb or placebo for one week. Cognitive performance and moods improved in those given 1600 mg of dried leaf. Displacement from nicotinic and muscarinic receptors was noted, *in vitro*, along with lack of cholinesterase inhibition.[753]

Patients with chronic stable angina often experience high levels of depression, anxiety, stress and insomnia. A DB, PC trial of 80 angina patients for eight weeks, found the Melissa group had significant reduction of all symptoms above.[754]

Female adolescents suffering PMS (premenstrual syndrome) related anxiety, depression and insomnia all did better with lemon balm than placebo in another study.[755]

For ADHD individuals constantly in a bad mood or depressed, combine it with green flowering oats and/or St. John's wort.

Remember lemon balm for SAD (seasonal affective disorder), combining well with latter herb.

DOSE- 20-30 drops three times daily of 1:4 fresh leaf tincture or equivalent. Infused tea as often as desired.

CAUTION- Large amounts MAY act as an antagonist to Synthroid and Levoxyl. Unlikely, but caution is advised. The herb is used in the treatment of acute hyperthroidism, sometimes combined with Bugleweed and/or Motherwort.

Linden (Tilia spp.)

Linden was originally an adjective from the Old English or Norse LIND, for tree. The root LI, from the Indo-European root means flax thread, with LENTUS coming to mean "flexible". Linné, the father of taxonomy, was Swedish and LINN, meant linden. Lyne may later have become lyme. Hence the use by some English herbalists, of the common name, lime flower.

The German verb LINDERN means, "to soothe."

Linden flowers and bracts are gathered and used in herbal teas for their sedative and relaxing quality, and cooling and drying nature.

The stalks of dried linden flowers are used in France for Tilleul tea.

The flowers have been used traditionally in France, and elsewhere for the symptomatic treatment of neurotic states, especially minor sleep disturbances, nervous vomiting and heart palpitations. This may be due to the binding of GABA receptors, similar to valerian.

It combines well with lemon balm, chamomile to reduce stress, irritability, anxiety and depression, including ADHD children.

An added advantage is the tea helps remove arterial plaque, associated with restriction of blood flow, and prevention of aneurism and clots.

Linden leaf bud extracts (gemmotherapy) have long been recommended for their ability to increase serotonin production in the brain. It has a soothing effect on the nervous system, making it useful for insomnia and anxiety.[756]

It treats a badly defined anguish neurosis (anticipative anguish), and works well on the nervous system of fragile people like children, pregnant women and the elderly. It is not hypnotic and induces sleep.[757]

A study on the bud extracts suggest they mimic GABA and benzodiazepine agonists by targeting hippocampal GABAergic synapses and inhibit network excitability by strengthening inhibitory output.[758]

DOSE- Linden flower infused tea is diaphoretic (causes sweating) when taken hot. Cool before drinking for insomnia. Linden flower and leaf tincture is taken at 30-40 drops twice daily.

Linden gemmotherapy is taken 20-30 drops twice daily.

CAUTION- Linden flower is contraindicated when taking SSRI medications such as Paxil, Zoloft, or Prozac.

Lobelia (*Lobelia inflata*)

Lobelia is named after Matthias de l'Obel, Flemish botanist, and physician to King James I of England. In 1570, he published an early Herbal under the Latinized name *Lobelius*, which tried to classify plants according to leaf shape.

Inflata refers to the inflated, hollow seed capsules. The medicinal herb is indigenous to North America.

By 1829, it was used in a pharmacy in Rome. The patent medicine, Bantron, utilized lobelia alkaloids in a stop-smoking medication, banned by the FDA in 1993.

The great Eclectic physician Dr. Ellingwood wrote. "Lobelia seems at once to supply a subtle but wholly sufficient force, power, or renewed vital influence, by which the nervous system and the essential vital force with the system again re-assert themselves and obtain complete control of the functional action of every organ.

From this influence, in a natural and sufficient manner, a complete harmonious operation of the whole combined forces is at once resumed, in some cases in an almost startling manner. The sympathetic nerves are either relaxed or stimulated as well as adjusted with the parasympathetic; depending upon the symptoms."[759]

Lobeline is almost chemically identical to the nicotine alkaloid; with potency from 1/5 to 1/20 that of nicotine.

I used a combination of lobelia, green-flowering oats, and skullcap as a Stop Smoking mixture in clinical practice.

The latter two herbs are included for calming and strengthening the nervous system.

In clinical practice I would ask the client to reduce cigarette intake to six daily at timed intervals. Then five cigarettes with 10 drops of lobelia tincture would be taken for a week; then four cigarettes and 10 drops twice daily, etc. Since lobelia is not addictive, it can be discontinued at any time.

Lobeline appears to prevent the re-uptake of dopamine, a way for the body to turn off neurotransmitters. Like nicotine, it stimulates the autonomic ganglia (nicotinic receptors), which is followed by depression.

However, lobeline possesses several significant differences from nicotine. It decreases the basal release of acetylcholine and reduces NMDA evoked acetylcholine release at low dosage. Nicotine does not. Nicotine does appear, however, to protect brain neurons from AD.[760]

A chief metabolite of nicotine is cotinine, which protects against AD and PD pathology.[761]

Lobeline binds to different nicotinic receptor sub-types, and is unaffected by the nicotine antagonist, mecamylamine. It releases serotonin mediated by uptake transporters, but not affected by mecamylamine.

Lobeline activates nicotinic channels at low dose, and inhibits them at high dosage. And although nicotine releases acetylcholine in the hippocampus and frontal cortex, this is not true for lobeline, which activates muscarinic receptors and is a weak AChE inhibitor.[762]

Lobeline inhibits dopamine uptake more than its release, but at very low concentrations it does release dopamine, by inhibiting the uptake into vesicles. At low levels it increases release of norepinephrine, but at higher doses, the opposite is true.

It may be useful in PD through protection of dopaminergic neurons.[763]

But unlike acetylcholine, it does not reduce the release of either by NMDA receptors, but blocks nicotine-induced release of norepinephrine from the locus coeruleus.[764]

Lobeline inhibits dopamine uptake and promotion of dopamine release from the storage vesicles within the pre-synaptic terminal via an interaction with the tetrabenazine-binding site on the vesicular monamine transporter. Early work suggests lobeline may have more potential in the treatment of methamphetamine abuse.[765]

Various derivatives of the herb appear to cross the blood-brain barrier by passing through basic amine transporters.

DOSE- 3-5 drops of 1:5 seed/leaf tincture as required in water.

CAUTION- Lobelia stimulates sympathetic nerve ganglia, and should not be used during pregnancy (uterine relaxant), lactation, or long term. Lobelia is contraindicated in dyspnea from enlarged or fatty heart, weak heart with valvular incompetence, sinus arrhythmia, pneumonia, asthma of cardiac decompensation, hydrothorax, and hydro-pericardium.

Disorders of various types due to cholinergic excess, and lobelia are contra-indicated. As little as four grams can be fatal. This is a highly unpredictable, but valuable herb. Caution with other herbs and drugs is advised.

Mistletoe (*Viscum album*)

Mistletoe has been used for centuries to treat epilepsy, hysteria, psychosis and headaches. Various extracts show central nervous system activity, including anti-epileptic, anxiolytic, anti-depressant, and sedative effects. Mistletoe increases level of brain-derived neurotrophic factor, prevents neuronal death induced by beta-amyloid; and weakly inhibits cholinesterase activity.[766]

A four-year old girl with absence epilepsy was treated with different anti-epileptic drugs and ketogenic diet, but failed to become seizure-free over a two-year span. She received herbal therapies as well as valproate, and then clobazam. Final cessation of seizures occurred after a dose increase of *Viscum album*, and she remained seizure free at her one-year follow-up.[767] More research is needed.

Oats (*Avena sativa*)

Oats in the milky stage, known as green-flowering oats, contain a relaxing nervine.

Oat may stem from the Celtic or Anglo-Saxon ATEN or ETAN "to eat." This later became Oat. Avena means, "nourishment", and comes from the Latin AVIDUS, meaning, "sought after." The Sanskrit word AVASA means nourishment.

Richer in zinc than any other plant, Oats soothe an exhausted nervous system. Green flowering oats are thymoleptic, especially associated with relieving depressive mental states.

Depression is a complex condition, and some differentiation may help direct the beginner.

For depression, with restlessness, look to scullcap and California poppy. For caffeine abuse and addiction, try combining oats with German chamomile.

Avenine, one of its alkaloids, stimulates the central nervous system, and is a wonderful cerebral restorative. Gramine, an indole alkaloid in the flowering tops, has a mildly sedative and hypnotic property. It combines well with valerian or scullcap for those individuals attempting withdrawal from addictions; or taken alone for convalescence after flu or viral infections, accompanied by nervous insomnia and exhaustion.

It also combines well wood betony for nerve weakness, and/or with scullcap to minimize attacks of petit mal epilepsy and other convulsive states. It does not seem to combine well with lady's slipper or passionflower.

Patients with multiple sclerosis report less nerve pain and fatigue, with a greater sense of wellbeing, but no definitive studies have been conducted.

Green oat extract, combined with scullcap is a specific for helping withdrawal from addictions of tobacco, alcohol and cocaine.

In one placebo-controlled clinical trial of 28 days, fresh green oat extracts resulted in tobacco smoking diminishment from 19.5 to 5.7 per day as compared to the placebo (16.5 to 16.7).[768]

As reported in the *British Medical Journal*, 10 chronic opium addicts with an average of over ten years dependence were given 2 ml doses of green flowering oats three times daily.

On the patient's own initiative, six gave up opium completely, 2 had reduced intake, and 2 showed no change. No serious withdrawal symptoms or side effects were noted.[769]

Children who exhibit nervous symptoms such as bedwetting, colic, allergies and hyperactivity, greatly benefit from green oat tincture. I have personally used green flowering oats with good success, treating children diagnosed with ADD or ADHD.

It reduces symptoms of withdrawal from Ritalin. It combines well with hawthorn berry for this purpose, especially in individuals suffering low-level, histamine-type allergies.

A company Frutarom selected optimal accessions of *Avena sativa* to produce an extract called EFLA955 Wild Green Oat Neuravena Special Extract.

In the process of their research, they used a CNS system to test for cognitive function, stress/burnout and chronic fatigue. This sets the bar a little higher for green oat extracts.

Two enzymes, closely related to mental health, have been identified and stabilized in this green oat product. The enzymes inhibit MAO-B and phospho-diesterase 4, associated with anti-depressant and cognitive enhancement capabilities.

MAO-B is responsible for metabolizing dopamine, and levels in the brain are important for mental health and cognitive function. Inhibitors of MAO-B are used to treat neurodegenerative conditions such as Alzheimer's and Parkinson's disease.

Inhibition is associated with mood enhancing, stimulating and neuro-protective properties.[770]

PDE 4 is responsible for the degradation of the key second messenger molecule cAMP, which is used for intracellular signal transduction, such as transferring effects of neurotransmitters like noradrenaline.

PDE 4 inhibitors increase cAMP levels in the brain, acting as signal enhancers. This mechanism is used in the treatment of depression and enhancing cognitive enhancement.

A study found 1600 milligrams daily of Neuravena® acutely improved attention and concentration and the ability to maintain task focus.[771]

A recent DB, PC, counterbalanced, cross-over study found Neuravena®, taken in a single dose increased the cognition and speed of performance in adults aged 40-65 years old, reporting age-related decline in memory.[772]

DOSE- 30-40 drops up to three times daily of fresh green oat tincture 1:5 in 45% alcohol. Neuravena is taken as directed.

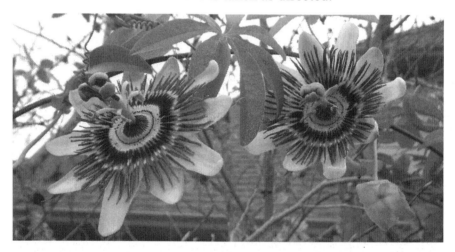

Passionflower/Maypop (*Passiflora incarnata*)

Passionflower derives from its association with the Passion of Christ. Maypop, Maracoc and Maycock are derived from the Powhatan name, MAHCAWQ.

The English herbalist Parkinson wrote in 1629, it "may be called in Latine, *Clematis Virginiana*." Incarnata means "in bodily form," or human representation.

Various parts of the flower have been ascribed to biblical connection. The leaf symbolizes the spear, the five petals and five sepals, the ten faithful apostles (Peter who denied, and Judas who betrayed are omitted). The five anthers represent the five wounds, the spiraled tendrils are the lash of the scourges. The column of the ovary is the pillar of the cross, the stamens the hammers. The three stigmas are the three nails, and the 72 radial filaments within the flower represent the crown of thorns. The style is the sponge used to moisten his lips with vinegar. The calyx is the glory, the white is purity and blue is heaven. The round fruit is the world Christ came to save.

The plant is native to the southern United States down into Central America. The leaves have been traditionally smoked for their calming effect. In Japan, passionflowers are called 'clock face flowers', as they resemble timepieces. In Tokyo and other large cities, passionflower is symbolic of early gay-lesbian protests over equal rights.

Passionflower leaf helps calm anxiety and irritability associated with poor sleep, and chronic stress.

It relieves advanced forms of twitching, trembling and spasms including epilepsy and Parkinson's tremor. I have used equal parts of passionflower and skullcap with good success in epilepsy, as well as severe nervous tension associated with mental exhaustion and depression.

The leaf contains anti-spasmodic and anti-convulsant agents, useful in excitable conditions, and is worthy of a trial for narcolepsy.

Passionflower is indicated in both acute and chronic forms of anxiety.

It inhibits the sympathetic nervous system and its cool, bittersweet energy helps reduce hypertension states of short or long standing.

It relieves tight muscles, congestive headaches, and reduces heart palpitations. Think of using passionflower in bronchitis, spasmodic asthma or whooping cough as a respiratory relaxant.

Harmine, one leaf constituent, was known as telepathine, and used by the Nazis in "truth serums."

295

These alkaloids are found in numerous psychotropic plants including *Banisteriopsis caapi* in Ayahuasca.

Matthew Wood notes. "Early experimentation indicated that it calms the cerebral cortex and has a special affinity to the medulla oblongata, the area of the brain stem that oversees sleep, temporary blood pressure fluctuations related to stress, and the vagus nerve— hiccough, vomiting, and respiration." [773]

Daniel Gagnon adds, "It is wonderful for the headstrong individual, the thinker and the chronic worrier". He notes to use caution in children under four years of age, as too high a dose can cause overexcitement and vomiting.

Passionflower tea was trialed on 41 participants in a DB, PC trial measuring subjective sleep benefit. Sleep quality showed a significant better rating with passionflower, compared to placebo.[774]

Passionflower may be a useful adjuvant in opiate withdrawal.[775] I would suggest combining with green flowering oats for improved benefit. A review of controlled clinical studies found passionflower, chamomile and valerian showed potential for use in anxious disease.[776]

The tincture may be helpful in epilepsy, based on a mouse study.[777] It ameliorates the post-ictal depression that follows seizures.

In fact, I found in clinical practice, a combination of fresh skullcap and passionflower leaf tinctures most efficacious for petit mal and other seizure disorders.

The benefits of the herb for drug withdrawal, insomnia, generalized anxiety disorder (GAD), ADHD and cardiac palpitations and hypertension may be due to modulation of both $GABA_A$ and $GABA_B$ receptors, and its effect on GABA uptake.[778]

One mouse study found, when amino acids were removed from the herbal extracts, GABA currents were absent.

Chrysin, a flavonoid in passionflower, is also found in male catkins of poplar trees. It appears to be an antagonist of the $GABA_B$ receptor, and is partial agonist to benzodiazepine receptors.

DOSE- twenty to thirty drops of dry leaf 1:5 tincture, up to three or four times as needed.

CAUTION- The herb may increase effects of prescription sedatives, anti-spasmodics and anxiolytics. Do not use concurrently with MAO drugs.

Chrysin has the known ability to disrupt thyroid function by blocking the enzymatic conversion of T4 to T3. Individuals with hyper or hypothyroid conditions should be aware.

Passionflower interacts with lorazepam in an additive or synergistic manner, suggesting concurrent treatment and dosage be approached with caution.

Maritime Pine (*Pinus pinaster*) bark is concentrated into a 1000:1 extract known as Pycnogenol. Over seventy human clinical trials have shown its benefit in various inflammatory conditions, due to powerful anti-oxidant and neuroprotective effects.

Several trials suggest efficacy in ADHD children, including one randomized, double-blind placebo controlled trial that found decreased dopamine, adrenaline and noradrenaline, and hyperactivity.[779]

Sixty-one children with ADHD were given pycnogenol, or placebo for four weeks in a DB, RC study. After one month, there was significant reduction of hyperactivity, improved attention and concentration. One month later, after termination of the supplement, a relapse of symptoms was noted.[780]

A mouse study found the supplement improved spatial memory and significantly decreased the number of plaques associated with Alzheimer's disease.[781]

It may be helpful in protecting dopaminergic neurons in neurodegenerative diseases including Parkinson's disease.[782]

Poppy, California (*Eschscholzia californica*)

California poppy is a beautiful golden-flowered annual, found on roadsides in its namesake floral emblem state. It is self-sowing and prolific.

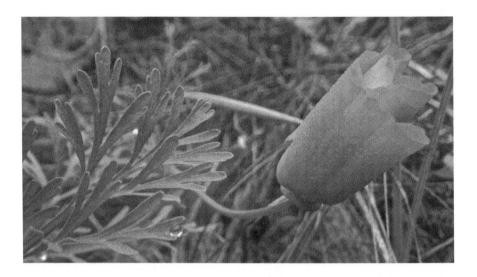

Poppy is thought to derive from the ancient Sumerian PA PA, the chewing noise of poppy seeds. Some authors believe it from the Celtic PAPA, meaning pap or porridge; and referring to the Celtic custom of mixing poppy juice with gruel for sleepless babies.

This became the Middle English PAPPE, a breast, in reference to the soporific milky juice that exudes from the plant. PAQER is from the ancient Egyptian for poppy seed.

It may derive from the Latin PAPPS, alluding to the thick, milky latex, or the Old English POPAEG and Middle English POPI, which means, sleep.

Johann F. G. von Eschscholtz was an Estonian doctor and biologist that explored the west coast of North America from 1815-1818, on voyages led by Otto von Kotzebue. The poppy was named, but misspelled, in his honor, following his death at age 38, by the botanist and shipmate, Ludolf Chamisso. The ports of Chamiss and Kotzebue were named on one of their voyages. They then sailed on to the various Pacific islands, one of which the captain named Eschscholtz Atoll. The name was changed in 1946 to Bikini Island, of nuclear waste infamy.

Early Spanish settlers called it COPA DEL ORA, and told a legend of the orange petals turning to gold, and filling the soil with the precious metal.

In fact, it has an affinity for copper rich soils and indicates the presence of this mineral. Other Spanish names are LA AMAPOLA, meaning flame flower and even DORMIDERA, the drowsy one, or little sleepy head.

It is a safe herb for young children (six years and older), with none of the narcotic or addictive properties associated with opium poppy.

In rat brains, protopine and allocryptopine enhance gamma-aminobutyric acid (GABA) binding to synaptic membrane receptors; indicating a benzo-diazepine like activity.

Work by Rolland et al,[783] found herbal tinctures attach to benzodiazepine receptors, and act as an analgesic on peripheral nerve receptors.

The herb combines with valerian, passionflower, green flowering oats and hops in a number of German preparations. In fact, it is one of the most prescribed herbs for anxiety in that country.

Southwest herbalist Charles Kane noted usefulness "to highly motivated individuals in diminishing or eliminating stronger opiate habits or other similar non-opiate pharmaceutical habits used for pain relief."

A DB, PC study of 264 patients (81% female) with mild to moderate anxiety were given a product containing California poppy, hawthorn berry and magnesium or placebo, for 90 days. The Hamilton anxiety scale showed benefit over placebo in final outcomes.[784]

Roots and aerial parts containing reticuline 9 and 14, inhibit butrylcholinesterase activity, suggestive of benefit in Alzheimer's disease.[785]

The related (S)-reticuline, from aerial parts, affects GABA-A receptors, suggesting a modulating effect.[786]

The two major papaverine alkaloids, eschscholtzine and californidine vary widely (from 1-10 fold) in plants from different growing regions and conditions.

The green seedpods possess the strongest properties, but herbalists use the whole plant, including flowers and root, which contain the highest level of alkaloids. The herb also contains berberine, mentioned under Supplements.

DOSE- 20-40 drops up to three times daily of 1:5 tincture.

CAUTION- Do not use California poppy during pregnancy or lactation, or in cases of glaucoma due to the sanguinarine content. Do not take concurrently with MAO inhibitors or anti-psychotics. Cryptopine is a uterine stimulant.

Purslane (*Portulaca oleracea*) is a common green, growing wild and cultivated for its rich source of Omega-3s. It contains dopamine, norepinephrine, and inhibits acetylcholinesterase.[787]

Red Oak (*Quercus robur*) wood extract (Robuvit®) has been found in clinical trials to help reduce post-mastectomy post-radiation arm lymphedema, reduce chronic fatigue and alleviate post-traumatic-stress disorder (PTSD).

Thirty-four individuals with chronic PTSD for three to seven years were given either 300 mg daily of the supplement or placebo for four weeks. In the oak group, reductions were noted in flashbacks (56%), emotional numbness (50%), recurrent nightmares (42%) and memory of traumatic events (38%). Sleep problems, irritability and fatigue were also significantly reduced.[788]

Rose root (*Rhodiola rosea*)

Roseroot was so named by Linnaeus due to its fresh, pink rhizome having a rose-like scent when cut or bruised.

The first mention of roseroot was recorded by Dioscorides in *De Materia Medica* in 1st century AD. "Rhodia radix grows in Macedonia being like to Costus, but lighter, and uneven, making a scent in ye bruising, like that of Roses.

It is of good use for ye aggrieved with headache, being bruised and layered on with a little Rosaceum, and applied moist to ye forehead, and ye temples."

I identified Roseroot as the number one medicinal herb of choice for commercialization in Alberta, in a report commissioned by the province. This was based on projected market demand, but also the plant's resiliency, surviving temperatures of minus 60 degrees

Celsius, and drought resistant. The plant requires fourteen hours or more of sunlight for its growing season, and thus cannot be easily cultivated in more southern climates.

Later, as chairman of *The Alberta Natural Health Agricultural Network*, I helped initiate, with other enthusiastic members, the *Rhodiola Project*, which began the cultivation of several million plants from 2004-07. Later, of course, several government bureaucrats took credit for its success. What else is new?

On a recent trip to Iceland, I saw wild roseroot everywhere, especially in little nooks and crannies amongst volcanic rock covered with moss and lichens.

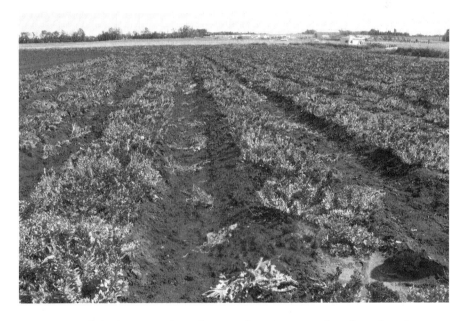

The perennial plant requires four to five years to develop the size of root, and adequate levels of rosavin and salidrosides, needed for medicinal efficacy.

It is classified an adaptogen, like ginseng, eleuthero, schisandra berry, and reishi mushroom; a substance that is "innocuous, causing minimal physiological disorder; non-specific in action; and increasing resistance and normalizing function in the body irrespective of the direction of the pathological change." An adaptogen must, by definition, adhere to these specifics.

Since then, over 800 studies have validated it use for anxiety, depression, Parkinson's disease and other issues surrounding brain health.

A recent review of 36 studies found improved learning and memory function, largely through anti-oxidant, cholinergic regulation, anti-inflammatory and improved cerebral metabolism.[789]

Rhodiola appears to combine well with saffron (below) in a mild to moderate depression study of 45 adults.[790]

It reduced anxiety, stress, anger, confusion and depression in a self-reported study of 80 mildly anxious participants.[791]

A review of its use for depression looked at two randomized DB, PC trials of 146 patients with major depression, and seven open-label studies of 714 individuals with stress-induced mild depression. The review concluded the herb demonstrates multi-target effects on various parts of the neuro-endocrine, neurotransmitter and molecular networks associated with possible beneficial effects on mood.[792]

Although possessing less anti-depressant effect versus sertraline, it showed significantly less adverse events and was better tolerated in a randomized trial of 57 subjects with major depressive disorder.[793]

Several animal studies suggest benefit of Rhodiola species in Alzheimer's disease, but no human clinical trials are published to date.

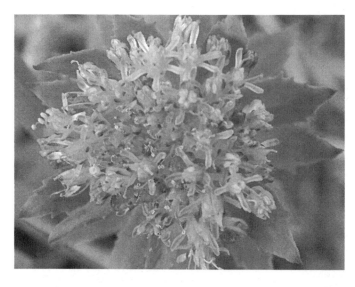

Rhodiola rosea modulates cortical plasticity (without excitability) in a study of 28 healthy volunteers, preventing a reduction in the efficacy of neuronal synapses.[794]

A mouse study found rosin, from *Rhodiola rosea*, suppressed L-glutamate-induced neurotoxicity and inflammation.[795]

DOSE- I personally make a 1:3 fresh root tincture at 70% alcohol and 10% glycerine. There are tablets in the market from Alberta grown roots that are also great. 100-200 mg daily.

CAUTION- Various other Rhodiola species, especially *R. crenulata*, are used for adulteration. Some products on market do not contain any rosavin, or salidroside; or have lower than 3% rosavins, suggested by clinical trials. Rosavin can be synthesized, so the author strongly advises consumers to avoid adulterated Asian product.

Caution is advised when combining this herb with anti-depressants and patients with bipolar conditions, due mainly to additive and stimulating effects. Some herbalist report the drying, astringent effects aggravate some clients.

Saffron (*Crocus sativus*) is one of my favorite spices. I lived for a period of time in Barcelona and paella became a favorite dish I still prepare on special occasions. It is expensive, as 75,000 hand-picked stigma makes a pound, which can sell for up to five thousand dollars.

It contains over 150 potentially active compounds, and was used in traditional herbal medicine for over 90 health conditions.

A 22-week, randomized DB controlled trial found benefit in mild to moderate Alzheimer's disease.[796]

Another trial compared saffron to memantine in a DB trial for moderate to severe AD, also with favorable results.[797]

Recent work suggests it has significant benefit in anxiety, depression and ADHD.

An eight-week, DB, PC randomized trial of 80 youth aged 12-16 with mild to moderate anxiety or depression were given a saffron extract or placebo. Self-reports found improved anxiety and depression, and reduction of headaches in those who received the herb.[798]

A number of clinical trials suggest saffron possesses anti-depressant properties similar to fluoxetine, imipramine and citalopram, with fewer side effects.[799]

A meta-analysis of 11 randomized trials, reported saffron has significant benefit on the severity of depression, and is non-inferior to anti-depressant drugs.[800]

Co-morbid depression-anxiety (CDA) in type two diabetic patients looked at saffron in a DB, PC, randomized study of 54 outpatients. Mild to moderate CDA, anxiety and sleep disturbance were all significantly relieved.[801]

One recent trial suggests short-term therapy with saffron showed efficacy equal to methylphenidate in children with attention-deficit/hyperactivity disorder (ADHD). The six week DB, randomized study involved 54 children aged 6-17.[802]

A study of 45 adults given a combination of rhodiola and saffron for mild to moderate depression for six weeks, found the Hamilton Rating Scale for depression decreased significantly.[803]

A combination of saffron and curcumin (Turmeric below) has been studied for efficacy in major depression.[804]

Saffron extract reduces blood glucose in type 2 diabetes.[805]

DOSE- 30 mg daily from concentrated extract. Tincture is made at 1:10 with 40% alcohol.

Saint John's Wort (*Hypericum perforatum*)

Hypericum has several origins, the most common being from the Greek HYPER meaning "over" and EIKON "image". The expression "over an apparition" comes from a belief the herb was obnoxious to evil spirits, and placed over religious images to ward them off. Hypericum lifts the human spirit over threatening internal images, disturbed imagination or internal dialogue.

Another ancient name was FUGA DEMONUM, meaning Devil's Scourge or Scare the Devil.

It may originate from the Greek, HYPERION, or Sun God. It is believed the Yperikon of Dioscorides, from HYPER "on, over or above", and EREIKE "heath or heather"; hence "among the heather". Perforatum means, "pierced" from the Latin PERFORO and refers to the tiny perforations in leaves.

In Russia, the plant is known as ZVEROBOI or beast killer, in reference to the skin photosensitivity experienced after ingestion by some animals.

I was informed, years ago, by an Ukrainian Catholic priest (former herbal student) the word is derived from a related language, translating as "wound healer."

In the late 1990s, I was invited to present on medicinal herbs at a conference in Manitoba, Canada. The herb, like elsewhere, is considered an invasive weed. When discussing my top ten herbs, I suggested that rather than destroying the herb, it be harvested for the commercial market. Several district agriculturalists approached me after my talk to express their displeasure with my ill-informed opinion. Sigh.

The next year a study, investigated the herb vs. Prozac (fluoxetine), the world's best selling anti-depressant. The study was funded, not by a pharmaceutical company, nor a manufacturer of SJW extract, but by a medical insurance company. After six weeks, the depression scores were deemed identical, in the randomized, double-blind trial. However, 72% side effects were reported for Prozac, vs. only 28% for the herb.[806]

The headlines in the news cited the herb was no better than prozac, exposing the bias of advertised media.

Nearly twenty years later, research is ongoing.

A meta-analysis looked at 5428 papers, and reviewed 27 clinical trials involving 3808 people comparing an SSRI drug and the herb for depression. For mild to moderate cases, it showed comparable efficacy and safety.[807]

A small study found it was only modestly effective in short-term treatment of irritability in autism spectrum disorder.[808] It is not recommended for obsessive-compulsive disorder (OCD).

A recent study found a single dose of the extract modulates cortical plasticity in 28 healthy adults.[809] This suggests increased interest and more research of this amazing plant.

DOSE- 1-3 300 mg capsules (standardized extract of 0.3% hypericin. A good tincture is prepared from fresh aerial parts at 1:1.5 with 60% alcohol. Use 4-6 inches of flowering tips.

CAUTION- The photosensitizing effect of hypericin was first noted in 1787. The only recorded research case of photo-toxicity was in patients receiving high doses of intravenous hypericin. The usual therapeutic doses of Hypericum are 30-50 times below the levels of phototoxicity. Sheep eating the herb in elevated Andes Mountains sometimes suffer sun-burned noses.

It should not be used concurrently with MAO inhibitors such as Furoxone, Marplan, Manerex, Nardil, Eldepryl or Parnate.

It may, however be an effective replacement for Selective Serotonin Reuptake Inhibitor (SSRI) drugs such as Prozac, Paxil, or Zoloft. This should be done over a period of time with the advise and support of a health practitioner.

The often-noted suggestion to avoid foods high in tyramine, is without foundation, as hypericin and hyperforin do not act as MAO inhibitors.

Hyperforin shows promise as an inhibitor of butrylcholinesterase, suggestive of benefit for AD.[810]

The herb may interact with L-dopa and 5 HTP, but no complete human studies have been conducted.

Saint John's wort is a significantly weaker inhibitor of cytochrome activity, than grapefruit juice.

It does, however, affect liver degradation of a number of medications including amitriptyline, cyclosporine, verapamil, digoxin, fexofenadine, indinavir, methadone, midazolam, nevirapine, phenprocoumon, simvastatin, tacrolimus, theophylline, warfarin and chemotherapy drugs such as irinotecan and imatinib.

Low hyperforin extracts show no clinical relevant interaction on cytochrome P450 enzymes and P-glycoprotein, suggesting much safer products will be available down the road.

It decreases efficacy of oxycodone significantly.[811] The herb is reportedly safe to use during pregnancy and breastfeeding.

Schisandra (*Schisandra chinensis*) berry is known as five-flavor berry or Wu Wei Zi in TCM. This refers to the balanced tastes of sweet, sour, bitter, pungent and salty. It possesses the attributes of an adaptogen, helping modify the HPA axis response to stress. The fruit has long history of herbal use for "tranquilizing the mind and overcoming anxiety."

Lignans in the fruit show benefit in age-associated neurodegenerative diseases, and improvement of cognitive function.[812]

Schisandra berry improves sleep time and quality, and up-regulates and modulates expression of $GABA_A$ in cerebral cortex, hippocampus and hypothalamus.[813]

In a metabolomic study, a total of 38 metabolites identified as potential biomarkers of AD, showed significant attenuation from ingestion of schisandra polysaccharide. Both phosphorylation of tau protein and deposition of beta-amyloid was reduced.[814]

Scullcap, Blue (*Scutellaria lateriflora*)
Scullcap, Marsh (*S. galericulata*)

Scutellaria is derived from the Latin SCUTELLA, meaning little dish, tray or saucer, referring to the bell-shaped, lipped calyx. *Galericulata* means "helmet shaped" another reference to the flower's appearance. Scullcap, or Skullcap, is named for the flower's resemblance a head or skull with a hood; think of a helmet with a raised visor. After going to seed, the inverted calyx closes over it, and hence a cap fitting the skull.

This became the plant signature, suggesting its use for ailments of the skull.

Scullcap is foremost a nervine and anti-spasmodic. In cases of nervous over-excitement, or whenever restlessness accompanies acute or chronic illness, Scullcap excels. In children, it soothes the nervous system and reduces teething pain.

Marsh scullcap is more bitter than its cousin, but both are astringent, cool, dry, relaxing and restorative.

Consider scullcap as a modulator of life energy and flow, useful when emotions and body feel stuck. It combines well with California poppy for nerve and muscle tension.

But while relaxing the nervous tension, it revives and fortifies the central nervous system. It is a specific for seizures and epilepsy, and combines well with cow's parsnip green seeds for sciatica, TMJ and facial pains. In recent years, it has been found scutellarin stimulates the absorption of the important vitamin niacin (B3).

Zhang et al[815], identified 10 flavonoids and 2 phenyl ethanoid glycosides showing anticonvulsant activity, and acute seizure amelioration in a rodent model.

Scullcap plays an important role in regulating the balance of adrenaline and noradrenalin, a hormonal function that can often appear as a nervous disorder. This may explain, in part, its usefulness, in reducing PMS symptoms.

It encourages the brain to produce endorphins, promoting sleep, while easing worry and anxiety.

It may be useful when experiencing anxiety and agitation while taking or withdrawing from entheogens, such as marijuana, psilobin and other psychoactive substances.

Scullcap is useful in the motor symptoms associated with Sydenham's chorea (formerly known as St. Vitus's dance) and nerve pain associated with the early stages of multiple sclerosis.

It may have application in anorexia nervosa, mild cases of Tourette syndrome (TS), and pain associated with fibromyalgia. In children with ADHD it is useful for irritability, repetitive movements, and outbursts of anger. For TS, it may be helpful for tremors, nervous tics and muscular spasms.

Scutellarein, wogonin, baicalein, and baicalin all contain phenyl benzopyrone nuclei, and bind to the benzodiazepine site of the GABA receptor.[816]

Baicalein is a potent inhibitor of GABA transaminase, and scutellarein inhibits succinic semialdehyde dehydrogenase; both of which increase GABA levels in the brain.[817]

Scutellarin, a related compound, possesses estrogenic and neuroprotective properties. This suggests benefit in post-menopausal symptoms as well as Alzheimer's disease (AD), due to *in vitro* inhibition of beta amyloid, and prevention of brain neuron cell death.

Scutellarein assists the brain to produce more endorphins and thereby enhance awareness and calmness. This suggests its use in panic attacks, stress-induced headaches and emotional trauma.[818]

Baicalin and Baicalein show potent inhibition of amyloid B protein-induced neurotoxicity, suggesting possible use in AD.[819]

Baicalin is transformed into baicalein by our intestinal bacteria, then absorbed in the intestine, and conjugated back into baicalin in blood plasma.[820]

Baicalin may protect dopaminergic neurons and increase brain dopamine levels, suggesting a novel, effective treatment for ADHD.[821]

Baicalein appears to protect and possibly treat Parkinson's disease.[822], and rescues synaptic plasticity and memory deficits in a mouse model of AD.[823]

It inhibits prolyl-oligopeptidase, associated with bipolar, schizophrenia and other related neuro-disorders.[824]

It appears to be a potent inhibitor of alpha synuclein, protects SH-SY5Y cells, and amyloid beta peptide induced toxicity in PC12 cells, suggesting benefit in both Alzheimer's and Parkinson's disease.

DOSE- 20-30 drops up to three times daily of fresh tincture prepared at 1:4 and 60% alcohol. Dried tincture is 1:5 at 45%.

NOTE: I have found the fresh plant tincture vastly superior to dry herb, whether in tincture, capsule or tea form.

CAUTION- Long-term use has been found to diminish sexual desire in males. Do not combine with blood-thinners or used during pregnancy. Curcumin, derived from tumeric root inhibits the absorption of baicalein.[825] Do not use concurrently.

Sensitive Plant (*Mimosa pudica*) is a semi-tropical leguminous shrub or tree, so named for folding its leaves when touched or at night for protection. In Ayurvedic medicine it is known as *Iajjalu* and mainly used for the management of type 2 diabetes.

The whole plant, both *in vitro* and *in vivo*, reduces LPS-induced pro-inflammatory mediators, confirming its traditional use for the prevention of inflammation.

Like passionflower, it contains vitexin that modulates cholinergic receptors, thus enhancing memory.[826]

The leaves, in a mouse study, possess anti-anxiety, anti-depressant and memory-enhancing activities. Dopamine and norepinephrine levels increased after only four weeks, and inhibition of acetylcholinesterase was noted.[827]

Another rodent study found the herb ameliorated cadmium-induced testicular damage, including regeneration of sperm count.[828] Its benefit on removing this heavy metal from humans has not been confirmed.

Alpha-glucosidase inhibition is comparable to acarbose, suggesting possible benefit in the management of diabetes.[829]

The content of myoinositol in the stems could play a role in glucose disposal into adipose tissue, and could have application in the treatment of obesity-associated type 2 diabetes mellitus.[830]

A recent product on the market is derived from the fat-soluble seed, and its sticky nature. The powder is taken in capsule form and opens in the intestine where its sticky texture helps remove parasites, bacterial fungal biofilm, and reportedly, heavy metals from the body. The product is taken at least one hour apart from food.

Sour Jujube or Sour Date (*Zizyphus jujuba* var. *spinosa*) seed is used in TCM for reducing anxiety, and helping with irritability and insomnia. It is known as *Suan Zao Ren*. The seeds modulate GABAergic activity and the serotonergic system.[831]

Moreover, the anxiolytic effects of an isolate of the seed, was comparable to diazepam, without the reduced locomotor activity.[832]

Seed tinctures ameliorate the memory deficits in Alzheimer's disease model mice, by regulating plasmin activity.[833]

DOSE- 10-30 drops twice daily of 1:5 seed tincture.

Tridax Daisy (*Tridax procumbens***)**

The naturally occurring flavone, 7,8-dihydroxyflavone (DHF) is found in the Tridax Daisy, a perennial native to Mexico and south, but invasive to temperate zones of America, including South Carolina, Florida, and as far north as Massachusetts.

It is a potent and selective molecule against of the main signaling receptor for brain derived neurotropic factor. It crosses the blood-brain barrier (BBB) and has shown promise in a wide variety of brain disorders including depression, Alzheimer's[834] disease, schizophrenia[835], Parkinson's disease[836], Huntington's disease[837], autism[838], epilepsy[839], ALS[840], diabetic glucose brain toxicity[841] and lead poisoning[842]. It protects against glutamate-induced[843] and methamphetamine-induced dopaminergic neurotoxicity[844].

Turmeric (*Curcuma longa***)** is a tropical plant related to ginger. The rhizome contains curcumin, which has numerous anti-inflammatory, anti-oxidant and neurotropic uses. It is, however, poorly soluble and bio-available even in most oil soluble forms.

One DB, PC study of 40 subjects with a bioavailable form of curcumin found improved memory and attention. The findings suggest symptom benefits were associated with decreases in amyloid plaque and tau accumulation.[845]

Curcumin binds up copper, inhibits acetylcholinesterase, and mediates the insulin-signaling pathway.[846]

Curcumin inhibits amyloid peptide-induced expression and may help ameliorate the inflammation and progression of Alzheimer's disease.[847]

A randomized, controlled study of curcumin effects on schizophrenia involving 36 patients, over 8 weeks, found it improved levels of brain neuron growth factor (BNGF).[848]

A randomized, DB, PC trials of 70 women with PMS ran for three months; capsules for seven days before menstruation and for three days after. The curcumin group symptoms were significantly less than placebo and possibly mediated through enhanced serum brain-derived neurotrophic factor.[849]

A new product on the market contains 95% tetrahydro-curcuminoids, and advertisements claim a 92% absorption rate. Make sure to take curcumin supplements with fats and oils for increased absorption. There are a wide variety of companies, all claiming their form is the most bioavailable. Theracurmin is one product that appears well absorbed in blood level studies.

DOSE- One to four capsules daily of a 20:1 turmeric extract.

CAUTION- The herb should be avoided, or used with caution by those with gall bladder inflammation or stone formation. Excessive use may increase iron deficiency anemia.[850]

Valerian (*Valeriana officinalis***)**

Valerian is derived from Latin VALERE, "to be healthy", VALOR for courage, or VALEO, "to be strong." Some authors suggest it may be named after Valeria, a part of Hungary, where *V. officinalis* grows wild. Others claim it is named after the Roman Emperor, Valerius Cordus. The Swedish name VÄNDELROT, refers to the plants used by Teutons, known as Vandals.

Valerian root has a tranquillizing and calmative effect on the central nervous system. This is useful in convulsions, fevers, and insomnia; in many cases halving the time to initially fall asleep.

It does not, however, interfere with activity and coordination in the manner of a true sedative, such as Wild Lettuce, but does reduce excessive surrounding noises that agitate when stressed out.

It is fundamentally a nerve and brain tonic, restoring memory, strengthening the spinal nerves and improving vision. In Germany, over 100 OTC sleep aids contain valerian, some especially formulated for children.

As a neuro-cardiac sedative, valerian root relieves anxiety states, but is useful in depression brought on by chronic stress. The herb is useful for overly sensitive individuals, and those who start choking or coughing as they start to fall asleep. It is somewhat grounding to individuals who feel they are floating in air in their sleep, or easily disrupted by light and sound.

Alcohol preparations contain more isovaltrate and are inverse agonists of adenosine A1 receptors, with CNS stimulating activity. Water extracts, on the other hand stimulate adenosine A1 receptors, bringing a sedative effect.

It is the perfect remedy for chronic stress and illness affecting the heart and nerves, or where fatigue and tension are present. It will promote rest and sleep when there is exhaustion, and when a person needs to recuperate. With extreme fatigue and exhaustion from severe, chronic, long-lasting stress however, it may act as a stimulant if taken in large amounts.

When first taking valerian, some people complain of feeling exhausted. What they are experiencing is relaxation- something foreign to the over-wrought and uptight individual. This will pass in a day or two, and they will sleep well and rise easily from bed.

Due to the affinity of valerian extracts and valepotriates with GABA and benzodiazepine receptors sites, the herb may help in programs for withdrawal from Valium and related diazepam drugs. Valerian has been shown to inhibit the production of an enzyme that breaks down GABA, which regulates and inhibits neuron activity. Hydroxy-valerenic and acetoxy-valerenic acid help prevent the breakdown of GABA. Valerian also increases the sensitivity of GABA receptor sites.

Another possibility is binding of valerian ligands to glutamate receptors.[851] Lipophilic fractions and didrovaltrate show affinity for barbiturate receptors.

Another possible mechanism of action is lignan (+)-hydroxypinoresinol, that shows high affinity for the $5\text{-}HT1_a$ receptor, suggesting serotonin involvement. Tricyclic N-(p-hydroxyphenethyl) actinidine is an acetylcholinesterase inhibitor, suggesting another possible mode of activity.

By inhibiting the breakdown of GABA, the increased neural activity preceding epileptic seizure may be moderated or prevented. Valerian, passion flower and scullcap are often useful in the prevention of seizure activity.

Valerenic acid inhibits enzymatic breakdown of GABA, and low levels of herbal extracts enhance benzodiazepine binding.

Valerian modulates cortical excitatory circuits in our brains, based on a DB, PC, randomized, cross-over study of 15 volunteers.[852]

Valerian root may be useful in some cases of obsessive-compulsive disorder. An eight- week randomized double-blind trial of 31 adults suffering OCD found significant benefit.[853]

Patients on dialysis suffer cognitive disorders twice the general population. A cross-over DB trial of 30 patients found valerian root improved their cognitive scores.[854]

Determining valerian dosage is tricky. The problem with high doses of Valerian is that there is an equal chance of producing the opposite effect, such as excitation, headache, and vision disturbance. Valerian is unpredictable and variable, especially in the dried form. A qualified herbalist or naturopath can help determine the best dosage.

Valerian should not be taken with any sleep inducing drugs, or barbiturates as it may potentiate their activity.

If you have low blood pressure, and/or sensitive liver and sluggish bile ducts, then Valerian may not be the herb for you. It tends to stimulate bile flow, and initiate more bile production, and thus cause nausea and stomach distress. In those individuals with low thyroid function, whether sub-clinical or not, valerian can be stimulating in larger quantities.

For those individuals suffering depression, it may not be your herb, unless combined with stimulating plant medicines.

It may, however, enhance the action of hops, California poppy, skullcap, lemon balm or vervain.

DOSE- Both the tea and tincture are unpleasant tasting to most people, in which case look for product standardized to 0.8% valerenic acids. Start at low dose and increase as needed.

CHAPTER 17

MEDICINAL MUSHROOMS

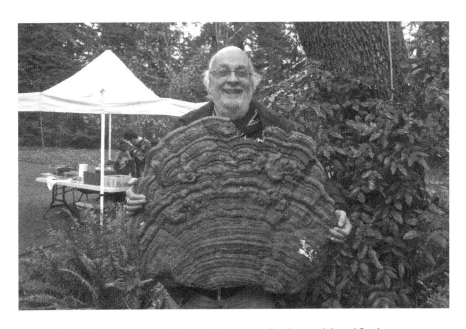

Over 5 million species of fungi have so far been identified on our planet, but only 600 have been seriously studied for medicinal benefit.

Nearly all the macrofungi mentioned in this chapter help reduce inflammation in the mind and body; and modulate the immune system.

Auto-immune conditions respond well to medicinal mushrooms due to their ability to up-regulate the immune system when deficient, or down-regulate whenever there is inflammation and the destruction of tissue.

All mushrooms contain various amounts of ergothioneine, a powerful anti-oxidant and anti-inflammatory compound.

Mushrooms and their isolated compounds reduce beta-amyloid neurotoxicity, inhibit acetylcholinesterase, stimulate neurite outgrowth, encourage nerve growth factor synthesis, and provide brain protection. They contain the unique sugar, trehalose that may be useful for Huntington's and Parkinson's disease.

The optimizing of immune function and reduction of inflammation in the body may be one of the keys to longevity and increased quality of life.

A study of dietary patterns and risk of Parkinson's disease suggests a high intake of vegetables, seaweed, pulses, fruit, fish and mushrooms may help decrease the progression.[855]

A number of edible mushrooms contain compounds with positive benefit on brain cells, both *in vitro* and *in vivo*. [856]

A recent study in Singapore of 663 seniors compared those eating mushrooms less than once a week, and those eating at least two portions. All other life-style associations were accounted for, and a direct correlation between mushroom consumption and delayed neurodegeneration was observed.[857]

Here are a few of the more recent studies on brain health and medicinal mushrooms. For readers interested in more information they can read *The Fungal Pharmacy* published by the author in 2011.[858]

For medicinal mushroom combinations related to specific brain health concerns, consult a practitioner with expertise.

Button mushrooms, including crimini and portobello (*Agaricus bisporus*) are found in every grocery store. Many are still subject to fungicides, so look carefully to ensure you are buying organic product. Many people still consume them raw in salads. This should be discouraged as they contain agaritine, a cumulative toxin. And besides, edible mushrooms taste much better sautéed in a little butter or coconut oil. The active compounds are not heat labile so nearly all mushrooms should be cooked.

One study found button mushrooms exhibit acetylcholinesterase inhibitory activity, suggesting a healthy dietary addition for preventing and treating senile dementia, and AD.

Portabella, button and shiitake mushrooms up-regulate IL-23 associated with colitis.[859]

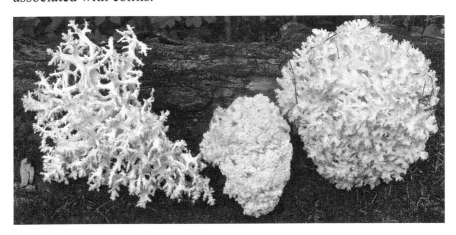

Lion's Mane (*Hericium erinaceus*) has been studied for its possible benefit in the treatment of brain and nerve-related conditions.[860] The ability of small molecules to cross the blood brain barrier and induce production of nerve growth factor is indeed, an exciting possibility for further research.

Various compounds, including water soluble hericenones and erinacines, have been found to induce synthesis of nerve growth factor (NGF) which is required by the brain for developing and maintaining important sensory neurons. These low molecular weight compounds travel through the blood-brain barrier intact. Erinacine A may be one of the most powerful, natural compounds yet identified that induces NGF.

Neurite outgrowth of brain, spinal cord and retinal cells has been observed in laboratory studies.

A study of one hundred patients in a Japanese rehab hospital looked at the effects of five grams of lion's mane powder or placebo for six months. There was significant benefit, in six of the seven patients identified with cognitive impairment.

317

In 2009, a study of twenty-nine patients aged fifty to eighty years old, with mild cognitive problems showed significant improvement a double-blind, placebo-controlled trial, at eight, twelve and sixteen weeks.[861]

Thirty women, suffering menopausal symptoms including sleep deprivation, depression and other complaints were given hericium or placebo cookies for four weeks. Four different subjective, clinical index scales were taken before and after. Concentration, irritation and anxiety tended to be lower than placebo group.[862]

Erinacin E is a highly selective agonist of kappa opioid receptor, and may relieve pain without the side effects associated with agonists such as morphine.

Lion's mane may have significant benefit in a wide range of neurological conditions, including prevention and/ or treatment of Parkinson's disease, Alzheimer's disease, depression, and various neuromuscular conditions.

Both erinacine A and S lessen AD pathology by reducing amyloid deposition and promoting neurogenesis. Erinacine A inhibits amyloid beta production.[863]

It is sure to be part of functional foods in the near future, to help maintain brain and nerve health.

The mushroom acts as a prebiotic, helping to grow and maintain healthy bacteria in the microbiome.

It is important to note that oven-dried Hericium products lose the ability to stimulate neurite outgrowth.

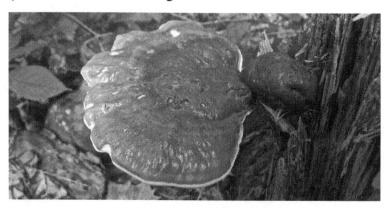

Reishi (*Ganoderma lucidum*) has been reported to encourage neurite growth and improve neuronal health benefits.

Reishi extracts contain neuro-active compounds that induce neuronal differentiation and prevent apoptosis (self-programmed death) of cells, albeit in a rat study.[864]

Various ganoderma species calm the spirit, a property known for thousands of years by Daoist monks.

Work by Phan et al[865] found water extracts of reishi, *Lignosus rhinocerotis, Grifola frondosa*, and ethanol extracts of *Cordyceps militaris* significantly promote brain neurite growth, and may be useful for brain and cognitive health.

Reishi and Hen of the Woods (*G. frondosa*) water extracts have been shown to promote nerve growth factor.[866]

A novel randomized DB, PC clinical study looked at children aged 3-5 years old. They were given either yogurt, or yogurt enriched with beta-glucans from reishi. The latter group showed significant improvement in lymphocyte counts, immunoglobulin A and natural killer cell counts.[867]

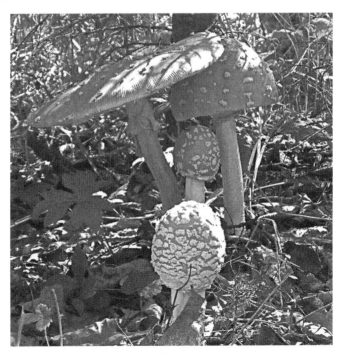

Fly Agaric (*Amanita muscaria*) is a favorite of photographers, and presented as the home of a hookah-smoking caterpillar conversing with Alice, in Wonderland. The yellow, orange or red cap with white spots, associated with flying reindeer led some authors to speculate about the mythology of Santa Claus. In Norse mythology, Odin rode an eight-legged horse that traveled the nine worlds of the gods, giants, elves and the underworld. The mushrooms are dried in looping bows by the fireplace, reminiscent of today's seasonal garlands. And of course, Santa climbs down the chimney, in the reverse manner of shaman climbing down yurt poles in Kamchatka.

Not to mention mischievous little elves making gifts for people.

The books, *Magic Mushrooms* by Carl Heinrich, and *Mushrooms in Christian Art* by John A. Rush, contain hundreds of medieval and Middle age photographs of paintings and tapestries linking the consumption of this mushroom with spiritual enlightenment. In many cases, the mushroom representations are quite obvious, once the association is made.

Two compounds, ibotenic acid, and muscimol target GABA receptors in the brain. Or more accurately, ibotenic acid activates NMDA (N-methyl-D-aspartic acid) receptors, and muscimol is a $GABA_a$ (gamma-amino-butryic acid A) agonist.

This disturbance allows glutamate and acetylcholine to dominate, thus increasing states of anxiety, sweating, drowsiness, and visual and auditory hallucinations. GABA is a neurotransmitter and NMDA is a glutamate receptor involved in learning, affecting the amygdala of our brain. Inactivation in the brain by these two substances inhibits fear response.

In clinical practice I kept files on 24 individuals suffering from Parkinson's disease and tremor. I observed eighteen clients (75%) experience total or partial relief of tremors, using a homeopathic preparation of the mushroom. It is drinkable ampoule available from holistic pharmacies under the name Agaricus-Injeel forte.

The related Caesar (*Amanita caesarea*) is a choice edible. It contains polysaccharides that show possible benefit in Alzheimer's disease, including improvement in cholingeric system. The sugars suppress beta-amyloid deposition and reduce oxidative stress by modulating levels of related enzymes.[868]

The Honey mushroom (*Armillaria ostoyae*) living in eastern Oregon is considered the largest living organism in the world. It covers over 880 hectares, and may be 2500 years old. The mycelium and rhizomorphs glow a blue-green phosphorescence, that exhibits maximum intensity around 7:30 p.m. Radiation from honey mushrooms will pass through cardboard and develop photographic plates.

Mycelium extracts show neuroprotective protection and treatment, reducing amyloid beta deposition and oxidative damage associated with Alzheimer's disease in one animal study.[869]

Honey mushroom exhibits anti-epileptic effect both *in vitro* and *in vivo*.[870]

King Bolete (*Boletus edulis*), also known as porcini, cepe and penny bun, is the most prized edible mushrooms around the world.

Both water and alcohol extracts inhibit the impulse of neurons. The mycelium contains 1274 mg/kg of GABA (gamma aminobutyric acid) that regulates nerve excitability and inhibits neurotransmitters. It reduces hypertension by affecting the activity of angiotensin-1-converting enzyme.[871]

Shaggy Mane (*Coprinus comatus*) is widespread, and deliquesces into inky mass when mature.

An extract of the fruiting body exhibits potent anti-acetylcholinesterase activity, comparable to the drug donepezil.[872]

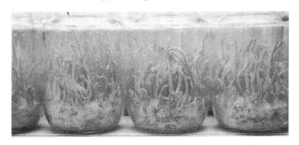

Cordyceps (*Cordyceps militaris*) fruiting bodies promote neurite growth, suggesting support in brain and cognitive health.

Cordycepin up-regulates brain derived neurotrophic factor (BDNF), and down-regulates serotonin levels and inflammation in the hippocampus, suggesting possible benefit in depression.[873]

Adenosine and cordycepin are closely related components in cordyceps fruiting bodies. Adenosine shows potential for the prevention and treatment of neurodegenerative disorders, related to glutamate oxidative stress.[874] The fruiting bodies contain trehalose.

Enoki (*Flammulina velutipes*) is easily found in grocery stores; identified by its bright white color and elongated stipes. Polysaccharides given to AD rats showed significantly improved cognitive ability after treatment.[875]

Birch Polypore (*Fomitopsis betulina*) fruiting body and mycelium contains compounds that reduce fatigue and soothe the mind. It can be thinly sliced, dried and added to smoking mixtures for relaxation. This may be due, in part, to content of various indole compounds, including L-tryptophan, 5-hydroxy-L-tryptophan and 5-methyltryptamine.[876]

Chaga (*Inonotus obliquus*)

Chaga is a sterile conk found on birch trees. It is presently being over-harvested and used by many people as a recreational beverage. It has great potential as a medicinal mushroom, but has yet to undergo a single human clinical trial.

One mouse study suggests methanol extracts significantly improve cognitive enhancement through anti-oxidant activity and inhibition of acetylcholinesterase.[877]

Polysaccharides from chaga show protective effects against AD, via modulation of oxidative stress, particularly NF-E2p45-related factor 2 signaling and reducing the deposition of beta-amyloid peptides and neuronal tangles induced phosphor-Tau in the brain.[878]

It contains oxalic acid that may precipitate kidney stones. Individuals taking blood thinners have noted sloughing of the mucus membranes in mouth and throat.

One of my favorite edible mushrooms *Lactarius deliciosus* is easily identified as it bleeds orange latex that soon turns green. It has a nutty flavor. The fruiting body contains tryptamine, tryptophan and melatonin, suggesting benefit for insomnia.

More research is warranted.

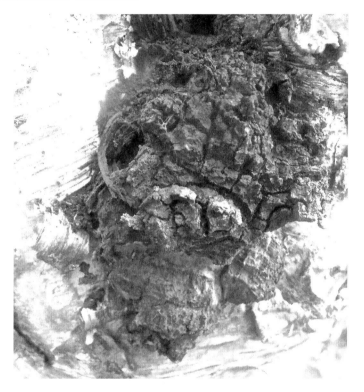

Oyster (*Pleurotus ostreatus*) mushroom polysaccharides may be helpful in AD due to alleviation of cognitive impairment, albeit in a rat model. Acetylcholinesterase activity was reduced, as well as formation of beta-amyloid peptides and tau phosphorylation.[879]

Parasol (*Macrolepiota procera*) mushroom is a choice edible and rich source of 5-hydroxytryptophan (5HTP), a widely used amino acid supplement for depression, sleep and migraine and tension type headaches. It is the precursor to serotonin, and generally sourced from the seed of *Griffonia simplicifolia*.

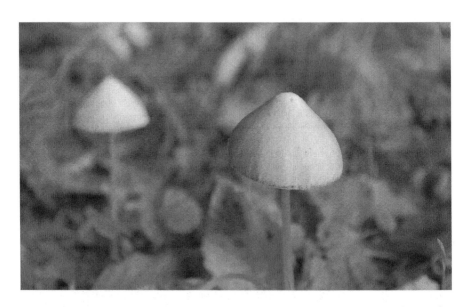

Psilocybe species

Various Psilocybe species have been utilized around the world as an entheogen by shaman, and other wisdom seekers. The noted Terence McKenna suggested human ancestors on the savannah of Africa may have sought out and ingested these entheogenic mushrooms, which increased their visual acuity, making them better hunters, and increased their lateral thought processes in the brain. Maybe.

In the mid 1950s, modern science identified psilocybin mushrooms in southern Mexico. Albert Hofmann, the Swiss scientist that discovered LSD, identified psilocybin and psilocyin in 1958. The chemical structure is similar to serotonin.

Life magazine published an article *Seeking the Magic Mushroom*, by Gordon Wasson in 1957, detailing his ingestion of psilocybin, two years earlier, during a ceremony conducted by María Sabina. It did not take long for beatniks and hippies, including celebrities like Bob Dylan, John Lennon and Mick Jagger to find their way to Sabina's small village.

This led to the widespread recreational use of the mushrooms by adolescents and young adults. At last count there are some 180 species of mushrooms, containing this compound, not all in the *Psilocybe* genera.

Moving ahead nearly fifty years, Roland Griffiths published a paper on a small clinical trial of 36 volunteers and the spiritual significance of psilocin ingestion.[880] This opened the door for another study in the same year, showing 22 of 26 patients suffering cluster headaches benefited from extended remissions.

Dr. Grob wrote several papers on the psychological benefit of treating anxiety in advanced stage cancer patients.[881]

Four randomized, controlled trials published between 2011 and 2014 found entheogenic assisted treatment can produce robust, and sustained improvements in cancer-related psychological and existential distress.

Other studies have followed looking at the benefits of psilocin for depression, post-traumatic stress disorder (PTSD), obsessive-compulsive disorder (OCD), and various addictions related to tobacco, and alcohol. At last count there have been three controlled trials suggesting psilocybin may decrease symptoms of anxiety and depression.

After psilobyin ingestion, cortisol levels spike and activate the executive control network of the brain, with subsequent increased control over emotional processes, and relief of negative thinking and persistent negative emotions.

Psychological support and psilocybin might support pessimism biases in treatment-resistant depression.

Work in England has found the mushrooms create a still point, allowing the brain to reset itself.[882] This may explain, in part, the benefits found with PTSD.

The mushrooms have a low risk of toxicity and dependence and can be very useful under controlled clinical settings. For some individuals, the benefits are best enjoyed out with nature.

Activation of serotonin receptor agonists produces potent anti-inflammatory effect via novel mechanisms; suggesting new potential benefits. A new study has found psilocybin appears to promote emotional empathy, with potential in the treatment of dysfunctional social cognition. Another study found it revives emotional responsiveness in depression, enabling patients to reconnect with their emotions.

A small trial of fifteen patients with treatment-resistant depression showed a change in personality, attitude and optimism.[883]

A vote on de-criminalizing psilocybin (Initiative 301) was held in Denver, Colorado on May 7, 2019. It narrowly passed with 50.56% support. Oakland, California soon followed.

Today, the practice of micro-dosing has been popularized for anxiety and depression, albeit no clinical trials have been conducted to date. Micro-dosing involves the ingestion of one-tenth the normal dose of an entheogenic journey, to sharpen the mind and relieve anxiety and depression. The psychologist James Fadiman introduced the idea a decade ago, and it soon became popular with productivity hacks in Silicon Valley's high tech community. A small study in the Netherlands of 38 participants found micro-dosing allowed for creation of more out-of-the-box alternative solutions, and improvement in the convergent thinking elements of creativity.

Caution: Individuals with genetic pre-disposition to schizophrenia, bi-polar and other related issues should not ingest these mushrooms.

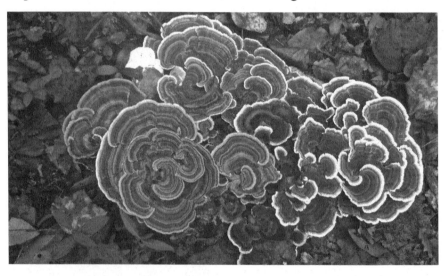

Turkey Tail (*Trametes versicolor*)

Turkey Tail is one of the most important medicinal mushrooms, with a wide variety of benefit in cancer, and various auto-immune conditions.

Turkey tail fruiting bodies and mycelium are effective inhibitors of acetylcholinesterase, suggesting anti-neurodegenerative activity. A recent study found it promotes a significant increase in dendritic length and branching, as well as total dendritic volume of immature neurons. This suggests a positive effect on hippocampal neurogenic reserve, and possible benefit in various human neurological conditions.

Polysaccharides from the mushroom may be a useful adjunctive therapy for the relief of morphine tolerance via activation of the cannabinoid type 2 receptor.[884]

Poria (*Wolfiporia cocos*) is a tuber-like mushroom used extensively in traditional Chinese medicine (TCM). Low alcohol tinctures provide memory promotion function, inhibit neuron cytotoxicity induced by beta-amyloid, and increase the expression of acetylcholine synthetase and muscarinic acetylcholine receptor in hippocampus.

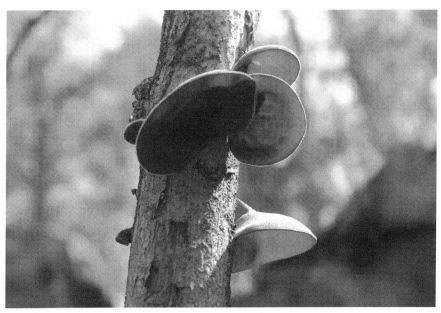

Wood Ear (*Auricularia polytricha*)

Wood Ear mushrooms, as water extracts, show anti-epileptic action against both electroshock and isoniazid induced seizures in mice.[885]

The mushroom is used in hot and sour soups, and has been shown to be a natural blood-thinner, and therefore contraindicated concurrently with warfarin and Coumadin.

The pharmaceutical drug Antabuse was developed from coprine, found in Inky Cap (*Coprinopsis atramentarius*) mushroom. The drug works by a violent form of aversion therapy, due to its ability to shut down liver enzymes involved in the breakdown of alcohol. It has saved lives. Caution is advised.

CHAPTER 18

HOMEOPATHY AND CELL SALTS

Homeopathy is a natural form of medicine used by over 200 million people worldwide. It is based on the principle of similar cures similar, and very small amounts will cure symptoms caused by ingesting larger amounts of the same substance. It is not placebo, but is under continuous attack by biomedicine critics for being "unscientific." The Gold standard of double-blind, placebo-controlled trials is cited as the only proof of efficacy, and yet numerous pharmaceuticals pass this standard, receive FDA or Health Canada approval, go to market and are later recalled, along with huge class action lawsuits when people begin dying.[886]

Hippocrates, the Father of Medicine, suggested above all do no harm.

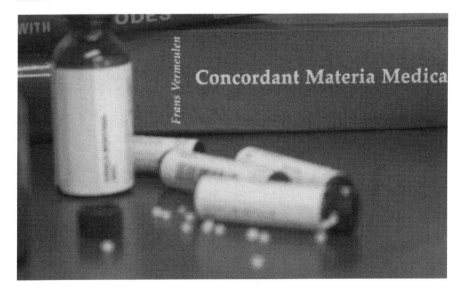

I shared office space with Dr. Robert Pearman ND for eight years. He was well versed in prescribing homeopathy, and I learned pretty much all I know under his tutelage.

Biomedicine and science in general have great difficulty with the concept of energetic medicine. Vibrational medicine, due to its subtle energetic influence on cellular health, is difficult to measure with yesterday's technology.

How can such dilute products influence cellular function?

Highly recommended viewings are *The Message of Water*[887] by *Emoto* and the 2004 film called *What the Bleep Do We Know*, both of which explain the new world of quantum physics in lay terms.

A book I also highly recommend is *Vibrational Medicine*, third edition, by Dr. Richard Gerber.

One study looked at 1562 patients with anxiety or depression. Those choosing to consult homeopaths reported less use of psychotrophic drugs and were marginally more likely to experience clinical improvement over those managed with conventional care.[888]

A study was conducted on 110 seniors (aged 65-93), with 87 suffering anxiety and depressive disorders. Those who used homeopathy were found more likely to have clinical improvement after 12 months than those in the conventional medicine or mixed prescriptions group.[889]

A randomized, PC, DB, double-dummy, superiority, three-arm trial of 133 peri- and postmenopausal women with major depression, found the homeopathic group had better outcomes than drug or placebo.[890]

A number of studies showing the benefit of homeopathy for depression, anxiety disorder, and addiction, along with psychiatric counseling, was recently published, albeit in German.[891]

One RCT study compared homeopathy to fluoxetine for moderate to severe depression, with favorable results.[892]

Several European countries are leading the way with integration of homeopathy and complementary medicine in the public-funded healthcare systems.

Generally speaking, the lower potencies from 6-12X are better for treating physical symptoms and higher (30-200X) potencies for mental and emotional issues. Consult your local homeopath for more definitive recommendations.

Cell Salts

The 12 Schuessler Cell Salts are available in 6X potency. I used them with good success in clinical practice. They can do no harm, and are often very useful adjuncts when treating brain health.

The following very brief descriptions are derived from a well-known homeopathic book that I have consulted for nearly fifty years.[893]

ALZHEIMER'S DISEASE

Alumina is useful when loss of memory is associated with confusion over personal identity. Decision-making is difficult, with mistakes in writing and speech. Time passes slowly. It may help the chronic constipation suffered by those with PD.

Anacardium is helpful for more immediate forgetfulness, related to what they have just seen or heard. Hallucinations, with patient thinking they are possessed of two persons or wills. Anxiety when they walking, as if being pursued. Suspicious, and lack confidence.

It helps those with impaired memory, depression and irritability, as well as diminished sight, smell and hearing. Irresistible desire to swear and curse, associated with Tourette syndrome.

Sulphur is for those who are very forgetful, or have difficulty thinking clearly. This type is nearly always irritable, depressed, thin and weak. A tell-tale symptom is a constant heat emanating from the top of head, and itch of skin made worse from heat of bed. Standing is difficult, and they may have aversion to being washed. Child-like peevishness may be present in grown adults.

Mercurius is indicated in the later stages, where care and attention to personal hygiene has declined. Slow in answering questions, and think they are losing reason. They can be mistrustful and weary of life. Tremors and trembling.

Calcarea Carb helps in cases of forgetfulness, slow mental processing and the inability to retain or process information. Apprehension toward evening, fear loss of reason or misfortune. They suffer an aversion to work or any exertion.

The 6X potency is a cell salt.

ANXIETY

Arsenicum album is a great remedy when exhaustion is combined with anxiety. There may be fear of death, or being left alone. Clients may think taking any medicine is useless. It may be helpful to those addicted to alcohol or nicotine. Hallucinations of sight and smell are often present. Sensitivity to disorder and confusion.

Kali phosphoricum (Kali Phos) is indicated in cases of anxiety, nervous exhaustion and fear. Extreme lassitude, hysteria and depression are often present. They are very nervous, and startle easily. Night terrors and loss of memory may be part of picture. Kali Phos is one of the great nerve remedies.

The 6X potency is a cell salt.

DEPRESSION

Aurum metallicum (Gold) helps alleviate feelings of worthlessness, low self-esteem and despair. It is most beneficial for people with high ideals, or lofty goals that experience life-changing experiences, and then feel they have failed. They may talk of suicide. Patients may suffer from hypertension.

Natrium muraticum (Nat Mur) Common Table Salt helps relieve depression associated with shock or grief. They may believe they have to be strong and controlled for other people. They can be irritable and get passionate about small matters. Thyroid or adrenal dysregulation may be involved. Tears do not come easily.

The 6X potency is a cell salt.

Pulsatilla is useful for those who are changeable like an April day. It may be useful in depressed side of bipolar conditions. They may weep easily or suffer religious melancholy. They like sympathy, but fear to be alone, in the dark, with the opposite sex, or fear ghosts. They are given to extremes of pain and pleasure.

Conium is for depression and fear, with mental confusion much worse after the loss of spouse, and the fear of being alone. It helps one to focus, concentrate and regain memory associated with grief. May suffer vertigo when lying down. Insomnia and trembling may be present.

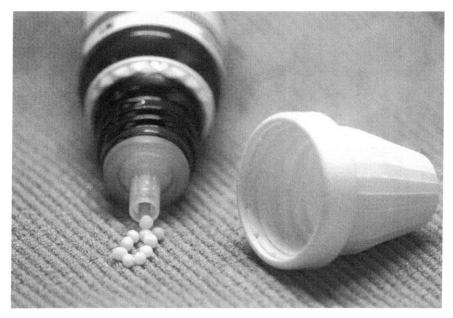

MEMORY

Nux moschata (Nutmeg) is useful when thoughts suddenly vanish while writing. They may appear absentminded and experience irresistible drowsiness. Think they have two heads.

Baryta carbonica is useful for memory loss associated with recent events. Senile dementia. Loss of confidence may be present, with child-like upset over trivial events. Brain feels loose.

Lycopodium is for loss of memory due to anxiety or depression. They are extremely sensitive and may suffer from loss of self-confidence. They have a weak memory and constantly fear breaking down under stress. Spelling and words are difficult.

Argentum nitricum is for those suffering long continual mental exertion. Myelitis and sclerosis of the brain and spinal cord are present. They tend to be fearful and nervous, with weak memory and errors of perception.

Thuja is a constitutional remedy useful for individuals who have difficulty finding the right words, or suffer other speech disorders related to left-brain dysfunction. The appearance of skin growths on the left side of body may help guide one to this important remedy.

PARKINSON'S DISEASE

Agaricus muscaria (*Amanita muscaria*)- for reduction of tremors of Parkinson's disease. See Medicinal Mushroom chapter.

Gelsemium provides relief from anxiety, trembling and loss of muscular control. Fatigue after slight exercise. There is a desire to be left alone, with an apathy regarding their illness. They will often startle awake at night, perhaps accompanied by screaming. I have used it for *Myasthenia gravis* with moderate success.

Rhus toxicodendron (Poison Ivy) helps limbs that are stiff and feel paralyzed. Cold air makes them worse. Trembling worse after exertion. Loss of power in hands and finger tips.

Heel is a well-known homeopathic company located in Baden-Baden, Germany. My wife and I enjoyed a pleasant day at the hot springs in the town, during our honeymoon.

They produce single remedies, but what I like about the company is the well-researched combinations, for various health conditions.

A few related to brain health that I found worked extremely well were *Psorinoheel* for endogenous depression or schizoid disorders, *Nervoheel* for exogenous forms, and *Ignatia Hommacord* for bipolar disorder. My favorite was *Cerebrum compositum* which I found was very effective in many cases of depression, ALS, multiple sclerosis, and Parkinson's disease. In one case, a patient in vegetative dystonia, confined to a hospital bed for three months, awoke less than ten minutes after one dose. Coincidence?

CHAPTER 19

FLOWER ESSENCES,
AND MUSHROOM ESSENCES

Flower and mushroom essences are prepared in sunlight and moonlight respectively. They are vibrational remedies that work on issues related to personality, mental and emotional patterns, and a deep-seated need for spirit and soul re-connection.

Flower essences were introduced and popularized by Dr. Edward Bach in England in the early 1930s. Further study and benefits have spread the benefit of flower essences around the world.

Today, there are numerous excellent flower essence companies around the world, including the *Flower Essence Society* in California and the *English Flower Essence Company* in the UK. The *Australian Bush Flower Essences*, developed by Ian White, are also exceptional.

Laurie, my wife and life partner, and I developed the *Prairie Deva Flower Essences* line some thirty years ago.[894] A recent re-print of the essences is now available on-line.

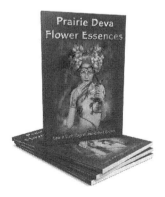
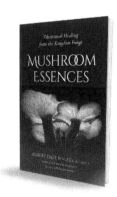

In 2016, I published a book on mushroom essences.[895] This is widely available in bookstores and on-line.

Short versions of their benefits for brain health are included here, with more complete description and uses of the flower and mushroom essences in the two books mentioned above.

Trained flower and mushroom essence practitioners can help individuals with their own personal journey.

ADDICTIONS

Alcohol- Sweet Clover, Dogbane, Water Plantain, Earth Star

Cocaine- Earth Star

Food (Anorexia nervosa, Bulimia)- Wolf Lichen

Nicotine- Nicotiana (FES), Sweet Clover, Earth Star

Opioids- Sweet clover, Earth Star, Cordyceps

Ritalin- Agaricus, Algae Maze

Shopping- Liberty Cap

Television, Video Games – Agaricus

ADHD- Attention Deficit Hyperactivity Disorder- Toadflax, Algae Maze

ALS- Field Bindweed

ALZHEIMER'S DISEASE- Field Bindweed, Comb Tooth

ANXIETY- Field Bindweed, Buckbean, Birch Polypore, Giant Puffball.

ASPERGER'S- Alum

AUTISM SPECTRUM DISORDER- Field Bindweed, Toadflax, Wood Ear

DEPRESSION- Alberta Wild Rose, Green Death Cap, Cinnabar, Birch Polypore, Fly Agaric.

DOPAMINE/SEROTONIN BALANCE- Wolf Lichen

OCD (Obsessive Compulsive Disorder)- Alum, Giant Puffball, Algae Maze

PARKINSON'S DISEASE- Field Bindweed, Fly Agaric

PTSD (Post Traumatic Stress Disorder)- Varnish Conk

SCHIZOPHRENIA- Wood Ear

TOURETTE- Alum

THE ESSENCES

Agaricus mushroom essence is useful for stress-related and fear-based modern illness. It can be useful on its own, or combined with Turkey Tail mushroom essence for addiction to television, computer games, smart phones and other devices.

It may be helpful to weaning off or reducing the use of Ritalin, Adderall and other stimulants, combining well with Algae Maze.

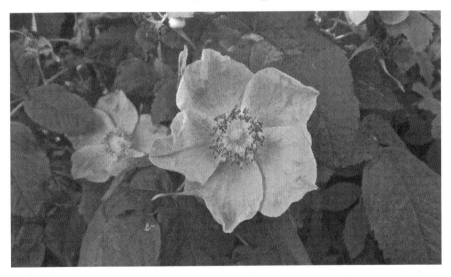

Alberta Wild Rose (*Rosa woodsii*) flower essence is for apathy, depression and issues surrounding long-term low self-esteem.

Algae Maze (*Cerrena unicolor*) mushroom essence helps with obsessive-compulsive disorder (OCD), or attention deficit hyperactivity disorder (ADHD). They appear initially like seeming opposite conditions, but there is often a strong overlap.

It combines well with Earth Star for nicotine addiction, and with Toadflax for ADHD.

Alum (*Heuchera richardsonii*) flower essence is indicated for individuals who feel limited by fixed ideas and behavior. This includes obsessive-compulsive disorders, as well as Aspberger and Tourette syndromes. It combines well with Giant Puffball or Algae Maze mushroom essence.

Birch Polypore (*Fomitopsis betulina*), formally *Piptoporus betulinus*, mushroom essence helps relieve anxiety, melancholy and depression.

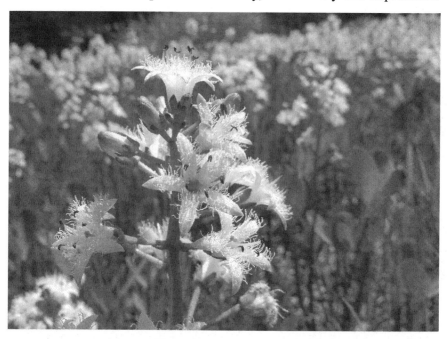

Bogbean/Buckbean (*Menyanthes trifoliata*) flower essence helps maintain a calmness and detachment in the presence of energetics emanating from others. It combines well with Peziza mushroom essence for various neuroses.

Cinnabar (*Pycnoporus cinnabarinus*) mushroom essence is related to issues of impatience, anger, temper and depression.

Comb Tooth (*Hericium coralloides*) mushroom essence is for cellular memory, including Alzheimer's disease.

Cordyceps (*Cordyceps militaris*) mushroom essence helps relieve dizziness, tinnitus and Meniere's disease. It combines well with Earth Star or Liberty Cap for opiate or other narcotic addictions.

Dogbane (*Apocynum androsaemifolium*) flower essence helps ease withdrawal from drugs and alcohol. For addictions to sex or pornography, it combines well with Giant Puffball.

It may help gambling addictions, combined with Liberty Cap.

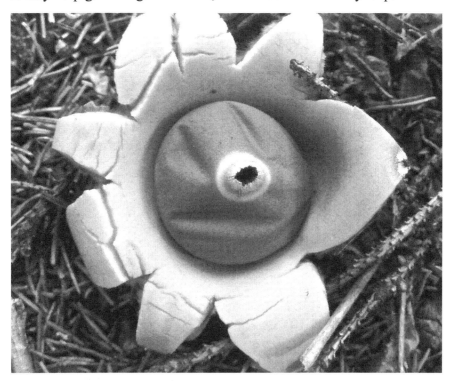

Earth Star (*Geastrum triplex*) mushroom essence is for addressing addictions to alcohol, cannabis, nicotine, heroin, cocaine, opioids and addictive pharmaceuticals. The individual may exhibit a Jekyll-and-Hyde personality.

Field Bindweed (*Convolvolus arvensis*) is related to the human nervous system. Unlike most plants, it turns from the sun in right to left direction (counter-clockwise), and is so insistent that it will choose to die, rather than adapt to the opposite direction.

The flower essence may be useful for various auto-immune conditions such as multiple sclerosis, ALS and myasthenia gravis. It may help in Alzheimer's and Parkinson's disease, as well as autism, combining well with Comb Tooth or Fly Agaric.

Fly Agaric (*Amanita muscaria*) mushroom essence, along with homeopathic dilutions, assists with the tremor of Parkinson's disease. It helps relieve Dupuytren's contracture, and reduce pain associated with various inflammatory joints and muscle pain.

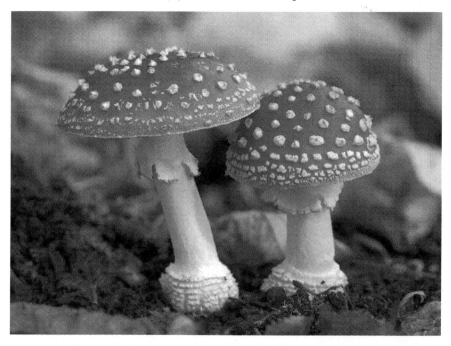

Giant Puffball (*Calvatia booniana*) mushroom essence is for anxiety, obsessive-compulsive disorders, as well as addiction to pornography.

Green Death Cap (*Amanita phalloides*) mushroom essence is for depression and paralysis of the will.

Liberty Cap (*Psilocybe semilanceata*) mushroom essence helps one deal with shopping addiction. In Parkinson's disease, the flood of too much dopamine can create shopping, sex, gambling and other hyperactive addictions.

Sweet Clover (*Melilotus officinalis*) flower essence is useful to those suffering memory loss, dementia and fear associated with brain trauma. This may include recovery from stroke and aneurism. It combines well with Agaricus mushroom essence for helping wean, or cut down Ritalin. It combines well with Dogbane for addictive patterns associated with opiates, tobacco and alcohol.

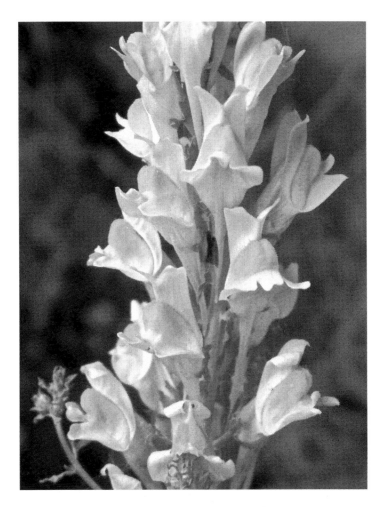

Toadflax (*Linaria vulgaris*) flower essence may help in cases of autism spectrum disorder, or in ADHD. For the latter combine with Algae Maze mushroom essence, and/or Alum flower essence.

For autism, a good combination would include Wood Ear mushroom essence, especially for issues surrounding the ability to listen.

Varnish Conk (*Ganoderma tsugae*) mushroom essence is helpful in cases of post-traumatic stress disorder (PTSD), or for individuals that are free-thinking and non-conformist. It is helpful for the mental illness, recently introduced in new edition of *Diagnostic and Statistical Manual of Mental Disorders* (DSM-5), as oppositional defiant disorder (ODD).

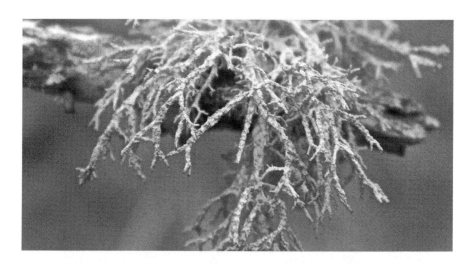

Wolf Lichen (*Letharia vulpina*) essence is for food addiction, or for cases of anorexia nervosa and/or bulimia.

Wood Ear (*Auricularia auricula*) mushroom essence is helpful for auditory hallucinations, schizophrenia and autism spectrum disorder (ASD). It is especially useful when tinnitus or Ménière's disease, affecting hearing and balance are present.

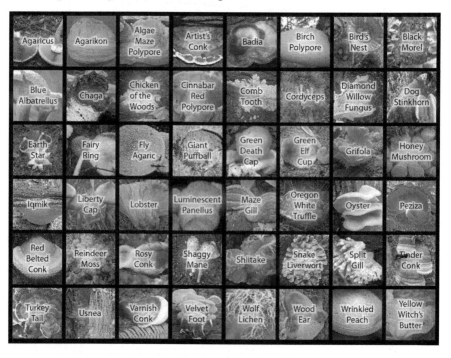

CHAPTER 20

AROMATHERAPY AND ESSENTIAL OILS

In 1988, I attended the first American Aromatherapy Association meeting in Napa Valley. There were only two Canadians in attendance, the other individual Rae Dunphy, a friend from Calgary. Rae is, sadly, no longer with us, but her contribution to the world of aromatherapy remains.

As a practicing clinical herbalist I became very excited about the possibilities associated with the medical use of essential oils.

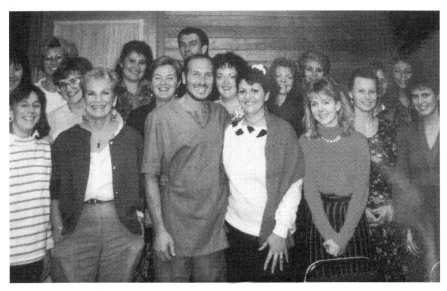

In 1990, Laurie and I invited Dr. Daniel Penoel, and wife Rosemary, to Edmonton for a four-day medicinal aromatic workshop. In France, over ten thousand medical doctors spend three additional years, after an initial seven years, in the study of essential oils. Pharmacies in the country create essential oil formulations for oral, rectal, vaginal or diffusion, to treat any medical condition. Entire wings of hospitals offer aromatherapy alternatives to their patients if so desired.

In North America, essential oils are diffused into the air, added to massage oils at 3-5% dilution, for pleasant, and therapeutic benefit.

I personally enjoy a daily aromatic steam or sauna, as part of my own healthcare protocol. Various essential oils (EOs) strongly influence our psychological and physiological health.

The Finnish sauna, and Indigenous sweat lodge provide physical, psychological and spiritual benefit.

Saunas can help alleviate depression[896] and remove heavy metals through the skin.

Of all the applications, oral ingestion of essential oils is by far the least effective, and most potentially dangerous application, despite what your MLM company may infer, or suggest.

Our line of essential oils, *Scents of Wonder* is now in its 30th year, and still brings me much joy, although I am long retired from clinical practice. My wife Laurie is a true 'Nose' in the aromatic sense, and at one time enjoyed creating fully natural perfumes for her clients. Her blends are truly magical.

Organic or wild-crafted essential oils are preferred and are produced either by cold expression (i.e. citrus peels) or steam distillation. Essential oils are produced from all parts of plants, including flowers, leaves, stems, roots, bark and seeds.

The basic route of inhalation is quite powerful, influencing the lungs, but more importantly the olfactory nerves and then olfactory bulb. This directly influences the hypothalamus and then the pituitary, as well as piriform cortex, amygdala, entorhinal cortex, striatum and hippocampus. In turn, the pituitary governs the functioning of the thyroid, adrenal and gonadal system, in short, the HPA axis.

Our olfactory receptor gene family comprises 1% of all genes.

Various essential oils will change brainwave patterns. Olfactory dysfunction is associated with depression, Parkinson's disease, AD and other neurodegenerative conditions.

See Chapter Four for Neurotransmitters and their related brain wave correlations.

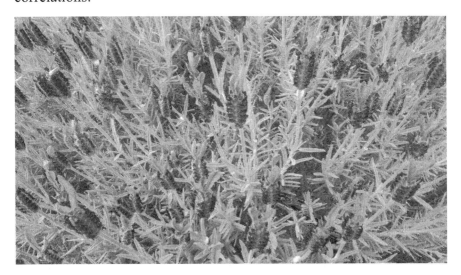

Lavender oil, for example, induces alpha wave activity fairly quickly.

Basil, black pepper, cardamon and rosemary induce beta wave patterns, associated with attention and alertness. Jasmine, neroli and rose induce delta patterns related to calmness and euphoria.[897] Siberian fir needle EO increases theta brain waves.

A recent study found postgraduate students with academic stress, responded to lavender oil by exhibiting theta brainwave activity.[898]

Sesquiterpenes in EOs increase the number of certain receptors in the brain and suggest possible treatment for AD, PD and schizophrenia spectrum disorder.[899]

Essential oils show benefit in reducing inhalant cravings. See Addictions Chapter 14.

Massage is both stimulating and sedating on body tissue. It can increase delta waves, associated with deep sleep, or increase alpha waves associated with relaxed and meditative states. Or decrease beta waves associated with alertness and stress. It stimulates the parasympathetic nervous system and may relieve depression due to increased dopamine and serotonin levels.

Small amounts definitely enhance or modify emotions, and may interact with receptors for neurotransmission and enzymes in both the peripheral and central nervous systems.

Work by Balacs[900] compared blood plasma concentrations of lavender oil after massage to effective levels of various psychoactive drugs. Linalool and linalyl acetate in lavender showed level of 100 nanograms/ml, compared to the antidepressant amitriptyline (200 ng/ml), the tranquilizer Chlorpromazine (100 ng/ml) and morphine (65 ng/ml).

Essential oils may work through the GABA receptors or sodium channels. An excellent review of EOs and their mode of action was published by Wang and Heinbockel[901]

Snoezelen is a Dutch concept developed in the 1970s for severely disabled people and later expanded the use for dementia patients. These rooms give the resident a combined experience of aroma, sound, texture and vision.[902,903]

This concept could be integrated into North American long-term dementia and AD care facilities, as an alternative to the over-medication and lack of interaction in present health care models.

It should be noted that a large number of essential oils, if taken orally, or, in some cases, simply smelling the oils will induce seizures or convulsions in those prone to epileptic events.

These include hyssop, pennyroyal, fennel, yarrow, Spanish lavender, wintergreen and many more.

I observed in clinical practice a great use for bergamot EO in patients with epilepsy. A few seconds or more before seizure, many people will experience a shift of vision or auric sense of the impending event. Quickly sniffing bergamot EO helped in many cases, prevent the seizure or convulsions from occurring, or lessened the severity or duration.

A large number of essential oils are contraindicated during pregnancy and breastfeeding.[904]

Essential oils will often evoke repressed memory, and may be helpful in psychotherapy, when childhood traumas have been buried, and continue to negatively influence mental and emotional health.

Aromatherapy massage has been found more beneficial than inhalation, in a systematic review of EOs for depression.[905]

Anxiety affects people in a variety of ways. A number of studies looking at stress relief in patients and hospital staff, identified lavender, sweet orange, bergamot, frankincense, rose, and neroli EOs as their scents of choice.[906]

Olfactory dysfunction is one marker for detecting Alzheimer's disease. Individuals testing positive for the apolipoprotein E (ApoE) e4 allele, are at higher risk, and is linked to olfactory decline.[907] This group, however, only comprises 5% of AD cases.

Poor olfaction in older adults is linked to higher rates of mortality. A community-based cohort study of 2289 adults aged 71 to 82 years found 1121 died by year 13; and those with poor olfaction had a 46% higher cumulative risk of death by year 10. Neurodegenerative disease was found in 22% of cases.[908]

Specific changes in olfactory function accompany children/adolescents with disorders of dopamine transmission, including attention deficit hyperactivity disorder, autism spectrum disorder, and schizophrenia.[909] Many essential oil show significant effects through anti-amyloid, antioxidant, anti-cholinesterase and memory enhancement.

It is essential to avoid health and beauty products containing fragrance. This generic term covers nearly four thousand potentially harmful chemicals listed under an "umbrella" transparency list, including 65 with known carcinogenic effect.

Here is a summary of some aromatic oils, used for various conditions associated with brain health.

Angelica (*Angelica archangelica*) root EO may be useful for nicotine addiction. One small study found inhaling the oil allowed subjects to wait an average of 53 minutes before having a cigarette.[910]

Angelica gigas EO, derived from the root, shows significant changes in absolute low beta (in both left temporal and parietal) activity, and may be useful for enhancing language learning in human brain.[911] It may also be effective in treating nicotine addiction, possibly through modulation of dopamine release in the nucleus accumbens.[912]

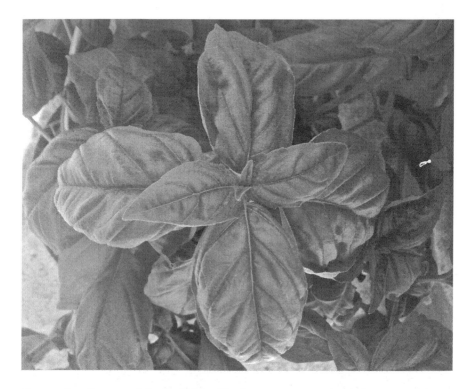

Sweet Basil essential oil (EO) alleviates memory impairment and hippocampal neurodegenerative changes induced by chronic stress.[913]

Bergamot (EO) has long been used to elevate mood. A study of 41 healthy females were tested in a random crossover study and measured for salivary cortisol. The bergamot group showed lower cortisol, as well as improved scores for fatigue and negative emotions.[914]

Bergamot is often diffused into mental health waiting rooms. One study on 57 women found fifteen minutes of exposure to the essential oil improved positive feelings compared to control.[915]

Bergamot oil EO shows neuroprotective effects and may be useful for anxiety disorders.[916]

The EO may be useful in cancer pain, mood disorders and stress-induced anxiety.

Black Pepper (*Piper nigrum*) essential oil inhalation shows great benefit in reducing nicotine withdrawal symptoms.[917]

Cataia or Craverio (*Pimenta pseudocaryophyllus*) EO contains over 93% (E)-methyl isoeugenol. It demonstrates anxyiolytic and anti-depressant properties via the serotonergic pathways.[918]

Chervil (*Anthriscus nemorosa*) EO, from aerial parts, has been found to possess anti-anxiety, anti-depressant, and cognitive benefit in a scopolamine-induced amnesia model in rats.[919]

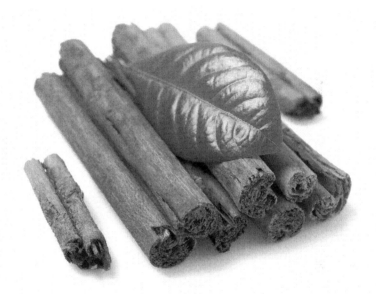

Cinnamon essential oil has been shown beneficial for attention problems, irritability and ADHD.[920]

Cinnamon leaf contains large amounts of eugenol. There is a link between the anti-depressant activity of eugenol and its monoamine amine oxidase A (MAOA) inhibition.[921] MAO is an enzyme that breaks down neurotransmitters such as adrenaline, dopamine norepinephrine and serotonin.

Cassia (*C. tamala*) EO reduces the biofilm and exopoly-saccharide layer of Candida fungal strains.[922]

Coriander seed EO increased anxiolytic-antidepressant behavior in beta-amyloid rat model of AD. Beta amyloid deposits were less in those treated with EO, probably due to suppression of oxidative stress.[923]

349

Clove bud (*Syzygium aromaticum*) leaf, bud and stem also are rich in eugenol and exhibit the same MAO inhibition as cinnamon.

The bud oil may be useful for depression, based on a rat study where they were exposed to chronic, unpredictable mild stress.[924]

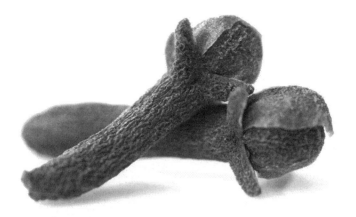

Cumin (*Cuminum cyminum*) EO contains cuminaldehyde which shows inhibition of alpha-synuclein fibrillation, associated with PD. It shows no toxic effect on normal brain cells.[925]

Eucalyptus EO can induce seizures, so extreme caution is advised in epileptic patients.[926]

Sweet fennel essential oil induced a seizure in one 38 year-old epileptic woman.[927]

Frankincense (*Boswellia* spp) has long been used by various religions to create meditative and mood-altering benefit during ceremony. Incensole and its acetate help alleviate anxiety or depression.[928]

Oral intake of *Boswellia serrata* gum resin, in a lecithin-based form, helps reduce symptoms of irritable bowel syndrome and ulcerative colitis in randomized clinical trials.[929,930]

Ginger EO, and specifically 6-gingerol, can be an effective remedy in prevention and treatment of AD. It showed enhancement of the immune system, increased antioxidant capacity, and protected against beta amyloid$_{25\text{-}35}$.[931]

Juniper berry EO inhalation showed improvement of amyloid-beta induced memory deficit in a rat model of AD.[932]

Lavender EO was tested on 97 patients with mild to moderate anxiety in a randomized DB study involving neutral and anxiety provoking film clips. Those taking lavender oil capsules showed reduced anxiety.[933]

One in ten Americans take sleeping pills, on a nightly basis. These include the harmful OTC anti-cholinergic drugs such as Benadryl, Dramamine, Excedrin PM, Nytol, Sominex, Tylenol PM. By blocking the cholinergic pathway (acetylcholine), people are creating eventual brain health dysfunction.

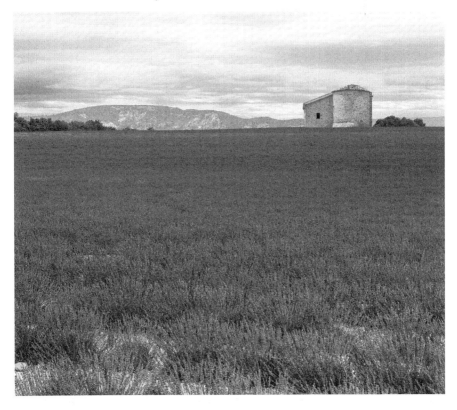

A controlled DB study compared lavender oil capsules and lorazepam and found comparable results for sleep and generalized anxiety, without the sedation and potential drug abuse associated with pharmaceuticals.[934]

In the 1980s, a nurse in Oxford England introduced lavender and/or marjoram EO into her ward of elderly patients. She reduced the drug bill by one-third by gradually replacing analgesia and night sedation with essential oils, either vaporized or in massage oil. Another hospital in Oxford offered the option of aromatherapy or sleep medication, and nearly all patients chose the former.[935]

Numerous studies have found lavender useful for insomnia.[936]

A Norwegian survey of 12 nurses found lavender EO reduced insomnia in all four residential homes for dementia patients.[937]

One study involved sleep patterns in children with autism spectrum disorder (ASD). Parents would apply a 2% lavender cream to their forearms before bedtime. Hours of sleep and waking were recorded for three weeks; the first for baseline, second with lavender, and third for washout. During the lavender week 8 of the 10 children had a dramatic reduction in number of times they awoke and needed attention.[938]

A six-week study involved 23 children with moderate to severe ADHD, enrolled in horse riding classes. Each child inhaled three drops of lavender EO for five minutes before their ride. Children, parents and teachers rated the results, showing the oil calmed the children and improved their focus.[939]

A Japanese randomized, controlled trial of 28 patients with dementia found two drops of lavender on their collar three times daily had measurable effect on symptoms.[940]

A Chinese clinical trial of 28 elderly found lavender, lemon, sweet orange and rosemary EO inhalation produced significant improvement in cognitive function.[941]

Sundowning is a disruptive behavior common in dementia patients between 3 pm and 6 pm. Lavender diffusion into a common room at a large residential long-term facility in Massachusetts found all ten patients, previously agitated at that time, became calmer.[942]

Lemon and other citrus peel EOs contain limonene. Recent work suggests limonene may help ameliorate drug-addiction related behaviors by regulating postsynaptic dopamine receptor supersensitivity.[943]

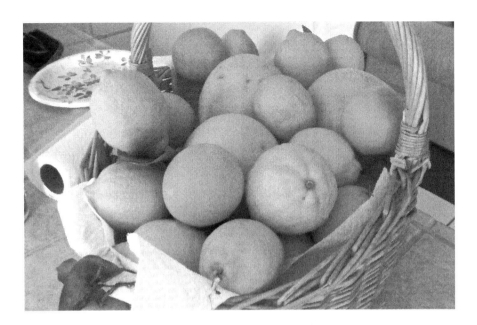

Lemon and rosemary EOs were diffused in the morning, and lavender and sweet orange in the evening, in a study of 28 elderly patients with dementia, including 17 with AD. It involved three periods of 28 days each of control, aromatherapy and washout. All patients showed significant improvement related to cognitive function after aromatherapy period, on both Gottfries-Brane-Steen scale and Touch Panel-type Dementia Assessment Scale.[944]

Lemon Balm (*Melissa officinalis*) EO shows potential for treating agitation in people with severe dementia. Melissa showed affinity for binding with $5HT_{1A}$ and the agonist binding site $GABA_A$ receptors. It also reduced social withdrawal times and increased the time of constructive activities of dementia patients.[945]

Both lemon balm and lavender reduce agitation associated with severe dementia.

A DB, PC controlled trial of the EO, involved a dilute oil that 72 AD patients applied to face and arms twice daily for 4 weeks. A 35% improvement in agitation was noted in Melissa group.[946]

Myrrh (*Commiphora myrrha*) EO contains sesquiterpenes that affect opioid agonists.[947] This suggests possible application and diffusion in opioid treatment centers.

Neroli (*Citrus aurantium* var. *amara*) EO has a sedative effect on mice and gerbils, the latter exhibiting anti-anxiety properties similar to the control drug Xanax.[948]

Both sweet orange and rose EOs were tested, olfactorally, on 20 female university students. A significant decrease in oxyhemoglobin concentration in the right prefrontal cortex, and an increase in "comfortable", "relaxed", and "natural" feelings was found; suggestive of both physiological and psychological relaxation.[949]

Patchouli EO reduces the biofilm and exopoly-saccharide layer of Candida fungal strains.[950]

Peppermint EO reduced the nausea associated with opiate and crack withdrawal in all eight patients. The oil was given 30 minutes before meals.[951]

Peppermint essential oil rich in menthol/menthone was tested orally in a DB, PC balanced cross-over study of 24 participants. The highest dose (100 uL) improved cognitive performance, and showed acetycholinesterase inhibition, and $GABA_A$/nicotinic receptor binding properties.[952]

Perilla (*Perilla frutescens*), as well as sage and peppermint EOs contain perillyl alcohol. The 6-hydroxydopamine (6-OHDA) model of Parkinson's is widely used to research the disease. In one study the compound demonstrated sufficient neuroprotection and restoration of mitochondrial membrane potential.[953]

Pine (*Pinus* sp.) needle oils contain alpha pinene, which in mouse studies was found to enhance non-rapid eye movement through GABAA-benzodiazepine receptors.[954]

Rosemary (*Rosmarinus* sp.) EO shows moderate AChE (acetylcholinesterase) inhibition, increases locomotor activity, motivates vigor, stimulates cerebral cortex, causes mood relaxation and increases alertness. This suggest benefit in management of neurodegenerative conditions such as AD, senile dementia and myasthenia gravis.[955]

Rosemary is very stimulating, and lavender more calmative.

Children and adults with attention deficit hyperactivity disorder (ADHD) are given stimulants such as Ritalin or Adderall. In one study of four children with ADHD attending piano lessons, lavender diffused into the air caused them to be more inattentive and restless. Rosemary EO increased attention and less restless behavior in three of the four.[956]

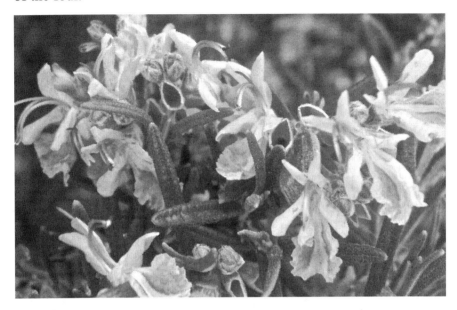

Short term and numerical memory on 79 school children (aged 13-17) showed positive results.[957]

The 1,8 cineole content of rosemary, found in blood plasma of healthy volunteers following inhalation, has been correlated with improved cognitive performance.[958]

Saffron (*Crocus sativus*) EO contains safranal, that shows anti-convulsant activity due to agonist activity on $GABA_A$ receptors.[959]

Sage (*Salvia officinalis*) EO was trialed in a single-blind randomized controlled trial of mood and cognition in healthy volunteers, with positive results.[960]

Lavender-leaved Sage (*Salvia lavandulaefolia*) has been used for centuries to improve memory and cognition. An *in vitro* study found the oil inhibits cholinesterase, suggesting benefit in AD.

Oral administration of EO in patients with mild to moderate AD, reported significant improvement in memory and cognition in a pilot, open-label study.[961]

355

A DB, PC balanced cross-over study examined cognitive/mood effect from a single oral dose of EO, and showed benefit in young healthy adults.[962] More research is needed.

Southern Burnet Saxifrage (*Pimpinella peregrina*) EO inhalation relieved scopolamine-induced memory deficits, depression and anxiety in a rat model of AD.[963]

Thymol and carvacrol, two main compounds in Thyme (*Thymus vulgaris*) EO, reversed the beta amyloid and scopolamine memory impairment in an animal model, suggesting possible benefit in AD and dementia.[964]

Valerian (*Valeriana officinalis*) EO contains the sesquiterpene valerenic acid, which has influence on GABA receptors[965] and lignan hydroxypinoresinol, that binds to benzodiazepine receptors.[966]

Bipolar disorder is increasing, perhaps due to better recognition and diagnosis. See Chapter 13.

Adjunct use of essential oils may be useful, but require testing and approval by the patient. If they like the odor, they may enjoy benefit from its use in diffusors, or as part of massage therapy.

EOs to consider in BD, include geranium, lavender, sandalwood, angelica root, rose, patchouli, ylang ylang, valerian, vetiver, spikenard, Melissa, bergamot and clary sage.

Oils to avoid are white camphor, hyssop, nutmeg, pennyroyal and tansy. These oils contain high levels of ketones that can cause negative effects on the brain.

A good review of the use of essential oils for the central nervous system by Dobetsberger & Buchbauer is worthy of a look.[967]

A recent paper on essential oils for AD in pre-clinical and clinical studies may be of interest to those in the mental health field.[968]

Vetivert EO may be useful in the treatment of ADHD and ADD, and relieve insomnia. A study of children with attention deficit and hyperactivity disorder had them inhale vetiver oil three times daily for 30 days. Improved brain wave patterns were observed in EEGs, as well as improved behavior and better class marks.[969]

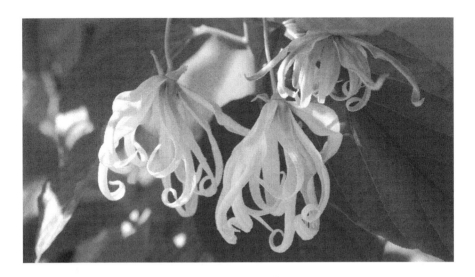

Ylang Ylang (*Cananga odorata*) EO was studied in a small group of ten women suffering cravings from substance abuse withdrawal. A few drops were applied to cotton and put under the pillow, or on a hanky to smell if they experienced a craving. It did not work for all, but four out of five in EO group believed smelling the oil relieved stress and anxiety in the moment.[970]

Ylang ylang EO given in massage oil for patients with epilepsy, remained in their consciousness for a period of time. Patient only had to think about the aroma of ylang ylang to prevent a seizure from occurring.[971]

A 5% blend of ylang ylang, roman chamomile and lavender was given to patients of alcohol addiction, to rub into throat and chest before bedtime. It appealed to women more than men, but a positive change of more than 50% of feeling less restless, was accompanied by reduced anxiety and less insomnia.[972]

An interesting study on alcohol addiction compared aromatherapy and auricular acupuncture. Ninety-nine participants were divided, with both groups having the same reduction in craving and withdrawal symptoms.[973]

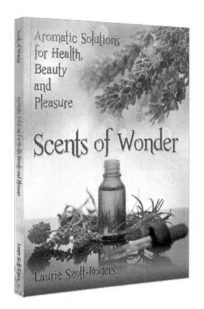

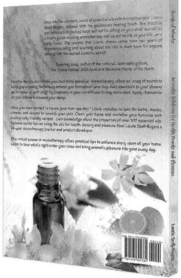

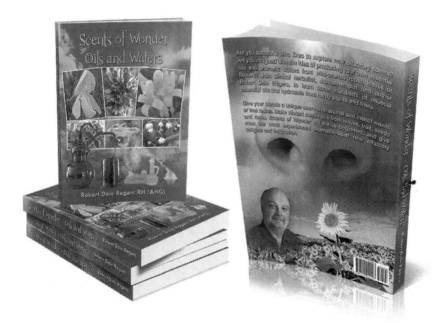

CHAPTER 21

THE FUTURE

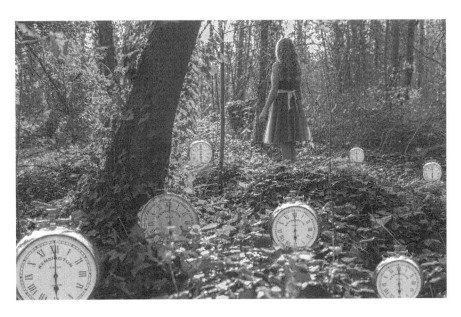

As mentioned in the introductory chapter, over 80% of what we know about the brain has been discovered in the past twenty years, and 80% of that in the last five years. We are making incredible progress in identifying the biochemistry involved in brain health and disease, but sorely lacking in low cost, natural solutions to the pending epidemic.

Here are some latest findings that may, or may not, translate into meaningful changes in the way we prevent and treat various neurological disorders.

Phoenixin is a recently discovered neuropeptide found in the brain, heart, lung and stomach, and involved in anxiety-related behavior.

The gut-brain connection is interesting as phoenixin may affect memory formation, depression, reproduction, food intake and anxiety-related disorders.[974]

One isoform Phoenixin-14 facilitates memory formation and prolongs memory retention, suggesting its use for enhancing memory and treating Alzheimer's disease.[975]

Both the saturated fatty acid palmitate and the endocrine-disrupting bisphenol A regulate Gpr173 expression, a putative phoenixin receptor, related to HPA axis, and reproductive health.[976]

What does this all mean? It suggests that this neuropeptide may play a key role in gut-brain information. Further research is needed.

The processed tuber of Aconite has long been used in TCM for pain relief. Due to the toxicity of the plant, various preparation involving salt and drying are necessary to avoid toxicity.

One alkaloid, with a different structure from aconitine alkaloids, is Ignavine, that specifically binds with the mu opioid, but not the k, opioid receptor. It exerts positive modulatory activity for morphine in cAMP assay.[977]

The boreal sponge *Geodia barretti* collected in cold waters off Norway, contains berettin and 8,9-dihydrobarettin. Both compounds inhibit acetylcholinesterase.[978] Geobarrettin B & C from same sponge may be useful for immune inflammation of the Th1 type.[979]

A marine sponge from waters off Madagasgar, *Fascaplysinopsis bergquist*, contains compounds that inhibit acetylcholinesterase and inhibit beta amyloid aggregation. Fascaplysin and 9-methylfascaplysin respectively show promise for aspects of AD.[980]

MODALITIES

Low intensity lasers are being investigated for treating Alzheimer's disease (AD). In this condition, amyloid and tau proteins build up in the brain leading to neurodegeneration.

A mouse study in Australia, introduced tau and amyloid plaque-caused human genes in brains and then used low level light therapy. This involved simply holding near-infrared light one to two centimeters above their head. This reduced tau and amyloid plaques by 70% in key brain areas.

Another animal study found light therapy improved damaged connections between neurons in AD by increasing brain-derived neurotropic factor (BDNF). Human studies would be useful.[981]

A systematic review of 15 preclinical trials found focused ultrasound was able to reduce amyloid-b plaques and tau phosphorylation in AD animals.

A recent focused ultrasound phase one safety trial opened the blood-brain barrier in five patients with early to moderate AD.

No serious clinical or adverse events were observed, but beta-amyloid levels before and after were unchanged.[982]

Neurotrack has developed the Imprint Cognitive Assessment Test, a five minute web-based assessment that tracks eye movements. It can detect hippocampus alterations, and help identify the beginning patterns of AD.

PoNS (Portable Neuromodulation Stimulator) is a small device named for the pons, a part of the brain stem. A team of neuroscientists invented the device to stimulate neuroplasticity in the brain, by modifying and correcting how neurons fire.

One part is put in the mouth, resting on the tongue like a flat, wide chewing gum, with 144 electrodes that fire electrical pulses.

These turn on the tongue's sensory neurons, but in a gentle manner. Its signals reach only 300 microns beneath the surface of the tongue, at 200 Hz, in a rhythm of three signals, a pause and then three more.

Why the tongue? Because it activates the whole human brain. The sense of smell and tip of tongue exploration have been used for ages. In fact, there are some 48 different sensory receptors on the tongue, 14 on tip of tongue alone, with 15-50 thousand nerve fibers.

Brain scans and EEG recording show that after 400 to 600 milliseconds, brain waves are stabilized.

This is not surprising as tongue diagnosis has been used in TCM for millennia. The governing vessels and the central vessel, meet at the tongue. Practitioners of martial arts, tai chi and qigong masters often place their tongue on the roof of the mouth to link these two energies. Several acupuncture points have been recently indentified on the tongue, and used in Hong Kong for Parkinson's, cerebral palsy, brain injury and other neurological issues. It has application for PD, multiple sclerosis and stroke recovery.

Vagus nerve stimulation shows promise for depression, but requires surgery. Deep brain stimulation has been used for PD and depression, but again surgery is required to plant electrodes deep inside the brain.[983]

Medical doctors are initially skeptical due to the generalized effect. However, to holistic practitioners, who have long valued the theory of vitalism; that you cannot separate mind and body, this is exciting, but no great surprise.

Transcranial Magnetic Stimulation (TMS) is FDA approved for depression and specific types of migraine. It is being trialed for off-label use in patients with Alzheimer's and shows modest, but promising results.

NanoSomiX offers a blood test that reveal your neural exosome levels, helping determine the level of cognitive damage and course of treatment for AD.

Professors Li and Dixon at the University of Alberta examined 6000 metabolites in saliva and identified three that may differentiate and identify senile dementia or AD at an earlier stage. The research is ongoing.

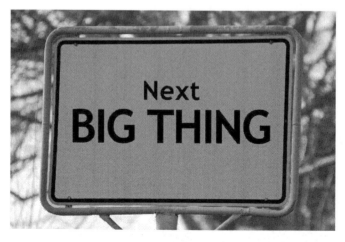

GENETICALLY ENGINEERED BACTERIA

Engineered bacteria are coming. Work by Zhongyi Chen at Vanderbilt has produced a chemical called NAPE that helps the brain feel satiated, decreasing food intake and body fat.[984]

Jeff Tabor at Rice University has re-engineered commensal *E. coli* to detect dysbiosis and then produce molecules that can correct it. He believes the delivery of these engineered bacteria could be as simple as programmed yogurt.[985]

Brain exercises can be divided into various categories including language and comprehension, verbal and visual memory, vision-spatial skills and abstract thinking. Although generally dismissed by many physicians, cognition remediation helps improve daily living, the relative quality of life, and reduce depression.

The development of epilepsy biosensors may well increase the quality of life for those afflicted. Work is underway on this technology and will likely be available for point of care application within the decade.[986]

Researchers no longer have to test drugs on rat neurons, but can use a Disease in a Dish model of investigation using stem cells. This could speed up the screening of therapies for ALS, sickle cell anemia, and Parkinson's disease.[987]

This work must proceed with care as two PD patients receiving stem cell neuron transplants developed dyskinesia, due to over-production of dopamine.[988]

Books by Robert Dale Rogers

www.amazon.com/author/robertdalerogers

www.selfhealdistributing.com - email: scents@telusplanet.net

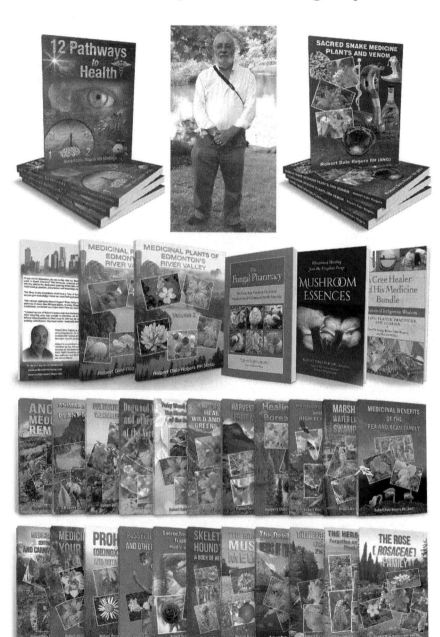

ABOUT THE AUTHOR

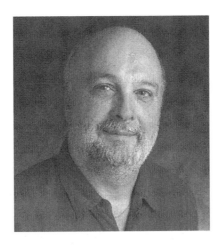

Robert Dale Rogers has been an herbalist for over forty-five years. He has a Bachelor of Science from the University of Alberta, where he is an assistant clinical professor in Family Medicine. He teaches plant medicine, including herbology and flower essences in the Earth Spirit Medicine Program at the Northern Star College of Mystical Studies in Edmonton, Alberta, Canada.

Robert is past chair of the Alberta Natural Health Agricultural Network and Community Health Council of Capital Health. He is a Fellow of the International College of Nutrition, past chair of the medicinal mushroom committee of the North American Mycological Association and served time on the editorial board of the International Journal of Medicinal Mushrooms. He writes the occasional article for Fungi magazine.

Robert co-initiated The Alberta Herb Gathering which is held every second year. Details can be found at www.albertaherbgathering.com

He lives on Millcreek Ravine in Edmonton with his beautiful and talented wife, Laurie Szott-Rogers and out of control cat Ceres.

You can email him at scents@telusplanet.net

or visit

www.selfhealdistributing.com

Books by Robert Dale Rogers

www.amazon.com/author/robertdalerogers

www.selfhealdistributing.com - email: scents@telusplanet.net

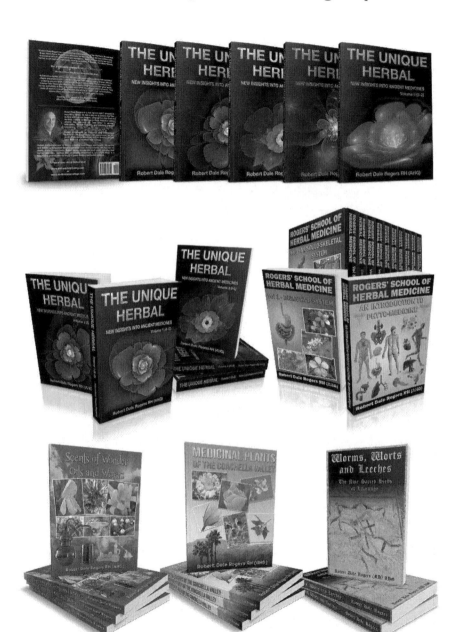

366

BIBLIOGRAPHY

Amen, Daniel G. 2015. *Change Your Brain Change Your Life*. Harmony Books. New York
_____. 2017. *Memory Rescue*. Tyndale Momentum. Tyndale House Publishing.
    Carol Stream, Illinois.
Anderson, Scott. 2017. The Psychobiotic Revolution. National Geographic. Washington
    DC.
Archer, Dale. 2015. *The ADHD Advantage*. Avery NY.
Boden, J. & S. Sinatra. 2012. *The Great Cholesterol Myth*. Four Winds Press Beverly, Mass.
Bredesen, Dale E. 2017. *The End of Alzheimer's: The First Program to Prevent and Reverse*
    Cognitive Decline. Avery NY.
Buckle, Jane. 2015. *Clinical Aromatherapy: Essential Oils in Healthcare*. Third Ed.
    Elsevier.
Burford-Mason, Aileen. 2017. *The Healthy Brain: Optimize Brain Power At Any Age*.
    Harper Collins Publishers Toronto.
Campbell-McBride, N. 2010. *Gut and Psychology Syndrome*. Medinform Pub. Cambridge
    UK.
Costandi, Moheb. 2016. *Neuroplasticity*. MIT Press Cambridge Mass.
Davis, Daniel, M. 2018. *The Beautiful Cure* Doubleday Canada.
Devi, G. 2017. *The Spectrum of Hope: An Optimistic and New Approach to Alzheimer's*
    Disease and other dementias. Workman Publishing NY.
Doidge, N. 2016. *The Brain's Way of Healing*. Penguin Books NY.
Honda, M. 2018. *Reverse Alzheimer's Disease Naturally*. Hatherleigh Press.
Ingram, Jay. 2014. *The End of Memory*. Harper Collins Pub Toronto
Jebelli, J. 2017. *In Pursuit of Memory*. Little, Brown & Co. NY
Jonsson, Bo & A. Saul. 2012. *The Vitamin Cure for Depression*. Basic Health Publications.
    Laguna Beach CA.
Junger, A. 2013. *Clean Gut*. Harper One. NY.
Kahn, J. 2013. *Angst- Origins of anxiety and depression*. Oxford University Press, NY.
Kellman, Raphael. 2014. *The Microbiome Diet*. Da Capo Lifelong Books. Boston MA.
Kharrazian, D. 2013. *Why Isn't My Brain Working?* Elephant Press. Carlsbad CA.
Kirsch, Irving. 2010. *The emperor's new drugs: Exploding the antidepressant myth*. Basic
    Books. New York.
Laake, Dana & Pamela Compart. 2013. *The ADHD and Autism Nutritional Supplement*
    Handbook. Fair Winds Press Beverly Mass.
Lewis, Cherry. 2017. *The Enlightened Mr. Parkinson*. Pegasus Books NY.
Lieberman, D. and Long, M. 2018. *The Molecule of More*. Benbella Books. Dallas TX.
Mosconi, Lisa. 2018. *Brain Food: The Surprising Science of Eating for Cognitive Power*.
    Avery Pub. NY.
Parashos, S.A., R. Wichmann & T. Melby. 2013. *Navigating Life with Parkinson Disease*.
    Oxford University Press. NY.
Penzel, Fred. 2017. *Obsessive-Compulsive Disorders* 2nd Ed. Oxford University Press. NY.

Rottenberg, J. 2014. *The Depths: The Evolutionary Origins of the Depression Epidemic.* Basic Books. Perseus Books Group NY.

Sawatsky, Jarem. 2017. *Dancing with Elephants.* Red Canoe Press Winnipeg MB

Schwartz, J. 2016. *Brain Lock- Free Yourself from Obsessive-Compulsive Behavior.* Harper Perennial NY.

Spinella, M. 2001. *The Psychopharmacology of Herbal Medicine.* MIT Press Cambridge Mass.

St. John, Noah. 2013. *The Book of Afformations* Hay House Inc., NY.

Penzel, Fred. 2017. *Obsessive-Compulsive Disorders. A Complete Guide to Getting Well and Staying Well.* Second Ed. Oxford University Press Sheridan Books.

Perlmutter, David. 2015. *Brain Maker.* Little, Brown and Company New York, NY.

Romm A., and T. Romm. 2000. *ADHD Alternatives: A Natural Approach to Treating Attention-Deficit Hyperactivity Disorder.* Storey Publishing. North Adams, Mass.

Sigman, Mariano. 2017. *The Secret Life of the Mind.* Little, Brown & Co. New York NY.

Schwartz, Michal. 2015. *Neuroimmunity.* Yale University Press. New Haven/London.

Temperman, L., P. Albanese, S. Stark & N. Zahlan. 2013. *The Dostoevsky Effect- Problem Gambling and the Origins of Addiction.* Oxford University Press. Don Mills Ontario.

NOTES

1   Oswald, A.J. & E. Proto. 2014. National Happiness and Genetic Distance: A Cautious Exploration. *IZA* discussion paper #8300. July.

2   Engemann, K. et al. 2019. Residential green space in childhood is associated with lower risk of psychiatric disorders from adolescence into adulthood. *Proc National Academy Science* 116(11): 5188-93.

3   Singh, R.B. et al. 2018. The gut-brain-axis and the heart. *MOJ Public Heath* 7(3): 129-138.

4   Gomm, W. et al. 2016. Association of proton pump inhibitors with risk of dementia. A pharmacoepidemiological claims data analysis. *JAMA Neurology* 73(4): 410-416.

5   Gray, S.I. et al. 2015. Cumulative use of strong anticholinergics and incident dementia: A prospective cohort study. *JAMA Internal Medicine* 175(3): 401-7.

6   Kaptchuk, T.J. & F.G. Miller. 2015. Placebo effects in medicine. *New England Journal of Medicine* 373(1) page 9.

7   Saver J. & J.L. Kalafut. 2001. Combination therapies and the theoretical limits of evidence-based medicine. *Neuroepidemiology* 20(2): 57-64.

8   Berensen, D. 2017. *The End of Alzheimer's*. Avery NY page 247.

9   Zelano, C. et al. 2016. Nasal respiration entrains human limbic oscillations and modulates cognitive function. The Journal of Neuroscience 36(49): 12448-467.

10 Erickson, K.I. et al. 2009. Aerobic Fitness is associated with hippocampal volume in elderly humans. Hippocampus 19: 1030-39.

11 Adan, A. 2012. Cognitive performance and dehydration. J Am College of Nutrition 31(2): 71-78.

12 The Environmental Working Group. 2009. *Toxic Chemical found in Minority Cord Blood*. News Release December 2.

13 Lazar, Sara et al. 2008. Meditation experience is associated with increased cortical thickness. Neuroreport 16(17): 1893-7.

14 Eladak, S. et al. 2015. A new chapter in the bisphenol A story: Bisphenol S and bisphenol F are not safe alternatives to this compound. *Fertility & Sterility* 103(1): 11-21.

15 Tiwari, S.K. et al. 2015. Bisphenol-A impairs myelination potential during the development in the hippocampus of the rat brain. *Molecular Neurobiology* 51(3): 1395-416.

16 Mosconi, Lisa. 2018. *Brain Food* Avery Books. New York

17 Ibid page 39

18 Waugh, D.T. 2019. Fluoride exposure induces inhibition of sodium-and potassium activated adenosine triphosphate (Na^+, K^+-ATPase) enzyme activity: Molecular mechanisms and implications for public health. Int Journal Environmental Research Public Health 16(8).

19 Parmar, K. et al. 2019. Variation in electroencephalography with mobile cell phone usage in medical students. *Neurol India* 67(1): 235-241.

20   Pall, M.L. 2016. Microwave frequency electromagnetic fields (EMFs) produce widespread neurpsychiatric effects including depression. *J Chem Neuroanatomy* 75 (Pt B): 43-51.

21   Tas, M. et al. 2014. Long-term effects of 900 MHz radiofrequency radiation emitted from mobile phone on testicular tissue and epididymal semen quality. *Electromagnetic Biology and Medicine* 33(3): 216-22.

22   Roggeveen, S et al. 2015. EEG changes due to experimentally induced 3G mobile phone radiation. *PLoS One* 10(6): e0129496.

23   Wilson, B.W. et al. 1990. Evidence for an effect of ELF electromagnetic fields on human pineal gland function. *Journal Pineal Research* 9(4): 259-269.

24   Marshall, T.G. & T.J.R. Heil. 2017. Electrosmog and autoimmune disease. *Immunol Research* 65(1): 129-135.

25   Maher, B.A. et al. 2016. Magnetite pollution nanoparticles in the human brain. *Proc Natl Acad Sci USA* 113(39): 10797-801.

26   Ibid page 45

27   Zhang, J. & Liu, Q. 2015. Cholesterol metabolism and homeostasis in the brain. *Protein and Cell* 6(4): 254-64.

28   Mosconi page 53

29   Ibid page 60

30   Schaeffer, E.L. et al. 2009. Phospholipase A2 activation as a therapeutic approach for cognitive enhancement in early-stage Alzheimer's disease. *Psychopharmacology* 202(1-3): 37-51.

31   Mosconi page 55

32   Ibid page 58

33   Mayor, S. 2019. Higher intake of cholesterol or eggs linked to increased risk of cardiovascular disease and death, finds study. *BMJ* 364:112-4.

34   Altic, L. et al. 2016. Validation of folate-enriched eggs as a functional food for improving folate intake in consumers. *Nutrients* 8(12).

35   Fernando, W. M. et al. 2015. *British Journal of Nutrition* 114(1): 1-14.

36   Hu, Yang I. et al. 2015. Coconut oil: nonalternative drug treatment against Alzheimer's disease. *Nutr Hosp* 32: 2822-27.

37   Newport, M. *The Coconut Oil & Low-Carb Solution.* Basic Health Pub pages261-2,

38   De la Rubia Orti, J.E. 2018. *Journal of Alzheimer's Disease* 65(2):577-87.

39   Campbell-McBride, N. 2012. *GAPS Gut and Psychology Syndrome.* Medinform Publishing Cambridge page 264.

40   Strom, B.L. et al. 2015. Statin therapy and risk of acute memory impairment. *JAMA Internal Medicine* 175(2): 1399-1405.

41   Bredesen, D. *The End of Alzheimers.* Avery NY page 142.

42   Alaedini, A. et al. 2007. Immune cross-reactivity in celiac disease: anti-gliadin antibodies bind to neuronal synapsin. *International Journal of Immunology*178(10): 6590-5.

43   Spinella, M. 2001. *The Psychopharmacology of Herbal Medicine.* MIT Press Cambridge Mass page 190.

44   Mosconi, L. page 73.

45   Tosukhowong, P. et al. 2016. Biochemical and clinical effects of whey protein supplementation in Parkinson's disease: a pilot study. *Journal of Neurol Sci* 367: 162-70

46   Song, W. et al. 2017. Cysteine-rich whey protein isolate (Immuncal®) ameliorates deficits in the GFAP.HMOX1 mouse model of schizophrenia. *Free Radical Biol Med* 110: 162-175.

47   Wan, W. et al. 2014. The potential mechanisms of amyloid-beta receptor for advanced glycation end-products interaction disrupting tight junctions of the blood-brain barrier in Alzheimer's disease. *International Journal of Neuroscience* 124(2): 75-81.

48   Varatharaj, A. & I. Galea. 2017. The blood-brain barrier in systemic inflammation. *Brain Behavior and Immunity* 60:1-12.

49   Westover, A.N. & L.B. Marangell. 2002. A cross-national relationship between sugar consumption and major depression. Depress Anxiety 16(3): 118-120.

50   Mosconi, L. page 89

51   Ibid page 88

52   Fagherazzi, G. et al. 2013. Consumption of Artificially and Sugar-Sweetened Beverages and Incident Type 2 Diabetes. American Journal of Clinical Nutrition 97(3): 517-23.

53   Abhilash, M. et al. 2013. Long-term consumption of aspartame and brain antioxidant defense status. *Drug Chem Toxicol* 36(2): 135-40.

54   Nettleton, J. et al. 2016. Reshaping the gut microbiota: impact of low calorie sweeteners and the link to insulin resistance? *Physiology and Behavior* 164 (pt B) 488-93.

55   Bokulich, N.A. et al. 2014. A bitter aftertaste: unintended effects of artificial sweeteners on the gut microbiome. *Cell Metabolism* 20(5): 701-3.

56   Mosconi, page 86

57   Phillips, M.C.L. et al. 2018. Low-fat versus ketogenic diet in Parkinson's disease: a pilot randomized controlled trial. *Mov Disord* 22(8): 1306-14.

58   Tanvetyanon, T. & G. Bepler. 2008. Beta-carotene in multivitamins and the possible risk of lung cancer among smokers versus former smokers: a meta-analysis and evaluation of national brands. *Cancer* 113(1): 150-7.

59   Lindbergh, C.A. et al. 2019. The effects of lutein and zeaxanthin on resting state functional connectivity in older Caucasian adults: a randomized controlled trial. *Brain Imaging Behaviour* doi: 10.1007/s11682-018-0034-y.

60   Mewborn, C.M. et al. 2018. Relation of retinal and serum lutein and zeaxanthin to white matter integrity in older adults: A diffusion tensor imaging study. *Arch Clin Neuropsychol* 33(7): 861-874.

61   Nataraj, J. et al. 2016. Lutein protects dopaminergic neurons against MPTP-induced apoptotic death and more dysfunction by ameliorating mitochondrial disruption and oxidative stress. *Nutr Neurosci* 19(6): 237-46.

62   Chen, D. et al. 2019. A review for the pharmacological effect of lycopene in central nervous system disorders. *Biomed Pharmacother* 111: 791-801.

63   D'Cunda, N.M. et al. 2018. Effect of long-term nutraceutical and dietary supplement use on cognition in the elderly: a 10-year systematic review of randomized controlled trials. British Journal of Nutrition 119(3): 280-298.

64   Blass, J.P. et al. 2001. Brain Metabolism and Brain Disease: Is metabolic deficiency the proximate cause of Alzheimer's Dementia? *Journal of Neuroscience Research* 66: 851-56.

65   Lee, J.H. et al. 2018. Dietary intake of pantothenic acid is associated with cerebral amyloid burden in patients with cognitive impairment. *Food Nutr Research* 62:1315.

66   Hermann, W et al. 2003. Vitamin B-12 status…in vegetarians. Am J Clin Nutr 78(1): 131-6.

67   Bagur, M.J. et al. 2017. Influence of diet in multiple sclerosis: a systematic review. *Adv Nutrition* 8(3): 463-72.

68   Morris, M.S. et al. 2007. Folate and vitamin B-12 status in relation to anemia, macrocytosis, and cognitive impairment in older Americans in the age of folic acid fortification. *Am J Clin Nutrition* 85: 193-200.

69   Laake,D.G. & P. Compart. *The ADHD and Autism Nutritional Supplement Handbook.* Fair Winds Press Beverly Mass page 66.

70   Shelton, R. 2013. Assessing effects of L-methylfolate in depression management: results of a real-world patient experience trial. *Prim Care Companion CNS Disord* 15(4).

71   Miller, A.L. 2008. The methylation, neurotransmitter and antioxidant connections between folate and depression. *Altern Med Rev* 13(3): 216-26.

72   Papakostas, G.I. et al. 2012. L-methylfolate as adjunctive therapy for SSRI-resistant major depression: results of two randomized, double-blind, parallel-sequential trials. *American Journal of Psychiatry* 169: 1267-74.

73   Rainero, I. 2019. Targeting MTHFR for the treatment of migraines. *Expert Opinion Therapeutic Targets* 23(1): 29-37.

74   Monacelli, F. et al. 2017. Vitamin C, aging and Alzheimer's disease. *Nutrients* 9(7).

75   Nam, S.M. et al. 2019. Ascorbic acid mitigates D-galactose-induced brain aging by increasing hippocampal neurogenesis and improving memory function. *Nutrients* 11(1) doi: 10.3390/nu11010176.

76   Wang Y. et al. 2013. Effects of vitamin C and vitamin D administration on mood and distress in acutely hospitalized patients. *Am J Clin Nutr* 98(3): 705-11.

77   Raygan, F. 2018. The effects of vitamin D and probiotic co-supplementation on mental health parameters. *Prog Neuropsychopharmacology Biol Psychiatry* 84(A): 50-55.

78   Ali, A. et al. Developmental vitamin D deficiency and autism: Putative pathogenic mechanisms. *Journal Steroid Biochem Mol Biol* 175: 108-118.

79   Wang, T. et al. 2016. Serum concentration of 25-hydroxyvitamin D in Autism Spectrum Disorder: A systematic review and meta-analysis. *European Child and Adolescent Psychiatry* 25(4): 341-50.

80   Morales, E. et al. 2015. Vitamin D in Pregnancy and Attention Deficit Hyperactivity Disorder-like Symptoms in Childhood. *Epidemiology* 26(4): 458-65.

81   Bagur, M.J. et al. 2017. Influence of diet in multiple sclerosis: a systematic review. *Adv Nutrition* 8(3): 463-72.

82   Patrick, R.P. & B.N. Ames. 2015. Vitamin D and the omega-3 fatty acids control serotonin synthesis and action, part 2: relevance for ADHD, bipolar disorder, schizophrenia, and impulsive behavior. *FASEB Journal* 29(6): 2207-22.

83   Littlejohns, T.J. et al. 2014. Vitamin D and the risk of dementia and Alzheimer disease. *Neurology* 83(10): 920-8.

84   Castle, M. et al. 2019. Three doses of vitamin D and cognitive outcome in older women: a double-blind randomized controlled trial. *The Journals of Gerontology Series A* doi.org/10.1093/gerona/giz041.

85   Mangialasche, F. et al. 2013. Serum levels of vitamin E forms and risk of cognitive impairment in a Finnish cohort of older adults. *Experimental Gerontology* 14(12): 1428.

86   Alisi, L. et al. 2019. The relationships between vitamin K and cognition: a review of current evidence. *Front Neurology* 10:239.

87   Popescu, D.C. et al. 2018. Vitamin K enhances the production of brain sulfatides during remyelination. *PLoS One* 13(8):e0203057.

88   Bolzetta, F. 2019. The relationship between dietary vitamin K and depressive symptoms in late adulthood: A cross-sectional analysis from a large cohort study. *Nutrients* 11(4).

89   Mosconi page 110

90   Honda, M. 2018. *Reverse Alzheimer's Disease Naturally*. Hatherleigh Press page 80-81.

91   Mold, M. et al. 2017. Aluminum in brain tissue in autism. *Journal of Trace Elements in Medicine and Biology* 46: 76-82.

92   Bakulski, K. et al. 2012. Alzheimer's disease and environmental exposure to lead: the epidemiologic evidence and potential role in epigenetics. *Current Alzheimer Research* 9: 563-573.

93   Buric, Ivana et al. 2017. What is the Molecular Signature of Mind-Body Interventions? *Frontiers in Immunology* volume 8 article 670.

94   Pantelyat, A. et al. 2016. Drum-PD: the use of a drum circle to improve the symptoms and signs of Parkinson's disease (PD). *Mov Discord Clin Pract* 3(3): 243-49.

95   Gershon, Michael. 1999. *The Second Brain: A Groundbreaking New Understanding of Nervous Disorders of the Stomach and Intestine*. Harper Perennial 1st Edition.

96   Montiel-Castro, A. J. et al. 2013. The microbiota-gut-brain-axis: neurobehavioral correlates, health and sociality. *Frontier Integrative Neuroscience* 7(70).

97   Kharrazian, D. 2013. *Why Isn't My Brain Working?* Elephant Press Carlsbad CA page 166.

98   Ibid page 170.

99   Roberts, R. C. et al. 2018. *The human brain microbiome; there are bacteria in our brains!* Session 594.08/yy23 November 6. SDCC Halls B-H.

100   Kessler, D. 2013. Antibiotics and Meat We Eat. *New York Times* March 27 Opinion page A27.

101   Slykerman, R.F. et al. 2017. Antibiotics in the first year of life and subsequent neurocognitive outcomes. *Acta Paediatrica* 106(1): 87-94.

102   Khalili, H. et al. 2013. Oral Contraceptives, Reproductive Factors and Risk of Inflammatory Bowel Disease. *Gut* 62(8): 1153-59.

103   Amen, Daniel G. 2015. *Change your Brain, Change your Life*. Revised & expanded. Harmony Books. Crown Pub. New York page 391-2.

104   Lambert, G.P. et al. 2012. Effect of aspirin dose on gastrointestinal permeability. *Int Journal of Sports Medicine* 33(6): 421-5.

105   Reuters. 2003. Daily Aspirin use linked with pancreatic cancer. *CNN.com/Health*. October 27.

106   Lanzini, A. et al. 2009. Complete recovery of intestinal mucosa occurs very rarely in adult celiac patients despite adherence to gluten-free diet. *Alimentary Pharmacology & Therapeutics* 29(12): 1299-308.

107   Kim, C.R. et al. 2018. Erucamide from Radish Leaves has an Inhibitory Effect Against Acetylcholinesterase and Prevents Memory Deficit Induced by Trimethyltin. *Journal of Medicinal Food* 21(8):769-776.

108   Li, M.M. et al. 2017. Antidepressant and anxiolytic-like behavioral effects of erucamide, a bioactive fatty acid amide, involving the hypothalamus-pituitary-adrenal axis in mice. *Neuroscience Letters* 640: 6-12.

109   Perlmutter, David. 2015. *Brain Maker*. Little, Brown & Co. NY page 194

110   Morris, M.C. et al. 2018. Nutrients and bioactives in green leafy vegetables and cognitive decline: Prospective study. *Neurology* 90(3): e214-222.

111 Shultz, S.R. et al. 2008. Intracerebroventricular injections of the enteric bacterial metabolic product propionic acid impair cognition and sensorimotor ability in the Long-Evans rat: Further development of a rodent model of autism. Behavioral Brain Research 200(1): 33-41.

112 Tana, C. et al. 2010. Altered profiles of intestinal microbiota and organic acids may be the origin of symptoms in irritable bowel syndrome. *Neurogastroenterology* 22(5): 512-9.

113 Stilling, R.M. 2016. The neuropharmacology of butyrate: The bread and butter of the microbiota-gut-brain axis. *Neurochem Int* 99: 110-132.

114 Valles-Colomer, M. et al. 2019. The neuroactive potential of the human gut microbiota in quality of life and depression. *Nature Microbiology*.

115 Campbell-McBride. 2010. *Gut and Psychology Syndrome*. Medinform Pub. Cambridge page 24.

116 Ibid page 46.

117 Gibson, G. 1999. *Colonic Microbiota, Nutrition and Health*. Kluwer Academic Publishers, Dodrecht.

118 Aslam, H. et al. 2018. Fermented foods, the gut and mental health: a mechanistic overview with implications for depression and anxiety. *Nutr Neurosci* 11:1-13.

119 Bell, V. et al. 2018. One Health, Fermented Foods, and Gut Microbiota. *Foods* 7(12).

120 Kim, C.S. & D.M. Shin. 2019. Probiotic food consumption is associated with lower severity and prevalence of depression: A nationwide cross-sectional study. *Nutrition* 63-64: 169-174.

121 Allonsius, C.N. 2017. Interplay between Lactobacillus rhamnosus GG and Candida and the involvement of exopolysaccharides. *Microb Biotechnol* 10(6): 1753-63.

122 Auclair, J. et al. 2015. *Lactobacillus acidophilus* CL 1285, *Lactobacillus casei* LBC80R, and *Lactobacillus rhamnosus* CLR2 (Bio-K+): Characterization, Manufacture, Mechanisms of Action and Quality Control of a Specific Probiotic Combination for Primary Prevention of Clostridium difficile infection. *Clin Infect Dis* 60 Suppl 2:S135-43.

123 Perez-Cornago, A. et al. 2016. Intake of high-fat yogurt, but not of low-fat yogurt or prebiotics is related to lower risk of depression in women of the SUN cohort study. *Journal of Nutrition* 146(9): 1731-9.

124 Anderson, S. 2017. *The Psychobiotic Revolution*. National Geographic Washington DC. pages 173-177.

125 Rousseaux, C. et al. 2007. *Lactobacillus acidophilus* modulates intestinal pain and induces opioid and cannabinoid receptors. *Nature Medicine* 13(1): 35-37.

126 Campana, R. et al. 2012. Antagonistic activity of *Lactobacillus acidophilus* ATCC 4356 on the growth and adhesion/invasion characteristics of human *Campylobacter jejuni*. *Current Microbiology* 64(4): 371-78.

127 Ishida, Y. et al. 2005. Clinical effects of Lactobacillus acidophilus strain L-92 on perennial allergic rhinitis: a double-blind, placebo-controlled study. *Journal Dairy Science* 88(2): 527-33.

128 Jose, P. & D. Raj. 2015. Gut Microbiota in Hypertension. *Current Opinion in Nephrology and Hypertension* 24(5): 403-9.

129 Taverniti, V. & S. Guglielmetti. 2012. Health-promoting properties of *Lactobacillus helveticus*. *Frontiers in Microbiology* 3: 392.

130 Benton, D. et al. 2007. Impact of consuming a milk drink containing a probiotic on mood and cognition. *European Journal of Clinical Nutrition* 61(3): 355-361.

131 Rao, A.V. et al. 2009. A randomized, double-blind, placebo-controlled pilot study of a probiotic in emotional symptoms of chronic fatigue syndrome. *Gut Pathogens* 1(1):6.

132 Cassani, E. et al. 2011. Use of probiotics for the treatment of constipation in Parkinson's disease patients. *Minerva Gastroenterologica E Dietologica* 57(2): 117-121.

133 Komatsuzaki, N. & J. Shima. 2012. Effects of live Lactobacillus paracasei on plasma lipid concentrations in rats fed an ethanol-containing diet. *Bioscience Biotechnology and Biochemistry* 76(2): 232-37.

134 Rudzki, L. et al. 2019. Probiotic *Lactobacillus plantarum* 299v decreases kynurenine concentration and improves cognitive functions in patient with major depression: a double-blind, randomized, placebo controlled study. *Psychoneuroendocrinology* 100: 213-222.

135 Chong, H.X. et al. 2019. Lactobacillus plantarum DR7 alleviates stress and anxiety in adults: a randomized, double-blind, placebo-controlled study. *Benef Microbes* 10(4): 355-373.

136 Hwang Y.H. et al. 2019. Efficacy and safety of *L. plantarum* C-29 fermented soybean (DW2009) in individuals with mild cognitive impairment: A 12-week, multi-center, randomized, double-blind, placebo-controlled clinical trial. *Nutrients* 11(2).

137 Varian, B. et al. 2017. Microbial lysate upregulates host oxytoxin. *Brain, Behavior and Immunity* 61: 36-49.

138 DiRienzo, D. 2014. Effect of probiotics on biomarkers of cardiovascular disease: implications for heart-healthy diets. *Nutrition Reviews* 72(1): 18-29.

139 Kamiya, T. et al. 2006. Inhibitory effects of *Lactobacillus reuteri* on visceral pain induced by colorectal distention in Sprague-Dawley rats. *Gut* 55(2): 191-6.

140 Capurso, L. 2019. Thirty years of *Lactobacillus rhamnosus* GG: A review. *Journal of Clinical Gastroenterology* 53 Supp 1:S1-S41.

141 Bravo, J. 2011. Ingestion of Lactobacillus strain regulates emotional behaviour and central GABA receptor expression in a mouse via the vagus nerve. *Proceedings of the National Academy of Sciences in the USA* 108(38): 16050-55.

142 Pärtty, A. et al. 2015. A possible link between early probiotic intervention and the risk of neuropsychiatric disorders later in childhood: A randomized trial. *Pediatric Research* 77(6): 823-28.

143 Akkasheh, G. et al. 2016. Clinical and metabolic response to probiotic administration in patients with major depression disorder: A randomized, doubl-blind, placebo-controlled trial. Nutrition 32(3): 315-20

144 Ghouri, Y.A. et al. 2014. Systematic review of randomized controlled trials of probiotics, prebiotics and synbiotics in inflammatory bowel disease. *Clinical & Experimental Gastroenterology* 7: 473-87.

145 Guyonnet, D. et al. 2007. Effect of a fermented milk containing Bifidobacterium animalis DN-173010 on the health-related quality of life and symptoms in irritable bowel syndrome in adults in primary care: A multicentre, randomized, double-blind, controlled trial. *Alimentary Pharmacology and Therapeutics* 26(3): 475-86.

146 Bercik, P. et al. 2010. Chronic gastrointestinal inflammation induces anxiety-like behavior and alters central nervous system biochemistry in mice. *Gastroenterology* 139(6): 2102-12.

147 Allen, A.P. et al. 2016. Bifidobacterium longum 1714 as a translational psychobiotic: Modulation of stress, electrophysiology and neurocognition in healthy volunteers. *Translational Psychiatry* 6(11) e939.

148 Wang, H. et al. 2019. *Bifidobacterium longum* 1714™ strain modulates brain activity of healthy volunteers during social stress. American Journal of *Gastroenterology* doi: 10.14309/ajg.000000000000000203.

149 Li, Y.D. et al. 2004. Effects of *Bifidobacterium breve* supplementation on intestinal flora of low birth weight babies. *Pediatrics International* 46(5): 509-15.

150 Fuller, R. 1991. Probiotics in Human Medicine. *Gut* 32(4): 439-42.

151 Guslandi, M et al. 2000. *Saccharomyces boulardii* in maintenance treatment of Crohn's disease. *Digestive Diseases and Sciences* 45(7): 1462-64.

152 Rogers, Robert. 2011. *The Fungal Pharmacy: The Complete Guide to Medicinal Mushrooms and Lichens of North America.* North Atlantic Books. Berkeley,CA.

153 Dominguez-Bello, M. G. et al. 2010. Delivery Mode Shapes the Acquistion and Structure of the Initial Microbiota across Multiple Body Habitats in Newborns. *Proc Nat Acad Sci* 107(26): 11971-75.

154 Perlmutter, David. 2015. *Brain Maker.* Little, Brown & Co. NY page 36.

155 Ibid page 149.

156 Marinho, A.C. et al. 2014. Monitoring the effectiveness of root canal procedures on endotoxin levels found in teeth with chronic apical periodontitis. *Journal of Applied Oral Science* 22(6): 490-5.

157 Perlmutter page 151.

158 Zhang, R. 2008. Circulating Endotoxin and Systemic Immune Activation in Sporadic Amyotrophic Lateral Sclerosis (ALS). *Journal of Neuroimmunology* 206(1-2).

159 Perlmutter page 173.

160 Ibid. page 193

161 Lee, Sang-Yeon et al. 2019. Association of chocolate consumption with hearing loss and tinnitus in middle-aged people based on the Korean National Health and Nutrition examination survey 2012-2013. *Nutrients* 11:746.

162 Acosta D., M. Wortmann. 2009. World Alzheimer Report in: *Alzheimer's Disease International.* Prince M. J. Jackson (Eds). London pp.1-92.

163 Risacher S.L., B.C. McDonald, E. F. Tallman. 2016. Association between anticholinergic medication use and cognition, brain metabolism, and brain atrophy in cognitively normal older adults. *Journal of the American Medical Association Neurology* 73(6):721-32.

164 Cai Xueya, N. Campbell, B. Khan, C. Callahan, M. Boustani. 2013. Long-term anticholinergic use and the aging brain. *Alzheimer's and Dementia* 9: 377-385.

165 Gomm W., K. von Holt, F. Thome, et al. 2016. Association of proton pump inhibitors with risk of dementia: A pharmacoepidemiological claims data analysis. *Journal of the American Medical Association Neurology* 73(4): 410-416.

166 Akter S., M.R. Hassian, M. Shahriar, et al. 2015. Cognitive impact after short-term exposure to different proton pump inhibitors: assessment using CANTAB software. *Alzheimer's Research and Therapy* 7: 79

167 Heading, R. et al. 2011. Prediction of response to PPI therapy and factors influencing treatment outcome in patients with GORD: A prospective pragmatic trial using pantoprazole. *BMC Gastroenterology* 11(52).

168 Dominy, S.S. et al. 2019. *Porphyromonas gingivalis* in Alzheimer's disease brains: Evidence for disease causation and treatment with small molecule inhibitors. *Sci Adv* 5(1).

169 Campbell-McBride page 43.

170 Kharrazian, D. 2013. *Why Isn't My Brain Working?* Page 240-1.

171 Schwartz, M. 2015. *Neuroimmunity.* Yale University Press. New Haven and London.

172 Ibid page 137

173 Garretti, F. et al. 2019. Autoimmunity in Parkinson's disease: the role of alpha-synuclein specific T cells. *Front Immunol* 10: 303.

174 Mischkowski, D. et al. 2019. A Social Analgesic? Acetominophen (Paracetamol) Reduces Positive Empathy. *Front Psychol* 10:538.

175 Kaufman D.W., J.P. Kelly, L. Rosenberg, et al. 2002. Recent patterns of medication use in the ambulatory adult population of the United States: the Slone survey. *Journal of the American Medical Association* 287:337-344.

176 Szekely, C. A., J. C. S. Breitner, A. L. Fitzpatrick, T. D. Rea, B. M. Psaty, L. H. Kuller, P. P. Zandi. 2008. NSAID use and dementia risk in the cardiovascular health study: Role of APOE and NSAID type. *Neurology* 70(1): 17-24.

177 Louveau, A et al. 2015. Structural and functional features of central nervous system lymphatic vessels. *Nature* 523: 337-341.

178 Jessen, N.A. et al. 2005. The Glymphatic System- A Beginner's Guide. *Neurochem Research* 40(12): 2583-99.

179 Shokri-Kojori, E et al. 2018. B-amyloid accumulation in the human brain after one night of sleep deprivation. *PNAS* 115(17): 4483-4488.

180 Killer, H.E. 2019. The importance of the lymphatic and the glymphatic system for glaucoma. *Klin Monbl Augenheilkd* 236(2): 142-144.

181 Spitzer, N. C. 2015. Neurotransmitter switching? No surprise. *Neuron* 86(5): 1131-1144

182 Shafi, M. et al. 1996. Nocturnal serum melatonin profile in major depression in children and adolescents. *Arch Gen Psychiatr* 53(11): 1009-13.

183 Baumgartner, L. et al. 2019. Effectiveness of melatonin for the prevention of intensive care unit delirium. *Pharmacotherapy* 39(3): 280-287.

184 Sandyk, R. 1992. The pineal gland and the clinical course of multiple sclerosis. *Int J Neurosci* 62: 65-74.

185 Halvorsen, A. et al. 2019. In utero exposure to selective reuptake inhibitors and development of mental disorders: a systematic review and meta-analysis. *Acta Psychiatr Scand* doi: 10.1111/acps.13030

186 Kumar, M. et al. 2019. Effect of selective serotonin reuptake inhibitors on markers of bone loss. *Psychiatry Research* 276: 39-44.

187 Lieberman, D. & M. Long. 2018. *The Molecule of More*. BenBella Books. Dallas TX. Page 16.

188 Ibid. page 46-7.

189 Sigman, Mariano. 2017. The Secret Life of the Mind. Little, Brown & Co. New York, Boston, London. Page 209.

190 Kharrazian, D. 2013. *Why Isn't My Brain Working?* Elephant Press Carlsbad CA. page 335.

191 Kharrazian, D. 2013. page 264.

192 Guang, Xi.Z. et al. 1997. Decreased beta-phenylethylamine in CSF in Parkinson's disease. *J Neurol Neurosurg Psychiatry* 63: 754-58.

193 Leonte, A. et al. 2018. Supplementation of gamma-aminobutryic acid (GABA) affects temporal, but not spatial visual attention. *Brain Cognition* 120: 8-16.

194 Kharrazian, D. 2013. page 208.

195 Jembrek, M. J., J. Vlainic. 2015. GABA Receptors: *Pharmacological Potential and Pitfalls*. 21(34): 4943-59.

196 Awad, R. et al. 2007. Effects of traditionally used anxiolytic botanicals on enzymes of the gamma-aminobutyric acid (GABA) system. *Canadian Journal of Physiology and Pharmacology* 85(9): 933-42.

197   LeWitt, P.A. et al. 2011. AAV2-GAD gene therapy for advanced Parkinson's disease: a double-blind, sham-surgery controlled, randomized trial. *The Lancet Neurology* 10(4): 309-319.

198   Benes, F.M. et al. 2007. Regulation of the GABA cell phenotype in hippocampus of schizophrenics and bipolars. *PNAS* 104:24.

199   Fatemi, S.H. et al. 2002. Glutamic acid decarboxylase 65 and 67 kDa proteins are reduced in autistic parietal and cerebellar cortices. *Biol Psychiatry* 52(8): 805-10.

200   Kharrazian, D. 2013. Page 233-4.

201   Ahangar, N. et al. 2016. Hypothermic activity of acetaminophen; involvement of GABAA receptor, theoretical and experimental studies. *Iran Journal of Basic Medical Science* 19(5): 470-5.

202   Noyer, C.M. et al. 1998. A double-blind, placebo-controlled pilot study of glutamine therapy for abnormal intestinal permeability in patients with AIDS. *American Journal of Gastroenterology* 93(6): 972-5.

203   Fernstrom, J.D. 2018. Monosodium Glutamate in the Diet Does Not Raise Brain Glutamate Concentrations or Disrupt Brain Functions. *Ann Nutr Metab* 73(5): 43-52.

204   Blaylock, R. L. 1996. *Excitotoxins: The Taste that Kills*. Health Press NM

205   Kraal, A.Z. et al. 2019. Could dietary glutamate play a role in psychiatric distress? Neuropsycholobiology 30: 1-7

206   Dean, W. & J. English. 1999. Lithium Orotate: the unique safe mineral with multiple use. *Vitamin Research News*. July.

207   Kharrazian, D. 2013. Page 324.

208   Blusztajn, J. K. et al. 2017. Neuroprotective Actions of Dietary Choline. *Nutrients* 9(8): 815.

209   Barbagallo Sangiorgi, G et al. 1994. *Ann NY Academy of Science* 717: 253-69.

210   Moreno, D.J. & M. Moreno. 2003. Cognitive improvement in mild to moderate Alzheimer's dementia after treatment with the acetylcholine precursor choline alfoscerete: a multicenter, double-blind, randomized, placebo-controlled trial. *Clin Ther* 25(1): 178-93.

211   Rivera, C.L. et al. 1988. Effects of ethanol and pantothenic acid on brain acetylcholine synthesis. *British Journal of Pharmacology* 95(1): 77-82.

212   Kaur, G. et al. 2016. Short update on docosapentaenoic acid: a bioactive long chain n-3 fatty acid. *Curr Opin Clin Nutr Metab Care* 19(2): 88-91.

213   Ivanovs, K. et al. 2017. Extraction of fish oil using green extraction methods: a short review. *Energy Procedia* 128: 477.483.

214   Ito, N. et al. 2018. Effects of composite supplement containing astaxanthin and sesamin on cognitive functions in people with mild cognitive impairment: a randomized, double-blind, placebo-controlled trial. *Journal Alzheimer's Disease* 62(4): 1767-75.

215   Lane, K. et al. 2014. Bioavailability and potential uses of vegetarian sources of omega-3 fatty acids: a review of the literature. *Crit Rev Sci Nutrition* 54(5): 572-9.

216   Su, G.Y. et al. 2019. Quercitin potentiates DHA to suppress lipopolysaccharide-induced oxidative/inflammatory responses, alter lipid peroxidation products, and enhance the adaptive stress pathways in BV-2 microglial cells. *International Journal of Molecular Science* 20(4).

217   Subbaiah, P.V. et al. 2016. Enhanced incorporation of dietary DHA into lymph phospholipids by altering its molecular carrier. *Biochim Biophys Acta* 186 (8 Pt A): 723-9.

218   Yalagala, P.C. et al. 2018. Dietary lysophosphatidylcholine-EPA enriches both EPA and DHA in the brain: Potential treatment for depression. *Journal of Lipid Research* doi: 10.1194/jlr.M090464.

219   Patrick, R.P. 2019. Role of phosphatydlcholine-DHA in preventing APOE4-associated Alzheimer's disease. *FASEB* 33(2): 1554-1564.

220   Martins, J.G. 2009. EPA but not DHA appears to be responsible for the efficacy of omega-3 long chain polyunsaturated fatty acid supplementation in depression. Evidence from a meta-analysis of randomized controlled trials. *Journal American College of Nutrition* 28(5): 525-42.

221   Parletta, N. 2016. Omega-3 and Omega-6 polyunsaturated fatty acid levels and correlations with symptoms in children with attention deficit hyperactivity disorder, autistic spectrum disorder and typically developing controls. *PLoS One* 2016 11:5.

222   Barragan, E. et al. 2017. Efficacy and safety of Omega-3/6 fatty acids, methylphenidate and a combined treatment in children with ADHD. *Journal of Attention Disorders* 21(5): 433-441.

223   Bloch, M. & A. Qawasmi. 2011. Omega-3 fatty acid supplementation in the treatment of children with attention deficit/hyperactivity disorder symtomatology: Systematic review and meta-analysis. *Journal American Academy Child Adolescent Psychiatry* 50(10): 991-1000.

224   Sinn, N. et al. 2008. Cognitive effect of polyunsaturated fatty acids in children with attention deficit hyperactivity disorder syndrome: A randomized controlled trial. *Prostaglandins Leukot Essential Fatty Acids* 78 (4-5): 311-26.

225   Gustafsson, P.A. et al. 2010. EPA supplementation improves teacher-rated behaviour and oppositional symptoms in children with ADHD. *Acta Paediatr* 99(10): 1540-9.

226   Mazahery, H. 2019. A randomized controlled trial of vitamin D and omega-3 long chain polyunsaturated fatty acids in the treatment of irritability and hyperactivity among children with autism spectrum disorder. *Journal Steroid Biochem Mol Biol* 187:9-16.

227   Keim, S.A. et al. 2018. w-3 and w-6 fatty acid supplementation may reduce autism symptoms based on parent report in preterm toddlers. *Journal of Nutrition* 148(2): 227-35.

228   Song, C. 2016. The role of omega-3 polyunsaturated fatty acids eicosapentaenoic and docosahexaenoic acids in the treatment of major depression and Alzheimer's disease: Acting separately or synergistically? *Prog Lipid Research* 62: 41-54.

229   Sarris, J. et al. 2012. Omega-3 for bipolar disorder: meta-analyses of use in mania and bipolar depression. *Journal Clinical Psychiatry* 73(1): 81-6.

230   Kahn, Jeffrey. 2013. *Angst: Origins of anxiety and depression.* Oxford University Press NY page 16.

231   Hunt, J. & D. Eisenberg. 2012. Mental health problems and help-seeking behavior among college students. *Journal of Adolescent Health* 46(1): 3-10.

232   Chae Y et al. 2013. Inserting needles into the body: a meta-analysis of brain activity associated with acupuncture needle stimulation. *The Journal of Pain: Official Journal of the American Pain Society* 14(3):215-22.

233   Jiang, X. et al. 2012. Maternal choline intake alters the epigenetic state of fetal cortisol-regulating genes in humans. *FASEB Journal* 26(8):3563-74.

234   Mills, J.L. et al. 2014. Maternal choline concentrations during pregnancy and choline-related genetic variants as risk factors for neural tube defects. *American Journal of Clinical Nutrition* 100: 1069-74.

235   Yu, C.P. et al. 2017. Effects of short forest bathing program on autonomic nervous system activity and mood states in middle-aged and elderly individuals. *Int J Environ Res Public Health* 14(8).

236   Amen, D. 2015. *Change Your Brain, Change Your Life.* Harmony Books NY. Page 327.

237   Belcaro, G. et al. 2018. Supplementation with Robuvit in post-traumatic stress disorders associated to high oxidative stress. *Minerva Med* 109(5): 363-368.

238   Ot'alora, G.M. et al. 2018. 3,4-methylenedioxymethamphetamine-assisted psychotherapy for treatment of chronic posttraumatic stress disorder: A randomized phase 2 controlled trial. *Journal of Psychopharmacology* 32(12): 1295-1307.

239   Mithoefer, M.C. et al. MDMA-assisted psychotherapy for treatment of PTSD: study design and rationale for phase 3 trials based on a pooled analysis of six phase 2 randomized controlled trials. *Psychopharmacology* doi: 10.1007/s00213-019-05249-5.

240   Willing, A.E. et al. 2019. Brazilian Jiu Jitsu training for US Service members and veterans with symptoms of PTSD. *Military Medicine* doi: 10.1093/milmed/usz074.

241   Herron, R.E. & B. Rees. 2018. The Transcendental Meditation program's impact on the symptoms of post-traumatic stress disorder of veterans: an uncontrolled pilot study. *Military Medicine* 183(1-2): e144-150.

242   Chen, L. et al. 2015. Eye movement desensitization and reprocessing versus cognitive-behavorial therapy for adult posttraumatic stress disorder: Systematic review and meta-analysis. *Journal of Nervous and Mental Disease* 203(6): 443-51.

243   Amen, D. page 144

244   Ibid page 144

245   Kumar, A. et al. 2018. A Comprehensive Review of Tourette Syndrome and Complementary Alternative Medicine. *Curr Dev Disord Rep* 5(2): 95-100.

246   Abi-Jaoude, E. et al. 2017. Preliminary Evidence on Cannabis Effectiveness and Tolerability for Adults with Tourette Syndrome. *Journal of Neuropsychiatry and Clinical Neuroscience* 29(4): 391-400.

247   Kompoliti, K. et al. 2009. Complementary and alternative medicine use in Gilles de la Tourette syndrom. *Mov Disord* 24(13): 2015-9.

248   Sanberg, P.R. et al. 1997. Nicotine for the treatment of Tourette's syndrome. *Pharmacology Ther* 74(1): 21-25.

249   Golden, S.H. 2004. Depressive symptoms and the risk of Type 2 diabetes. *Diabetes Care* 27: 429-35.

250   Addolorato, G. et al. 2004. Regional Cerebral Hypoperfusion in Patients with Celiac Disease. *The American Journal of Medicine* 116(5): 312-7.

251   Kirsch, I. et al. 2008. Initial severity and antidepressant benefits: a meta-analysis of data submitted to the Food and Drug Administration. *PLoS Medicine* 5(2): e45.

252   Kemper, K.J. & K.L. Hood. 2008. Does pharmaceutical advertising affect journal publication about dietary supplements? *BMC Complement Altern Med* 8(11).

253   Trivei, M.H. et al 2006. Evaluation of outcomes with citalopram for depression using measurement-based care in STAR*D: Implications for clinical practice. *American Journal of Psychiatry* 163: 28-40.

254   Yaffe, K. et al. 2012.Depressive symptoms and cognitive decline in non-demented elderly women. *Archives of General Psychiatry* 56(5): 425-30.

255   Amen, Daniel. 2017. *Memory Rescue.* Tyndale Pub Carol Stream, Illinois page 170-1.

256 Fancourt, D. et al. 2016. Effects of group drumming interventions on anxiety, depression, social resilience and inflammatory immune response among mental health service users. *PLoS* doi:org/10.1371/journal.pone.0151136

257 Haggerty, J.J. et al. 1986. Organic brain syndrome associated with marginal hypothyroidism. *American Journal of Psychiatry* 143(6): 785-86.

258 Shames, R. & K. Shames. 2011. *Thyroid Mind Power: The proven case for hormone-related depression, anxiety and memory loss.* Rodale Press NY.

259 Dao, M.C. et al. 2016. *Akkermansia muciniphila* and improved metabolic health during a dietary intervention in obesity: relationship with gut microbiome richness and ecology. *Gut* 65(3): 426-36.

260 Ruljancic, N. et al. 2007. Serum cholesterol concentration in psychiatric patients. *Biochemia Medica* 17(2): 197-202.

261 Merialdi, M. & J. Murray. 2007. The changing face of preterm labor. *Pediatrics* October 1.

262 Alpert, J.E. & M. Fava. 1977. Nutrition and Depression: The role of Folate. *Nutrition Review* 55: 145-9.

263 Frizel, D. et al. 1969. Plasma Magnesium and Calcium in Depression. *British Journal of Psychiatry* 115: 1275-77.

264 Sarris, J. et al. 2015. Is S-adenosyl methionine (SAMe) for depression only effective in males? A re-analysis of data from a randomized clinical trial. *Pharmacopsychiatry* 48(4-5): 141-4.

265 Terman, M. & J. Terman. 1995. Treatment of seasonal affective disorder with a high output negative ionizer. *Journal of Altern Complement Med* 1(1): 87-92.

266 Lubarda, J. et al. 2019. How is postpartum depression currently diagnosed and managed? Insights from a virtual patient simulation. *CNS Spectr* 24(1): 189-90.

267 Dowlati, Y. et al. 2017. Selective dietary supplementation in early postpartum is associated with high resilience against depressed mood. *Proc Natl Acad Sci U.S.A.* 114(13): 3509-14.

268 Aoyagi, S.S. et al. 2019. Association of late-onset postpartum depression of mothers with expressive language development during infancy and early childhood: The HBC study. *Peer J* doi: 10.7717/peerj.6566.

269 Gould, J.F. et al. 2017. Perinatal nutrition interventions and post-partum depressive symptoms. *J Affect Disord* 224: 2-9.

270 Sparling, T.M. et al. 2017. The role of diet and nutritional supplementation in perinatal depression: a systematic review. *Matern Child Nutr* 13(1).

271 Hsu, M.C. et al. 2018. Omega-3 polyunsaturated fatty acid supplementation in prevention and treatment of maternal depression: Putative mechanism and recommendation. *J Affect Disord* 238: 47-61.

272 Hoge, A. et al. 2019. Imbalance between Omega-6 and Omega-3 polyunsaturated fatty acids in early pregnancy is predictive of postpartum depression in a Belgian cohort. *Nutrients* 11(4).

273 Yan, J. et al. 2017. Association between duration of folic acid supplementation during pregnancy and risk of postpartum depression. *Nutrients* 9(11).

274 Van Ravesteyn, L.M. et al. 2017. Interventions to treat mental disorders during pregnancy: A systematic review and multiple treatment meta-analysis. *PLoS One* 12(3).

275 Fard, F.E. et al. 2017. Effects of zinc and magnesium supplements on postpartum depression and anxiety: a randomized controlled clinical trial. *Women Health* 57(9): 1115-28.

276   Vaziri, F. et al. 2016. A randomized controlled trial of vitamin D supplementation on perinatal depression: in Iranian pregnant mothers. *BMC Pregnancy Childbirth* 16:239.

277   Sheikh, M. et al. 2017. The efficacy of early iron supplementation on postpartum depression, a randomized double-blind, placebo-controlled trial. *European Journal of Nutrition* 56(2): 901-8.

278   Kianpour, M. et al. 2016. Effect of lavender scent inhalation on prevention of stress, anxiety and depression in the postpartum period. Iran *J Nurs Midwifery Res* 21(2): 197-201.

279   Gao, J.M. et al. 2019. The association between *Toxoplasma gondii* infection and postpartum blues. *J Affect Disord* 250: 404-9.

280   Scherer, S.W. et al. 2015. Whole-genome Sequencing of Quartet Families with Autism Spectrum Disorder. *Nature Medicine* doi: 10.1038/nm.3792

281   Grandin, Temple & R. Panek. 2013. *The Austistic Brain: Thinking Across the Spectrum.* Houghton Mifflin Harcourt Boston NY page 64.

282   Ibid. page 66.

283   Braunschweig, D. et al. 2013. Autism-specific maternal auto-antibodies recognize critical proteins in developing brain. *Translational Psychiatry* 3: e277.

284   Mortazavi, Gh. et al. 2016. Increased release of mercury from dental amalgam fillings due to maternal exposure to electromagnetic fields as a possible mechanism for the high rates of autism in the offspring: Introducing a hypothesis. *Journal Biomed Phys Eng* 6(1): 41-46.

285   Mazza, M. et al. 2014. Affective and cognitive empathy in adolescents with Autism Spectrum Disorder. *Frontiers in Human Neuroscience* 8:791.

286   Vojdani, A. et al. 2004. Immune response to dietary proteins, gliadin and cerebellar peptides in children with autism. *Nutritional Neuroscience* 7(3): 151-161.

287   Laake, D.G. & P. Compart. 2013. *The ADHD and Autism Nutritional Supplement Handbook.* Fair Winds Beverly Mass page 160-1.

288   Gorrindo,P. et al. 2012. Gastrointestinal Dysfunction in Autism: Parental Report, Clinical Evaluation, and Associated Factors. *Autism Research* 5(2):101-8.

289   Piwowarczyk, A. et al. 2018. Gluten- and casein-free diet and autism spectrum disorders in children: a systematic review. *Eur J Nutr* 57(2): 433-40.

290   Adams, J.B. et al. 2018. Comprehensive nutritional and dietary intervention for autism spectrum disorder- a randomized, controlled 12 month trial. *Nutrients* 10(3).

291   Hsaio, E. Y. et al. 2013. Microbiota Modulate Behavioral and Physiological Abnormalities Associated with Neurodevelopmental Disorders. *Cell* 155(7): 1451-63.

292   Bartz, J. & E. Hollander. 2008. Oxytocin and experimental therapeutics in autism spectrum disorders. *Progress in Brain Research, Advances in Vasopressin and Oxytocin—from Genes to Behaviour to Disease* 170, ed. Inga D. Neumann an Rainer Landgraf. Elsevier 451-62.

293   Pärtty, A. et al. 2015. A possible link between early probiotic intervention and the risk of neuropsychiatric disorders later in childhood: A randomized trial. *Pediatric Research* 77(6): 823-28.

294   Kaluzna-Czaplinska, J. et al. 2017. Tryptophan status in autism spectrum disorder and the influence of supplementation on its level. *Metab Brain Disease* 32(5): 1585-93.

295   deMagistris, L. et al. 2010. Alterations of the intestinal barrier in patients with autism spectrum disorders and their first-degree relatives. Journal of *Pediatric Gastroenterology and Nutrition* 51(4): 418-24.

296   Rossignol, D.A. et al. 2009. Hyperbaric treatment for children with autism: a multicenter, randomized, double-blind, controlled trial. *BMC Pediatrics* 9:21.

297   Lierberman, D. & M. Long. *The Molecule of More*. BenBella Books Dallas TX. Page 136.

298   Abrams, D.A. et al. 2013. Underconnectivity between voice-selective cortex and reward circuitry in children with autism. *Proceedings of the National Academy of Sciences* 110(29): 12060-65.

299   Modahl, C. et al. 1998. Plasma oxytocin levels in autistic children. *Biological Psychiatry* 43(4): 270-7.

300   Pretzsch, C.M. et al. 2019. Effects of cannabidiol on brain excitation and inhibition systems: a randomized placebo-controlled single dose trial during magnetic resonance spectroscopy in adults with and without autism spectrum disorder. *Neuropsycholpharmacology* doi: 10.1038/s41386-019-0333-8,

301   Yadav, S. et al. 2017. Comparative efficacy of alpha-linolenic acid and gamma-linolenic acid to attenuate valproic acid-induced autism-like features. *Journal Physiol Biochem* 73(2): 187-198.

302   Gogou, M. & G. Kolios. 2017. The effect of dietary supplements on clinical aspects of autism spectrum disorder: A systematic review of the literature. *Brain Dev* 39(8): 656-664.

303   Xia, R.R. 2011. Effectiveness of nutritional supplements for reducing symptoms in autism-spectrum disorder: a case report. *Journal Altern Complement Med* 17(3): 271-4.

304   Boris, M. et al. 2004. Association of MTHFR gene variants with autism. *Journal of American Physicians and Surgeons* 9(4): 106-8.

305   Mousavinejad, E. et al. 2018. Coenzyme Q10 supplementation reduces oxidative stress and decreases antioxidant enzyme activity in children with autism spectrum disorders. *Psychiatry Research* 265: 62-69.

306   Sweetman, D.U. et al. 2019. Zinc and vitamin A deficiency in a cohort of children with autism spectrum disorder. *Child Care Health Dev* doi: 10.1111/cch.12655.

307   Ali, A. et al. 2018. Developmental vitamin D deficiency and autism: putative pathogenic mechanisms. *J Steroid Biochem Mol Biol* 175: 108-118.

308   Al-Salem, H.S. et al. 2016. Therapeutic potency of bee pollen against biochemical autistic features induced through acute and sub-acute neurotoxicity of orally administered propionic acid. *BMC Complement Altern Med* 16:120.

309   Mahmood, U. et al. 2018. Dendritic spine anomalies and PTEN alterations in a mouse model of VPA-induced autism spectrum disorder. *Pharmacology Research* 128: 110-121.

310   Kratz, S.V. et al. 2017. The use of CranioSacral therapy for autism spectrum disorders: benefits from the viewpoints of parents, clients and therapists. *J Bodyw Mov Ther* 21(1): 19-29.

311   Kaplan, R.S. & A.L. Steele. 2005. An analysis of music therapy program goals and outcomes for clients with diagnoses on the autism spectrum. *Journal of Music Therapy* 42(1): 2-19.

312   DeMichele-Sweet, M.A. & R. Sweet. 2010. Genetics of psychosis in Alzheimer's disease: a review. *Journal of Alzheimer's Disease* 19(3): 761-780.

313   Fabiani, C. et al. 2018. A novel pharmacological activity of caffeine in the cholinergic system. *Neuropharmacology* 135: 464-473.

314   Kowalksi, K. & A. Mulak. 2019. Brain-gut-microbiota axis in Alzheimer's disease. *J Neurogastroenterol Motil* 25(1): 48-60.

383

315 Itzhaki, R.F. et al. 2017. Herpes simplex virus type 1 and Alzheimer's disease: possible mechanisms and signposts. *FASEB Journal* 31(8): 3216-26.

316 Itzhaki, R.F. et al. 2018. Corroboration of a major role for *Herpes simplex* virus type 1 in Alzheimer's disease. *Front Aging Neurosci* 10:324.

317 Kivipelto, M. & K. Håkansson. 2017. A rare success against Alzheimer's. *Scientific American* April 32-34.

318 Sheline, Y. et al. 2014. An antidepressant decreases CSF amyloid-beta production in healthy individuals and in transgenic AD mice. *Science Translational Medicine* 6:236re4.

319 Stilling, R. & J. Cryan. 2016. Host Response: A trigger for Neurodegeneration? *Nature Microbiology* doi: 10.1038/nmicrobiol.2016.129

320 Moreno-Jimenez, E. et al. 2019. Adult hippocampal neurogenesis is abundant in neurologically healthy subjects and drops sharply in patients with Alzheimer's disease. *Nature Medicine* doi: 10.1038/s41591-019-0375-9.

321 Sato, K. et al. 2019. Lower serum calcium as a potentially associated factor for conversion of mild cognitive impairment to early Alzheimer's disease in the Japanese Alzheimer's disease neuroimaging initiative doi: 10.3233/JAD-181115.

322 Newport, M. 2015. *The Coconut oil & low-carb solution for Alzheimer's, Parkinson's, and other diseases*. Basic Health Pub page 234.

323 Clarke, T. et al. 2012. Oral 28-day and developmental toxicity studies of (R)-3-hydroxybutyl (R)- 3-hydroxybutyrate. *Regulatory Toxicology and Pharmacology* 63: 196-208.

324 Oleson, S. et al. 2018. Apolipoprotein E genotype moderates the association between dietary polyunsaturated fat and brain function: an exploration of cerebral glutamate and cognitive performance. *Nutr Neurosci* 22:1-10.

325 Yurko-Mauro, K. et al. 2010. Beneficial effects of docosahexaenoic acid on cognition in aged-related cognitive decline. *Alzheimer's & Dementia* May 3.

326 Heo, J.H. et al. 2013. The possible role of antioxidant vitamin C in Alzheimer's disease treatment and prevention. *Am Journal Alzheimers Disease Other Dementia* 28(2): 120-5.

327 Mandal, P.K. et al. 2019. Cognitive improvement with glutathione supplement in Alzheimer's disease: A way forward. *J Alzheimer's Disease* doi: 10.3233/JAD-181054.

328 Tamtaji, O.R. et al. 2018. Probiotic and selenium co-supplementation, and the effects on clinical, metabolic and genetic status in Alzheimer's disease: A randomized, double-blind, controlled trial. *Clin Nutr* doi: 10.1016/j.cinu.2018.11.034.

329 Vaz, F.N.C. et al. 2018. The relationship between copper, iron and selenium levels and Alzheimer's disease. *Biol Trace Elem Res* 181(2): 185-191

330 Epperly, T. et al. 2017. Alzheimer Disease: Pharmacologic and nonpharmacologic therapies for cognitive and functional symptoms. *Am Fam Physician* 95(12): 771-8.

331 Oberman, L. & A. Pascual-Leone. 2013. Changes in plasticity across the lifespan: cause of disease and target for intervention. *Progress in Brain Research* 207: 91-120.

332 Lanza, G. 2018. Shiatsu as an adjuvant therapy for depression in patients with Alzheimer's disease: A pilot study. *Complement Ther Med* 38: 74-78.

333 Kuo, L.C. et al. 2019. Ginkgolide A prevents the amyloid-beta-induced depolarization of cortical neurons. *J Agric Food Chemistry* 67(1): 81-89.

334 Caraci, F. et al. 2017. Clinically relevant drug interactions with Anti-Alzheimer's drugs. *CNS Neurol Disord Drug Targets* 16(4): 501-513.

335 Svensson, E. et al. 2015. Vagotomy and subsequent risk of Parkinson's disease. *Annals of Neurology* 78(4): 522-9.

336   Gunnarsson, L.G. & L. Bodin. 2019. Occupational exposures and neurodegenerative diseases- A systematic literature review and meta-analyses. *Int J Environ Res Public Health* 16(3). pii:E337.

337   Kim, J.H. et al. 2019. Decreased dopamine in striatum and difficult locomotor recovery from MPTP insult after exposure to radiofrequency electromagnetic fields. *Sci Rep* 9(1): 1201.

338   Mostile, G. 2017. Iron and Parkinson's disease: A systematic review and meta-analysis. *Mol Med Rep* 15(5): 3383-3389.

339   Girota, T. et al. 2017. Levodopa responsive Parkinsonism in patients with hemochromatosis: Case presentation and literature review. *Case Rep Neurol Med* 2017:5146723.

340   Pesch, B. et al. 2019. Impairment of motor function correlates with neurometabolite and brain iron alterations in Parkinson's disease. *Cells* 8(2).

341   Bartzokis, G. et al. 1999. MRI evaluation of brain iron in earlier- and later-onset Parkinson's disease and normal subjects. *Magn Reson Imaging* 17(2) 213-22.

342   Wang, H.B. et al. 2018. Antiviral effects of ferric ammonium citrate. *Cell Discovery* 4(14).

343   Bartzokis, G et al. 2011. Gender and iron genes may modify associations between brain iron and memory in healthy aging. *Neuropsychology* 36(7): 1375-84.

344   Scheperjans, F. et al. 2015. Gut Microbiota are related to Parkinson's disease and clinical phenotype. *Movement Disorders* 30(3): 350-8.

345   Rong, H. et al. 2019. Similarly in depression, nuances of gut microbiota: evidences from a shotgun metagenomics sequencing study on major depressive disorder versus bipolar disorder with current major depressive episode patients. *Journal Psychiatric Research* 113: 90-99.

346   Cassani, E. et al. 2011. Use of probiotics for the treatment of constipation in Parkinson's disease patients. *Minerva Gastroenterologica E Dietologica* 57(2): 117-121.

347   Lieberman, D & M. Long. 2018. *The Molecule of More*. BenBella Books Dallas TX.

348   Friedman, Joseph. 2013, Making the Connection between Brain and Behavior: Coping with Parkinson's Disease 2nd Ed. DemosHealth NY.

349   Lieberman page 87.

350   Singh, J.A. & J.D. Cleveland. 2019. Gout and the risk of Parkinson's disease in older adults: a study of U.S. Medicare data. *BMC Neurol* 19(1): 4.

351   Fan, D. et al. 2018. Blackcurrant increases cyclic glycine-proline in cerebrospinal fluid and has potential to treat Parkinson's disease. *Nutrients* 10(6): 714.

352   Alamri, Y. 2018. The use of dietary supplements and perceived quality of life in patients with Parkinson's disease. *J Clin Neuroscience* 56: 137-8.

353   Friedman page 143-4.

354   Doidge, N. 2016. *The Brain's Way of Healing*. Penguin Books NY page 92.

355   Ibid page 83.

356   Ibid page 87.

357   Newport, M. 2015. *The Coconut oil & low-carb solution for Alzheimer's, Parkinson's, and other diseases*. Basic Health Pub page 98.

358   Srivastav, S. et al. 2017. Important medicinal herbs in Parkinson's disease pharmacotherapy. *Biomed Pharmacother* 92: 856-63.

359   Mischley, L.K. et al. 2017. Role of Diet and Nutritional supplements in Parkinson's disease progression. *Oxid Med Cell Longevity* 2017:6405278.

385

360 Yang, L. et al. 2009. Combination therapy with coenzyme Q10 and creatine produces additive neuroprotective effects in models of Parkinson's and Huntington's diseases. *Journal of Neurochemistry* 109(5): 1427-39

361 Sloley, B.D. et al. 2000. Identification of kaempferol as a monoamine oxidase inhibitor and potential neuroprotectant in extracts of Ginkgo biloba leaves. *J Pharm Pharmacol* 52(4): 451-9.

362 Mazzio, E. et al. 2013. High throughput screening to identify natural human monoamine oxidase B inhibitors. *Phytotherapy Research* 27(6): 818-28.

363 Chaurasiva, N.D. 2019. Selective inhibition of human monoamine oxidase B by acacetin 7-methyl ether isolated from *Turnera diffusa*. *Molecules* 24(4).

364 Schirinzi, T. et al. 2019. Dietary vitamin E as a protective factor for Parkinson's disease: clinical and experimental evidence. *Front Neurol* 10: 148.

365 Mandel, S. et al. 2004. Iron and alpha-synuclein in the substantia nigra of MPTP-treated mice: effect of neuroprotective drugs R-apomorphine and green tea polyphenol (-)-epigallocathecin-3-gallate. *Journal of Mol Neuroscience* 24(3): 401-16.

366 Lebeau, A. et al. 2001. Baicalein protects cortical neurons from beta-amyloid induced toxicity. *Neuroreport* 12(10): 2199-202.

367 Baum, L. 2004. Curcumin interaction with copper and iron suggests one possible mechanism of action in Alzheimer's disease animal models. *Journal of Alzheimer's Disease* 6(4): 367-77; discussion 443-9.

368 Zhang, X. et al. 2019. Prioritized brain selenium retention and selenoprotein expression: Nutritional insights into Parkinson's disease. *Mech Ageing Dev* 180: 89-96.

369 Song, R. et al. 2017. The impact of Tai Chi and Qigong mind-body exercises on motor and non-motor function and quality of life in Parkinson's disease: a systematic review and meta-analysis. *Parkinsonism Relat Disorders* 41:3-13.

370 Dos Santos, D.M. et al. 2018. Effects of dance practice on functional mobility, motor symptoms and quality of life in people with Parkinson's disease: a systematic review with meta-analysis. *Aging Clin Exp Research* 20(7): 727-735.

371 Noh, H. et al. 2017. Effectiveness and safety of acupuncture in the treatment of Parkinson's disease: A systematic review and meta-analysis of randomized controlled trials. *Complement Ther Med* 34: 86-103.

372 Zhang, S. et al. 2018. Bee venom therapy: Potential mechanisms and therapeutic applications. *Toxicon* 148: 64-73.

373 Porterfield, A. et al. 2015. What genetics reveals about Traditional Chinese Medicine. *General Literacy Project* 11:1.

374 Honda, M. 2018. *Reverse Alzheimer's Disease Naturally*. Hatherleigh Press page 18.

375 Newport, M. 2015. *The Coconut oil & low-carb solution for Alzheimer's, Parkinson's, and other diseases*. Basic Health Pub page 98-99.

376 Nabavi, S.F. et al. Natural compounds used as therapies targeting to amytrophic lateral sclerosis. *Curr Pharm Biotechnology* 16(3): 211-8.

377 Chico, L. et al. 2018. Amyotrophic lateral sclerosis and oxidative stress: A double-blind therapeutic trial after curcumin supplementation. *CNS Neurol Disord Drug Targets* 17(10): 767-779.

378 Sarkar, S. et al. 2007. Trehalose, a novel mTOR-independent autophagy enhancer, accelerates the clearance of mutant huntingtin and alpha-synuclein. *Journal Biol Chem* 282(8): 5641-52.

379   Ramachandran, S. & S. Thangarajan. 2016. A novel therapeutic application of solid lipid nanoparticles encapsulated thymoquinone (TQ-SLNs) on 3-nitroproponic acid induced Huntington's disease-like symptoms in wistar rats. *Chem Biol Interact* 256: 25-36.

380   Zanforlin, E. et al. 2017. The medicinal chemistry of natural and semisynthetic compounds against Parkinson's and Huntington's diseases. *ACS Chem Neurosci* 8(11): 2356-2368.

381   Zhang, H. et al. 2017. Recent advances in discovery and development of natural products as source for anti-Parkinson's disease lead compounds. *European Journal Med Chem* 141: 257-272.

382   Campbell-McBride, N. 2010. *Gut and Psychology Syndrome*. Medinform Pub Cambridge page 77.

383   Ahn, J.E. et al. 2018. Iron supplements in nursing home patients associated with reduced carbamezepine absorption. *Epilepsy Res* 147: 115-8.

384   Tello, I. et al. 2013. Anticonvulsant and neuroprotective effects of oligosaccharides from Lingzhi or Reishi medicinal mushroom, Ganoderma lucidum (Higher basidiomycetes). *International Journal of Medicinal Mushrooms* 15(6): 555-68.

385   Omrani, S. et al. 2019. The effect of omega-3 fatty acids on clinical and paraclinical features of intractable epileptic patients: a triple blind randomized clinical trial. *Clin Transl Med* 8(1):3.

386   Ibrahim, F.A.S. et al. 2018. The differential effects of eicosapentaenoic acid (EPA) and docosahexaenoic acid (DHA) on seizure frequency in patients with drug-resistant epilepsy- A randomized, double-blind, placebo-controlled trial. *Epilepsy Behav* 87: 32-8.

387   Campbell-McBride page 82.

388   Roehl, K. et al. 2019. Modified ketogenic diets in adults with refractory epilepsy: efficacious improvements in seizure frequency, seizure severity, and quality of life. *Epilepsy Behav* doi: 10.1016/j.yebeh.2018.12.010.

389   Falco-Walter, J.J. et al. 2019. Do certain subpopulations of adults with drug-resistant epilepsy respond better to modified ketogenic diet treatments? Evaluation based on prior resective surgery, type of epilepsy, imaging abnormalities, and vagal nerve stimulation. *Epilepsy Behav* doi: 10.1016/j.yebeh.2019.01.010.

390   Caraballo, R.H. et al. 2014. Ketogenic diet in patients with Lennox-Gastaut syndrome. *Seizure* 23(9): 751-5.

391   Sharma, S. et al. 2015. Use of modified Atkins diet in Lennox Gastaut syndrome. *J Child Neurol* 30(5): 576-9.

392   Wilson, M.P. et al. 2019. Disorders affecting vitamin B6 metabolism. *Journal Inherit Metab Dis* doi: 10. 1002/jimd.12060.

393   Coughlin, C.R. 2nd et al. 2015. Triple therapy with pyridoxine, arginine supplementation and dietary lysine restriction in pyridoxine-dependent epilepsy: Neurodevelopmental outcome. *Mol Genet Metab* 116(1-2): 35-43.

394   Nabavi, S.F. et al. 2015. Neuroprotective effects of chrysin: from chemistry to medicine. *Neurochem International* 90: 224-231.

395   Gómez-Equilaz, M. et al. 2018. The beneficial effect of probiotics as a supplementary treatment in drug-resistant epilepsy: a pilot study. *Benef Microbes* 9(6): 875-881.

396   Panebianco, M. et al. 2017. Yoga for epilepsy. *Cochrane Database Syst Rev* 10:CD001524.

397   Yimer, E.M. et al. 2019. The effect of metformin in experimentally induced animal models of epileptic seizure. *Behav Neurol* doi: 10.1155/2019/6234758.

398 Gudjonsson, G.H. et al. 2012. An epidemiological study of ADHD symptoms among young persons and the relationship with cigarette smoking, alcohol consumption and illicit drug use. *J Child Psycho Psychiatry* 53(3): 304-312.

399 Clemow, D.B. et al. 2017. Misuse of Methylphenidate. *Curr Top Behav Neurosci* 34: 99-124.

400 Romm, A. & T. Romm. 2000. *ADHD Alternatives.* Storey Pub. North Adams Mass.

401 Vaa, T. 2014. ADHD and relative risk of accidents in road traffic: A meta-analysis. *Accident; Analysis and Prevention* 62: 415-25.

402 Antshel, K.M. et al. 2003. Developmental Timing of Exposure to Elevated Levels of Phenylalanine is Associated with ADHD Symptom Expression. *Journal Abnorm Child Psychol* 31(6):565-74.

403 Neiderhofer, H. et al. 2006. A preliminary investigation of ADHD symptoms in persons with celiac disease. *Journal of Attention Disorders* 10(2): 200-204.

404 Bateman, B. et al. 2004. Food Additives increase hyperactivity in Children. *Arch Dis Child* 89(6): 506-11.

405 Del-Ponte, B. et al. 2019. Sugar consumption and attention-deficit/hyperactivity disorder (ADHD): a birth cohort study. *Journal Affect Disord* 243: 290-96.

406 Wei, H.T. et al. 2019. Risks of bipolar disorder, depressive disorder, and traumatic brain injury among siblings of patients with attention-deficit hyperactivity disorder. *J Affect Disord* 245: 335-9.

407 Milte, C.M. et al. 2015. Increased erythrocyte eicosapentaenoic acid and docosahexanoic acid are associated with improved attention and behavior in children with ADHD in a randomized controlled three-way crossover trial. *Journal of Attention Disorders* 19(11): 954-64.

408 Ghanizadeh, A. 2013. A systematic review of magnesium therapy for treating attention deficit hyperactivity disorders. *Archives of Iranian Medicine* 16(7): 412-7.

409 Hirayama, S. et al. The effect of phosphatidylserine administration on memory and symptoms of Attention-Deficit Hyperactivity Disorder: A randomized, double-blind, placebo-controlled clinical trial. *Journal of Human Nutrition and Dietetics* 27 (supp 2) 284-91.

410 Lyon, M.R. et al. 2011. The effects of L-theanine (suntheanine) on objective sleep quality in boys with Attention Deficit Hyperactivity Disorder (ADHD): A randomized, double-blind, placebo-controlled clinical trial. *Alternative Medicine Review* 16(4): 348-54.

411 Toren, P. et al. 1996. Zinc deficiency in Attention-Deficit Hyperactivity Disorder. *Biological Psychiatry* 40(12): 1308-10.

412 Gordon, H.A. et al. 2015. Clinically significant symptom reduction in children with attention-deficit/hyperactivity disorder treated with micronutrients: an open-label reversal design study. *J Child Adolesc Psychopharm* 25(10): 783-98.

413 Sagiv, S.K. et al. 2010. Prenatal organochlorine exposure and behaviors associated with attention deficit hyperactivity disorder in school-aged children. *Am Journal Epidemiol* 171: 593-601.

414 Alexander, J. 2012. Docosahexaenoic acid for reading, cognition and behavior in children aged 7-9 years: a randomized, controlled trial (the DOLAB Study). *PLoS One* September 6.

415 Akhondazedeh, S. et al. 2004. Zinc sulfate as an adjunct to methylphenidate for the treatment of attention deficit hyperactivity disorder in children: a double blind and randomized trial. *BMC Psychiatry* 4:9.

416 Huss, M. et al. 2010. Supplementation of polyunsaturated fatty acids, magnesium and zinc in children seeking medical advice for attention-deficit/hyperactivity problems—an observational cohort study. *Lipids Health Dis* 9:105.

417 Hoebert, M. et al. 2009. Long-term follow-up of melatonin treatment in children with ADHD and chronic sleep onset insomnia. *J Pineal Research* 47: 1-7.

418 Camargo, C.H. & A. Bronzini. 2015. Tourette's syndrome in famous musicians. *Arq Neuropsiquiatr* 73(12): 1038-40.

419 Doidge, N. *The Brain's Way of Healing*. Penguin pages 280-352.

420 Tan, O. et al. 2016. Obsessive-compulsive adults with and without childhood ADHD symptoms. *Atten Defic Hyperact Disord* 8(3): 131-8.

421 Bianco-Vieira, T. et al. 2019. The impact of attention deficit hyperactivity disorder in obsessive-compulsive disorder subjects. *Depress Anxiety* doi: 10.1002/da.22898.

422 Fuss, J. et al. 2019. Compulsive sexual behavior disorder in obsessive-compulsive disorder: Prevalence and associated comorbidity. *Journal Behav Addiction* 13:1-7.

423 Blum, A.W. et al. 2019. Links between sexuality, impulsivity, compulsivity, and addiction in a large sample of university students. *CNS Spectr* 15: 1-7.

424 Swartz, J. 2016. *Brain Lock- Free Yourself from Obsessive-Compulsive Behavior*. Harper Perennial NY.

425 Rodrigo, L. et al. 2018. Efficacy of a gluten-free diet in the Gillies de la Tourette syndrome: A pilot study. *Nutrients* 10(5).

426 Kharrazian, D. 2013. *Why Isn't My Brain Working?* Elephant Press Carlsbad CA page 303.

427 Grant, J.E. et al. 2009. N-acetylcysteine, a glutamate modulator, in the treatment of trichotillomania: a double-blind, placebo-controlled study. *Arch Gen Psychiatry* 66(7): 756-63.

428 Ghanizadeh, A. et al. 2017. Efficacy of N-acetylcysteine augmentation on obsessive-compulsive disorder: A multicenter randomized double blind placebo controlled clinical trial. *Iran Journal Psychiatry* 12(2): 134-141.

429 Taylor, L.H. & K.A. Kobak. 2000. An open-label trial of St. John's wort (*Hypericum perforatum*) in obsessive-compulsive disorder. *Journal of Clinical Psychiatry* 61(8): 575-8.

430 Pakseresht, S. et al. 2011. Extract of valerian root (*Valeriana officinalis* L.) vs. placebo in treatment of obsessive-compulsive disorder: a randomized double-blind study. *J Complement Integr Med* 8(1).

431 Sayyah, M. et al. 2010. Comparison of *Silybum marianum* (L.) Gaertn. with fluoxetine in the treatment of Obsessive-Compulsive Disorder. *Prog Neuropsycholpharmacol Biol Psychiatry* 34(2): 362-5.

432 Lieberman, D. & M. Long. 2018. *The Molecule of More*. BenBella Books. Dallas TX. Page 113.

433 Fuglewicz, A.J. et al. 2017. Relationship between toxoplasmosis and schizophrenia: a review. *Adv Clin Exp Med* 26(6): 1031-36.

434 Torrey, E.F. & R.H. Yolken. 2003. Toxoplasma gondii and Schizophrenia. *CDC Prevention* 9:11.

435 Cambell-McBride, N. 2012. GAPS: Gut and Psychology Syndrome. Medinform Pub. Cambridge UK page 71.

436 Ibid page 72.

437 Strassman, Rick. 2001. *DMT The Spirit Molecule*. Park St Press Rochester VT.

438 Bigelow, L. 1974. Effects of aqueous pineal extract on chronic schizophrenia. *Biological Psychiatry* 8:5-15.

439 Jiang, X. et al. Surgical resection of pineal epidermoid cyst contributed to relieving schizophrenia symptoms. *World Neurosurgery* 113: 304-7.

440 Stahl, B.A. et al. 2018. The taurine transporter Eaat2 functions in ensheathing glia to modulate sleep and metabolic rate. *Curr Biol* 28(22): 3700-08.

441 Sherman, J.A. 2012. Evolutionary origin of bipolar disorder-revised. EOBD-R. *Med Hypotheses* 78(1): 113-122.

442 Merinkangas, K. et al. 2011. Prevalence and Correlates of Bipolar Spectrum Disorder in the World Mental Health Survey Initiative. *Arch Gen Psychiatry* 68(3): 241-51.

443 Gao, Y. et al. 2018. Ethanol normalizes glutamate-induced elevation of intracellular sodium in olfactory neuroepithelia progenitors from subjects with bipolar illness but not nonbipolar controls: Biological evidence for the self-medication hypothesis. *Bipolar Disorders* doi: 10.1111/bdi.12737.

444 Lieberman page 190.

445 Shen, Y.C. et al. 2019. Association of hysterectomy with bipolar risk: A population-based cohort study. *Depression Anxiety* doi: 10.1002/da.22904.

446 Lieberman page 196.

447 Ibid page 192-3.

448 Ohlund, L. et al. 2018. Reasons for lithium discontinuation in men and women with bipolar disorder: a retrospective cohort study. *BMC Psychiatry* 18(1): 37.

449 Rogers, R. et al. 2003. *Herbal-Drug Interactions*. Capital Health. Mediscript Communications.

450 Schrauzer, G.N. & K.P. Shrestha. 1990. Lithium in drinking water and the incidences of crimes, suicides and arrests related to drug addictions. Biol Trace Elem Res 25(2): 105-13.

451 Liaugaudaite, V. et al. 2017. Lithium levels in the public drinking water supply and risk of suicide: A pilot study. *Journal of Trace Elements in Medicine and Biology* 43: 197-201.

452 Zhang, Q. et al. 2016. Timosaponin derivative YY-23 acts as a non-competitive NMDA receptor antagonist and exerts a rapid anti-depressant-like effect in mice. *Acta Pharmacol Sin* 37(2): 166-76.

453 Buckle, J. 2015. *Clinical Aromatherapy: Essential Oils in Healthcare*. Elsevier page 299-300.

454 Du, J.P. et al. 2017. Fast-onset antidepressant potentials of essential oil of herbs. *Zhongguo Zhong Yao Za Zhi* 42(10): 2006-16.

455 Özdin, S. et al. 2018. Early maladaptive schemas in patients with bipolar and unipolar disorder. *Int J Psychiatry Clin Pract* 22(2): 151-6.

456 Maruani, J. & P.A. Geoffroy. 2019. Bright light as a personalized precision treatment of mood disorders. *Front Psychiatry* 10:85.

457 Costi, S. et al. 2019. Lithium continuation therapy following ketamine in patients with treatment resistant unipolar depression: a randomized controlled trial. *Neuropsychopharmacology* doi: 10.1038/s41386-019-0365-0.

458 Rogers, R. 2016. *Mushroom Essences: Vibrational Healing from the Kingdom Fungi*. North Atlantic Books Berkeley, CA page 163.

459 Kalayasiri, R. et al. 2018. A novel approach of substitution therapy with inhalation of essential oils for the reduction of inhalant craving: A double-blinded randomized controlled trial. *Psychiatry Res* 261: 61-7.

460 Lieberman, D. & M. Long. *The Molecule of More*. BenBella Books Dallas TX page 47.

461 Durazzo, T.C. et al. 2014. Smoking and increased Alzheimer's disease risk: A review of potential mechanisms. *Alzheimer's and Dementia* 10 (S3):S122-45.

462 Mattioli, L. & M. Perfumi. 2006. Evaluation of Rhodiola rosea L. extract on affective and physical signs of nicotine withdrawal in mice. *Swed Dent Journal* 20(2): 55-60.

463 Catania, M. et al. 2003. Hypericum perforatum attenuates nicotine withdrawal signs in mice. *Psychopharmacology* 169(2): 186-9.

464 Rungruanghiranya, S. et al. 2012. Efficacy of fresh lime for smoking cessaton. *J Med Assoc Thai* 95 (Suppl 12):76-82.

465 Ding, J. et al. 2004. Alcohol intake and cerebral abnormalities on Magnetic Resonance Imaging in a community-based population of middle-aged adults. The Atherosclerosis Risk in Communities (ARIC) Study. *Stroke* 35(1): 16-21.

466 Topiwala, A. et al. 2017. Moderate alcohol consumption as risk factor for adverse brain outcomes and cognitive decline: longitudinal cohort study. *British Medical Journal* doi: doi.org/10.1136/bmj.j2353.

467 Berntsen, S. et al. 2015. Alcohol consumption and mortality in patients with mild Alzheimer's disease: a prospective cohort study. *BMJ Open* 5(12).

468 Connor, J. 2017. Alcohol consumption as a cause of cancer. *Addiction* 112(2).

469 Lieberman page 102.

470 Gao, Y. et al. 2018. Ethanol normalizes glutamate-induced elevation of intracellular sodium in olfactory neuroepithelia progenitors from subjects with bipolar illness but not nonbipolar controls: Biological evidence for the self-medication hypothesis. *Bipolar Disorders* doi: 10.1111/bdi.12737.

471 Koopmann, A. et al. 2018. The impact of the appetite-regulating, orexigenic peptide ghrelin on alcohol use disorders: A systematic review of preclinical and clinical data. *Biol Psychol* 131: 14-30.

472 Kushner, S. et al. 2013. Declinol, a complex containing kudzu, bitter herbs (gentian, tangerine peel) and bupleurum, significantly reduced alcohol use disorders identification test (AUDIT) scores in moderate to heavy drinkers: A pilot study. *Journal Addict Res Ther* 4(3): 153.

473 Mansoor, K. et al. 2018. An open prospective pilot study of a herbal combination "Relief" as a supportive dietetic measure during alcohol withdrawal. *Neuro Endocrinol Lett* 39(1): 1-8.

474 Lieberman page 191.

475 Cruz, J.I. & S.A. Nappo. 2018. Is Ayahuasca an option for the treatment of crack cocaine dependence? *Journal Psychoactive Drugs* 50(3): 247-255.

476 Coleman, J.A. et al. 2019. Serotonin transporter-ibogaine complexes illuminate mechanisms of inhibition and transport. *Nature* doi: 10.1038/s41586-019-1135-1.

477 Mojtabai, R. et al. 2019. Misuse of prescribed opioids in the United States. *Pharmacoepidemiol Drug Safety* 28(3): 345-353.

478 Boggis, J.S. & K. Feder 2019. Trends in and correlates of tranquilizer misuse among adults who misuse opioids in the United States, 2002-2014. *Drug Alcohol Depend* 198: 158-161.

479 Foley, M. et al. 2019. Associations of state-level rates of depression and fatal opioid overdose in the United States, 2011-2015. *Social Psychiatry and Psychiatric Epidemiology* 54(1): 131-134.

480 Hadland, S.E. et al. 2019. Association of pharmaceutical industry marketing of opioid products with mortality from opioid-related overdoses. *JAMA Network Open* 2(1):e186007.

481 Doidge, N. *The Brain's Way of Healing.* Penguin Books NY page 29.

391

482   Ibid pages 1-32.

483   Halpenny, G.M. 2017. Mitragyna speciosa: Balancing Potential Medical Benefits and Abuse. *ACS Med Chem Lett* 8(9): 897-899.

484   Henningfield, J.E. et al. 2018. The abuse potential of kratom according to 8 factors of the controlled substances act: implications for regulation and research. *Psychopharmacology* 235(2): 573-589.

485   Kruegel, A.C. & O. Grundmann. 2018. The medicinal chemistry and neuropharmacology of kratom: A preliminary discussion of a promising medicinal plant and analysis of its potential for abuse. *Neuropharmacology* 134 (Pt A): 108-120.

486   Nissan, H.P. et al. 2007. A red clover (*Trifolium pratense*) phase II clinical extract possesses opiate activity. *Journal of Ethnopharmacology* 112(1): 207-10.

487   Ling, W. et al. 2015. Pratensein attenuates amyloid-beta-induced cognitive deficits in rats: enhancement of synaptic plasticity and cholinergic function. *Fitoterapia* 101: 208-17.

488   Belofsky, G. 2004. New geranyl stilbenes from *Dalea purpurea* with *in vitro* opioid receptor affinity. *Journal Natural Products* 67(1): 26-30.

489   Dixon, M. et al. 2006. *Gambling: Behavior theory, research and application.* Context Press Reno, NV.

490   Temperman, L., P. Albanese, S. Stark, N. Zahlan. 2013. *The Dostoevsky Effect: Problem Gambling and the Origins of Addiction.* Oxford University Press page 159.

491   Grant, J.E. et al. 2019. Gambling and its clinical correlates in university students. *International Journal Psychiatry Clin Pract* 23(1): 33-39.

492   Gentile, D. 2009. Pathological video-game use among youth ages 8 to 18: A national study. *Psychological Science* 20(5): 594-602.

493   Noguerira, M. et al. 2019. Addictive Video Game Use: An Emerging Pediatric Problem? *Acta Med Port* 32(3): 183-188.

494   Kardaras, N. 2016. *Glow Kids: How screen addiction is hijacking our kids—and how to break the trance.* St. Martin's Press, Macmillan Pub NY.

495   Merchant, R.E. & C.A. Andre. 2001. A review of recent clinical trials of the nutritional supplement *Chlorella pyrenoidosa* in the treatment of fibromyalgia, hypertension and ulcerative colitis. *Altern Ther Health Med* 7(3): 79-91.

496   Souza, J.Q. et al. 2016. *Chlorella vulgaris* reduces the impact of stress on hypothalamic-pituitary-adrenal axis and brain c-fos expression. *Psychoneuroendocrinology* 65: 1-8.

497   Hwang, J.H. et al. 2011. Spirulina prevents memory dysfunction, reduces oxidative stress damage and augments antioxidant activity in senescence-accelerated mice. *Journal Nutr Sci Vitaminol* (Tokyo) 57(2): 186-91.

498   Pabon, M.M. et al. 2012. A spirulina-enhanced diet provides neuroprotection in an alpha-synuclein model of Parkinson's disease. *PLoS One* 7(9):e45256.

499   Perez-Juarez, A. et al. 2016. Neuroprotective effect of *Arthrospira* (*Spirulina*) *platensis* against kainic acid-neuronal death. *Pharm Biol* 54(8): 1408-12.

500   Koh, E.J. et al. 2018. *Spirulina maxima* extract prevents cell death through BDNF activation against amyloid beta 1-42 induced neurotoxicity in PC12 cells. *Neuroscience* 673: 33-38.

501   McCarty, M.F. & S. Lloki-Assanga et al. 2018. Co-administration of phycocyanobilin and/or phase 2-inducer nutraceuticals for prevention of opiate tolerance. *Curr Pharm Des* 24(20): 2250-54.

502 Scoglio, S. et al. 2014. Selective monamine oxidase B inhibition by an *Aphanizomenon flos-aquae* extract and by its constitutive active principles phycocyanin and mycosporine-like amino acids. *Phytomedicine* 21(7): 992-7.

503 Nuzo, D. et al. 2018. Effects of the Aphanizomenon flos-aquae extract (Klamin®) on a neurodegeneration cellular model. *Oxid Med Cell Longev* 2018: 9089016.

504 Lance, E. et al. 2018. Occurrence of b-N-methylamino-L-alanine (BMAA) and Isomers in aquatic environments and aquatic food sources for humans. *Toxins* (Basel) 10(2): 83.

505 Lin, J et al. 2017. Fucoxanthin, a marine carotenoid, attenuates beta-amyloid oligmer-induced neurotoxicity possibly via regulating the P13K/Akt and the ERK pathways in SH-SY5Y cells. *Oxid Med Cell Longev* 2017: 6792543.

506 Kim, S.O. et al. 2010. The ethyl alcohol extract of Hizikia fusiforme inhibits matrix metalloproteinase activity and regulates tight junction related proteins expression in Hep3B human hepatocarcinoma cells. *Journal of Medicinal Food* 13(1): 31-38.

507 Silva, J. et al. 2019. Antioxidant and neuroprotective potential of the brown seaweed Bifurcaria bifurcata in an in vitro Parkinson's disease model. *Mar Drugs* 17:2.

508 Silva, J. et al. 2018. Neuroprotective effects of seaweeds against 6-hydroxidopamine induced cell death on an in vitro human neuroblastoma model. *BMC Complementary Alternative Medicine* 18(1): 58.

509 Harris, C.B. et al. 2013. Dietary pyrroloquinone quinone (PQQ) alters indicators of inflammation and mitochondrial-related metabolism in human subjects. *Journal Nutr Biochem* 24(12): 2076-84.

510 Nakano, M. et al. 2016. Effects of antioxidant supplements (BioPQQ™) on cerebral blood flow and oxygen metabolism in the prefrontal cortex. Adv *Exp Med Biol* 923: 215-222.

511 Itoh, Y. et al. 2016. Effect of the antioxidant supplement pyrroloquinone quinone disodium salt (BioPQQ) on cognitive functions. *Adv Exp Med Biol* 876: 319-325.

512 Lu, J. et al. 2018. Mitochondrial regulation by pyrroloquinoline quinone prevents rotenone-induced neurotoxicity in Parkinson's disease models. *Neurosci Lett* 687: 104-110.

513 Ferreira, G.C. & M.C. McKenna. 2017. L-carnitine and Acetyl-L-carnitine roles and neuroprotection in developing brain. *Neurochem Res* 42(6): 1661-75.

514 Sergi, G. 2018. Effects of acetyl-L-carnitine in diabetic neuropathy and other geriatric disorders. *Aging Clin Exp Research* 30(2): 133-8.

515 Fernandes, S. et al. 2015. Methamphetamine promotes alpha-tubulin deacetylation in endothelial cells: the protective role of acetyl-l-carnitine. *Toxicol Lett* 234(2): 131-8.

516 Montgomery, S. A. et al. 2003. Meta-analysis of double blind randomized controlled clinical trials of acetyl-L-carnitine versus placebo in the treatment of mild cognitive impairment and mild Alzheimer's disease. *International Clinical Psychopharmacology* 18: 61-71.

517 Veronese, N. et al. 2018. Acetyl-l-carnitine supplementation and the treatment for depressive symptoms: A systematic review and meta-analysis. *Psychosomatic Medicine* 80(2): 154-159

518 Bigio, B. et al. 2016. Epigenetics and energetic in ventral hippocampus mediate rapid antidepressant action: Implications for treatment resistance. *Proc National Academy of Science U.S.A* 113(28): 7906-11.

519 Brennan, B.P. et al. 2013. A placebo-controlled trial of acetyl-L-carnitine and alpha lipoic acid in the treatment of bipolar depression. *J Clin Psychopharmacology* 33(5): 627-35.

520 Sanders, L. et al. 2017. Alpha-lipoic acid as adjunctive treatment for schizophrenia: an open-label trial. *J Clin Psychopharmacology* 37(6): 697-701.

521 Kim, N.W. et al. 2016. Adjunctive alpha-lipoic acid reduces weight pain compared with placebo at 12 weeks in schizophrenic patients treated with atypical antipsychotics: a double-blind randomized placebo controlled study. *International Clin Psychopharmacol* 31(5): 265-74.

522 De Sousa, C.N.S. et al. 2019. Alpha-lipoic acid in the treatment of psychiatric and neurological disorders: a systematic review. *Metab Brain Dis* 34(1): 39-52.

523 Kulikova, O.I. et al. 2018. Neuroprotective effect of the carnosine-alpha lipoic acid nanomicellar complex in a model of early-stage Parkinson's disease. *Regul Toxicol Pharmacol* 95: 254-9.

524 Namvarpour, Z. et al. 2018. Protective role of alpha-lipoic acid in impairments of social and stereotyped behaviors induced by early postnatal administration of thimerosal in male rat. *Neurotoxicol Teratol* 67:1-9.

525 Bernard, S. et al. 2001. Autism: a novel form of mercury poisoning. *Med Hypotheses* 56(4): 462-71.

526 Ripps, H. & W. Shen. 2012. Review: Taurine: a 'very essential' amino acid. *Molecular Vision* 18:2673-86.

527 Gebara, E. et al. 2015. Taurine increases hippocampal neurogenesis in aging mice. *Stem Cell Research* 14(3): 369-79.

528 Paula-Lima, A.C. et al. 2005. Activation of GABA(A) receptors by taurine and muscimol blocks the neurotoxicity of beta-amyloid in rat hippocampal and cortical neurons. *Neuropharmacology* 49(8): 1140-8.

529 Oja, S.S & P. Saransaari. 2013. Taurine and epilepsy. *Epilepsy Research* 104(3): 187-194.

530 Goodman, H.O. et al. 1980. Taurine transport in epilepsy. *Clinical Chemistry* 26(3).

531 Kendler, Barry S. 1989. Taurine: An overview of its role in preventive medicine. *Preventive Medicine* 18(1): 79-100.

532 Tsolaki, M. 2019. Future strategies of management of Alzheimer's disease. The role of homotaurine. *Hell J Nucl Med 22*(Suppl): 82-94.

533 Bossù, P. et al. 2018. Anti-inflammatory effects of homotaurine in patients with amnestic mild cognitive impairment. *Front Aging Neurosci* 10:285.

534 Ricciardi, L. et al. 2015. Homotaurine in Parkinson's disease. *Neurol Sci* 36(9): 1581-7.

535 Jongkees, B.J. et al. 2015. Effect of tyrosine supplementation on clinical and healthy populations under stress or cognitive demands- a review. *Journal of Psychiatr Research* 70: 50-57.

536 Salter, C.A. et al. 1989. Dietary tyrosine as an aid to stress resistance among troops. *Military Machine* 154(3): 144-146.

537 Bloemendaal, M. et al. 2018. Neuro-cognitive effects of acute tyrosine administration on reactive and proactive response inhibition in healthy older adults. *eNeuro* 5(2).

538 Gelenberg, A.J. et al. 1980. Tyrosine for the treatment of depression. *American Journal of Psychiatry* 1347(5):622.

539 Carvalho-Silva, M. et al. 2019. Omega-3 fatty acid supplementation can prevent changes in mitochondrial energy metabolism and oxidative stress caused by chronic administration of L-tyrosine in the brain of rats. *Metab Brain Dis* doi: 10.1007/s11011-019-00411-6.

540 Harmer, C.J. et al. 2001. Tyrosine depletion attenuates dopamine function in healthy volunteers. *Psychopharmacology* 154(1): 105-11.

541   Gedgaudas, Nora. 2011. *Primal Body, Primal Mind*. Healing Arts Press Rochester VT page 267.

542   Matthews, R.T. et al. 1999. Creatine and cyclocreatine attenuate MPTP neurotoxicity. *Exp Neurol* 157(1): 142-49.

543   Klivenyi, P.I. et al. 1999. Neuroprotective effects of creatine in a transgenic animal model of amyotrophic lateral sclerosis. *Nat Med* 5(3): 347-50.

544   Tanja, S. et al. 2006. The creatine kinase/creatine connection to Alzheimer's disease: CK inactivation, APP-CK complexes, and Focal Creatine deposits. *Journal Biomed Biotech* 2006:35936.

545   Campistol, J. 2016. Epilepsy in inborn errors of metabolism with therapeutic options. *Semin Pediatr Neurol* 23(4): 321-31.

546   Fons, C. & J. Campistol. 2016. Creatine defects and central nervous system. *Semin Pediatr Neurol* 23(4): 285-289.

547   Yang, Z.Y. et al. 2015. Proton magnetic resonance spectroscopy revealed differences in the glutamate + glutamine/creatine ratio of the anterior cingulated cortex between healthy and pediatric post-traumatic stress disorder patients diagnosed after 2008 Wenchuan earthquake. *Psychiatry Clinical Neuroscience* 69(12): 782-90.

548   Adriano, E. et al. 2018. Di-acetyl creatine ethyl ester, a new creatine derivative for the possible treatment of creatine transporter deficiency. *Neurosci Letters* 665: 217-223.

549   Ostojic, S.M. 2017. Dietary guanidinoacetic acid increases brain creatine levels in healthy men. *Nutrition* 33: 149-156.

550   Mehrazad-Sabar, Z. et al. 2018. Effects of l-carnosine supplementation on sleep disorders and disease severity in autistic children: a randomized, controlled clinical trial. *Basic Clin Pharmacol Toxicol* 123(1): 72-77.

551   Fujita, T. & K. Sakurai. 1995. Efficacy of glutamine-enriched enteral nutrition in an experimental model of mucosal ulcerative colitis. *British Journal of Surgery* 82(6): 749-51.

552   Chang, W.K. et al. 1999. Effect of glutamine on Th1 and Th2 cytokine responses of human peripheral blood mononuclear cells. *Clin Immunol* 93(3): 294-301.

553   Sogut, I. et al. 2017. Prenatal alcohol-induced neuroapoptosis in rat brain cerebral cortex: protective effect of folic acid and betain. *Childs Nervous System* 33(3): 407-17.

554   Zheng, Y. et al. 2016. Dietary phosphatylcholine and risk of all-cause, and cardiovascular-specific mortality among US women and men. *American Journal of Clinical Nutrition* 104(1): 173-80.

555   Fioravanti, M. & A.E. Buckley. 2006. Citicoline (Cognizin) in the treatment of cognitive impairment. *Clinical Interventions in Aging* 1(3): 247-51.

556   Nemkova, S.A. et al. 2018. Cognitive and emotional disorders in university students and teachers: the possibility of treatment with recognan (citicoline). *Zh Nevrol Psikhiatr Im S S Korsakova* 118(12): 11-18.

557   McGlade, E. et al. 2015. The effect of citicoline supplementation on motor speed and attention in adolescent males. *Journal of Attention Disorders* July 15.

558   Aminzadeh, A. & A. Salarinejad. 2019. Citicoline protects against lead-induced oxidative injury in neuronal PC12 cells. *Biochem Cell Biol* doi: 10.1139/bcb-2018-0218.

559   Brown, E.S. et al. 2015. A randomized, double-blind, placebo-controlled trial of citicoline for cocaine dependence in bipolar I disorder. *American Journal of Psychiatry* 172(10): 1014-21.

560 Glade, M.J. et al. 2015. Phosphatidylserine and the human brain. *Nutrition* 31(6): 781-6.

561 Kim, H.Y. et al. 2014. Phosphotidylserine in the brain: metabolism and function. *Prog Lipid Research* 56: 1-18.

562 Zhang, Y.Y. et al. 2015. Effects of phosphatidylserine on memory in patients and rats with Alzheimer's disease. *Genet Mol Research* 14(3): 9325-33.

563 Moré, M.I. et al. 2014. Positive effects of soy lecithin-derived phosphatydlserine plus phosphatidic acid on memory, cognition, daily functioning, and mood in elderly patients with Alzheimer's disease and dementia. *Adv Ther* 31(12): 1247-62.

564 Parnetti, L. et al. Multicentre study of l-alpha-glyceryl-phosphocholine vs ST200 among patients with probable senile dementia of Alzheimer's type. *Drugs Aging* 3(2): 159-64.

565 Gedgaudas, Nora. 2011. *Primal Body, Primal Mind.* Healing Arts Press Rochester VT page 260.

566 Page, K.A. et al. 2009. Medium-chain fatty acids improve cognitive function in intensively treat type 1 diabetic patients and support in vitro synaptic transmission during acute hypoglycemia. *Diabetes* 58(5): 1237-44.

567 Yang, X. et al. 2016. Neuroprotection of Coenzyme Q10 in Neurodegenerative Diseases. *Curr Top Med Chem* 16(8): 858-66.

568 Adams, J.B. et al. 2018. Comprehensive nutritional and dietary intervention for autism spectrum disorder- a randomized controlled 12-month trial. *Nutrients* 10(3).

569 Shoeibi, A. et al. 2017. Effectiveness of coenzyme Q10 in prophylactic treatment of migraine headache: an open label, add-on, controlled trial. *Acta Neurol Belgium* 117(1): 103-9.

570 Parohan, M. et al. 2019. Effect of coenzyme Q10 supplementation on clinical features of migraine: a systematic review of dose-response meta-analysis of randomized controlled trials. *Nutritional Neuroscience* 6:1-8.

571 Sanoobar, M. et al. 2016. Coenzyme Q10 as a treatment for fatigue and depression in multiple scerlosis patients: A double-blind randomized clinical trial. *Nutri Neurosci* 19(3): 138-43.

572 Lourens, W. 2019. Could coenzyme Q10 be the treatment for Dupuytren's disease? *BMJ Case Report* 12(3).

573 Hara, Y. et al. 2017. Evaluation of the neuroprotective potential of N-acetylcysteine for prevention and treatment of cognitive aging and dementia. *Journal Prev Alzheimers Disease* 4(3): 201-6.

574 Aaseth, J. et al. 2016. Treatment strategies in Alzheimer's disease: a review with focus on selenium supplementation. *Biometals* 29(5): 827-39.

575 Karas Kuzelicki, N. 2016. S-Adenosyl methionine in the treatment of depression and other psychiatric disorders. *Drug Dev Research* 77(7): 346-56.

576 Sharma, A. et al. 2017. SAMe for neuropsychiatric disorders: A clinician-oriented review of research. *Journal of Clinical Psychiatry* 78(6).

577 De Berardis, D. et al. 2018. A comprehensive review of the efficacy of S-Adenosyl-L-methionine in major depressive disorder. *CNS Neurol Disord Drug Targets* 15(1): 35-44.

578 Apud, J.A. & D.R. Weinberger. 2007. Treatment of cognitive deficits associated with schizophrenia: potential role of catechol-0-methyltransferase inhibitors. *CNS Drugs* 21(7): 535-7.

579 Bastos, P. et al. 2017. Catechol-0-Methyltransferase (COMT): An update on its role in cancer, neurological and cardiovascular diseases. *Rev Physiol Biochem Pharmacol* 173: 1-39.

580 Tanaka, M. et al. 2004. Trehalose alleviates polyglutamine-mediated pathology in a mouse model of Huntington disease. *Nat Med* 10(2): 148-54.

581 Abeysundera, H. & R. Gill. 2018. Possible SAMe-induced mania. *BMJ Case Rep* doi: 10.1136/bcr-2018-224338.

582 Remington, R. et al. Maintenance of cognitive performance and mood in individuals with Alzheimer's disease following consumption of a nutraceutical formulation: A one-year, open-label study. *Journal of Alzheimers Disease* 51(4): 991-5.

583 Panjwani, A.A. et al. 2018. Crucifers and related vegetables and supplements for neurologic disorders: what is the evidence? *Current Opin Clin Nutr Metab Care* 21(6): 451-7.

584 Huang, C. et al. 2019. Effects of sulforaphane in the central nervous system. *European Journal of Pharmacology* 853: 153-168.

585 Lynch, R. et al. 2017. Sulforaphane from Broccoli reduces symptoms of autism: A follow-up cases series from a randomized double-blind study. *Glob Adv Health Med* doi: 10.1177/2164957X17735826.

586 Egner, P.A. et al. 2014. Rapid and sustainable detoxification of air-borne pollutants by broccoli sprout beverage: results of a randomized clinical trial in China. *Cancer Prevention Research* 7(8): 813-23.

587 Singh, K. & A. W. Zimmerman. 2016. Sulphoraphane treatment of young men with autism spectrum disorder. *CNS Neurol Disord Drug Targets* 15(5): 597-601.

588 Gorji, N. et al. 2018. Almond, hazelnut and walnut, three nuts for neuroprotection in Alzheimer's disease: a neuropharmacological review of their bioactive constituents. *Pharmacol Research* 129: 115-127.

589 Bahaeddin, Z. et al. 2017. Hazelnut an neuroprotection: improved memory and hindered anxiety in response to intra-hippocampal amyloid-beta injection. *Nutr Neurosci* 20(6): 317-326.

590 Mazokopakis, E.E. & M.I. Liontiris. 2018. Commentary: Health concerns of brazil nut consumption. *J Altern Complement Med* 24(1): 3-6.

591 Medeiros-Linard, C.F.B. et al. 2018. Anacardic acids from cashew nuts prevent behavorial changes and oxidative stress induced by rotenone in a rat model of Parkinson's disease. *Neurotox Research* 34(2): 250-262.

592 Matsumura, S. et al. 2016. Inhibitory activities of sesame seed extract and its constituents against beta-secretase. *Nat Prod Commun* 11(11): 1671-74.

593 Yu, J. et al. 2019. The effects of pinoresinol on cholinergic dysfunction-induced memory impairments and synaptic plasticity in mice. *Food Chem Toxicol* 125: 376-82.

594 Kumar, P. et al. 2009. Sesamol attenuates 3-nitropropionic acid-induced Huntington-like behavorial, biochemical and cellular alterations in rats. *Journal Asian Natural Products Research* 11(5): 439-50.

595 Panzella, L. et al. 2018. Anti-amyloid aggregation activity of black sesame pigment: toward a novel Alzheimer's disease preventive agent. *Molecules* 23(3).

596 Manini, P. et al. 2016. Efficient binding of heavy metals by black sesame pigment towards innovative dietary strategies to prevent bioaccumulation. *Journal Agric Food Chem* 64(4): 890-7.

597 Chang, C.F. et al. 2016. Therapeutic effect of berberine on TDP-43-related pathogenesis in FTLD and ALS. *Journal of Biomed Sci* 23(1): 72.

598 Lee, D.Y.W. et al. 2017. Asymmetric total synthesis of tetrahydroproto-berberine derivatives and evaluation of their binding affinities at dopamine receptors. *Bioorg Med Chem Lett* 27(6): 1437-40.

599 Jiang, W. et al. 2015. Therapeutic potential of berberine on Huntington's disease transgenic mouse model. *PLos One* 10(7).

600 Menke, A. et al. 2015. Prevalence of and trends in diabetes among adults in the United States. *JAMA* 314(10): 1021-9.

601 Fitzgerald, J.C. et al. 2017. Metformin reverses TRAP1 mutation-associated alterations in mitochondrial function in Parkinson's disease. *Brain* 140(9): 2444-2459.

602 Luo, C. et al. 2019. Effect of metformin on antipsychotic-induced metabolic dysfunction: the potential role of gut-brain axis. *Front Pharmacology* 10:371.

603 Koenig, A.M. et al. 2017. Effects of the insulin sensitizer metformin in Alzheimer's disease: Pilot data from a randomized, placebo-controlled crossover study. *Alzheimer Dis Assoc Disord* 31(2): 107-113.

604 Praharaj, S.K. et al. 2016. Metformin for lithium-induced weight gain: A case report. *Clin Psycholpharmacol Neurosci* 14(1): 101-3.

605 Zheng, W. et al. 2019. Combination of metformin and lifestyle intervention for antipsychotic-related weight gain: A meta-analysis of randomized controlled trials. *Pharmacopsychiatry* 52(1): 24-31.

606 Keshavarzi, S et al. Protective role of metformin against methamphetamine induced anxiety, depression, cognitive impairment and neurodegeneration in rat: The role of CREB/BDNF and Akt/GSK3 signaling pathways. *Neurotoxicity* 72: 74-84.

607 Honda, M. 2018. *Reverse Alzheimer's Disease Naturally*. Hatherleigh Press. Page 21.

608 Ying, W. 2007. NAD+ and NADH in brain functions, brain diseases and brain aging. *Front Bioscience* 12: 1863-88.

609 Satoh, A. et al. 2017. The brain, sirtuins and ageing. *Nat Rev Neurosci* 18(6): 362-74.

610 Lee, C.F. et al. 2019. Targeting NAD$^+$ metabolism as interventions for mitochondrial disease. *Sci Rep* 9(1): 3073.

611 Kim, Y. J. et al. 1996. The effects of plasma and brain magnesium concentrations on lidocaine-induced seizures in the rat. *Anesth Analg* 83(6): 1223-8.

612 Slutsky, I. et al. 2010. Enhancement of learning and memory by elevating brain magnesium. *Neuron* 65(2): 165-77.

613 McKee, J.A. et al. 2005. Analysis of the brain bioavailability of peripherally administered magnesium sulfate: A study in humans with acute brain injury undergoing prolonged induced hypermagnesemia. *Crit Care Med* 33(3): 661-6.

614 Liu, G. et al. 2016. Efficacy and safety of MIMFS-01, a synapse density enhancer, for treating cognitive impairment in older adults: A randomized, double-blind, placebo controlled trial. *Journal Alzheimers Disease* 49(4): 971-90.

615 Tarleton, E. et al. 2017. Role of magnesium supplementation in the treatment of depression: a randomized clinical trial. *PLoS One* doi: org/10.1371/journal.pone.0189967.

616 Abumaria, N. 2013. Magnesium supplement enhances spatial-context pattern separation and prevents fear overgeneralization. *Behav Pharmacol* 24(4): 255-63.

617 Forsleff, L. et al. 1999. Evidence of functional zinc deficiency in Parkinson's disease. *Journal Altern Complement Med* 5(1): 57-64.

618 Gedgaudas, Nora. 2011. *Primal Body, Primal Mind*. Healing Arts Press Rochester VT page 324-5.

619 Zellner, T. et al. 2016. Dementia, epilepsy and polyneuropathy in a mercury-exposed patient: investigation, identification of an obscure source and treatment. *BMJ Case Rep* doi: 10.1136/bcr-2016-216835.

620   Jung, J.W. 2005. Effects of chronic *Albizia julibrissin* treatment on 5-hydroxytrypamine1A receptors in rat brain. *Pharmacol Biochem Behav* 81(1): 205-210.

621   Liu, J et al. 2017. Anti-Anxiety Effect of SAG from Albizia julibrissin Durazz (Leguminosae). *Molecules.* 22(8).

622   Winston, D. & S. Maimes.2007. *Adaptogens: Herbs for Strength, Stamina and Stress Relief.* Healing Arts Press Rochester, VT page 213.

623   Ebrahimzadeh, M. A. et al. 2017. Attenuation of brain mitochondria oxidative damge by *Albizia julibrissin* Durazz: neuroprotective and antiemetic effects. *Drug Chem Toxicol* 18:1-8.

624   Dutta K. et al. 2018. Protective effects of *Withania somnifera* extract in SOD1^{G93A} mouse model of amyotrophic lateral sclerosis. *Exp Neurol* 309:193-204.

625   Chengappa, K.N.R. et al. 2018. Adjunctive Use of a Standardized Extract of Withania somnifera (Ashwagandha) to Treat Symptom Exacerbation in Schizophrenia: A Randomized, Double-Blind, Placebo-Controlled Study. *Journal of Clinical Psychiatry* 79(5).

626   Chengappa, K.N. et al. 2013. Randomized placebo-controlled adjunctive study of an extract of withania somnifera for cognitive dysfunction in bipolar disorder. *Journal of Clinical Psychiatry* 74(11): 1076-83.

627   Anju, T.R. et al. 2018. Altered muscarinic receptor expression in the cerebral cortex of epileptic rats: restorative role of *Withania somnifera*. *Biochem Cell Biol* 96(4): 433-40.

628   Savage, K. et al. 2018. GABA-modulating phytomedicines for anxiety: A systematic review of preclinical and clinical evidence. *Phytotherapy Research* 32(1): 3-18.

629   Pandey, A. et al. 2018. Multifunctional neuroprotective effect of Withanone, a compound from *Withania somnifera* roots in alleviating cognitive dysfunction. *Cytokine* 102: 211-221.

630   Choudhary, D. et al. 2017. Efficacy and Safety of Ashwagandha (Withania somnifera (L.) Dunal) Root Extract in Improving Memory and Cognitive Functions. *Journal of Diet Suppl* 14(6): 599-612.

631   Wadhwa, R. et al. 2016. Nootropic potential of Ashwagandha leaves: beyond traditional root extracts. *Neurochem Int* 95: 109-18.

632   Caputi, F.F. et al. 2019. Evidence of PPARγ-mediated mechanism in the ability of *Withania somnifera* to attenuate tolerance to the antinociceptive effects of morphine. *Pharmacol Research* 139: 422-430.

633   Manchanda, S. & G. Kaur. 2017. *Withania somnifera* leaf alleviates cognitive dysfunction by enhancing hippocampal plasticity in high fat induced obesity model. *BMC Complementary and Alternative Medicine* 17(1):136.

634   Kongkeaw, C et al. 2014. Meta-analysis of randomized controlled trials on cognitive effects of *Bacopa monnieri* extract. *Journal of Ethnopharmacology* 151(1): 528-535.

635   Nemetchek, M.D. et al. 2017. The Ayurvedic plant *Bacopa monnieri* inhibits inflammatory pathways in the brain. *Journal of Ethnopharmacology* 197: 92-100.

636   Sekhar, V. C. et al. 2018. Insights into the molecular aspects of neurprotective Bacoside A and Bacopaside I. *Current Neuropharmacology* doi: 10.2174/1570159X1 6666180419123022.

637   Srivastav, S. et al. 2017. Important medicinal herbs in Parkinson's disease pharmacotherapy. *Biomed Pharmacotherapy* 92: 856-63.

638   Aguiar, S. & T. Borowski. 2013. Neuropharmacological review of the nootropic herb *Bacopa monnieri* 16(4): 313-26.

639   Singh, B. et al. 2016. Comparative evaluation of extract of Bacopa monnieri and *Mucuna pruriens* as neuroprotectant in MPTP model of Parkinson's disease. *Indian Journal Exp Biol* 54(11): 758-66.

640   Downey, L.A. et al. 2013. An acute, double-blind, placebo-controlled crossover study of 320 mg and 640 mg doses of a special extract of *Bacopa monnieri* (CDRI 08) on sustained cognitive performance. *Phytotherapy Research* 27(9): 1407-13.

641   Calabrese, C. et al. 2008. Effects of a standardized *Bacopa monnieri* extract on cognitive performance, anxiety, and depression in the elderly: a randomized, double-blind, placebo-controlled trial. *Journal of Alternative and Complementary Medicine* 14(6): 707-13.

642   Stough, C. et al. 2013. Examining the cognitive effects of a special extract of *Bacopa monniera*: A review of ten years of research at Swinburne University. *Journal of Pharmacy and Pharmaceutical Science* 16(2): 254-58.

643   Ghaziuddin, M. & M. Al-Owain. 2013. Autism spectrum disorders and inborn errors of metabolism: an update. *Pediatric Neurology.* 49(4): 232-6.

644   Ray, R.S. & A. Katyal. 2016. Myeloperoxidase: Bridging the gap in neurodegeneration. *Neurosci Behav Rev* 68:611-620.

645   Bowtell, J.L. et al. 2017. Enhanced task-related brain activation and resting perfusion in healthy older adults after chronic blueberry supplementation. *Applied Physiology Nutr Metab* 42(7): 773-779.

646   Boespflug, E.L. et al. 2018. Cognitive neural activation with blueberry supplementation in mild cognitive impairment. *Nutrition Neurosci* 21(4): 297-305.

647   Barfoot, K.L. et al. 2018. The effects of acute wild blueberry supplementation on the cognition of 7-10-year-old schoolchildren. *European Journal of Nutrition* 1843-6.

648   Spohr, L. Combined actions of blueberry extract and lithium on neurochemical changes observed in an experimental model of mania: exploiting possible synergistic effects. *Metab Brain Disease* doi: 10.1007/s11011-018-0353-9.

649   Li, Q. et al. Pterostilbene inhibits amyloid-B induced neuroinflammation in a microglia cell line by inactivating the NLRP3/caspase-1 inflammasome pathway. *Journal Cell Biology* 119(8): 7053-62.

650   Song, J. et al. 2010. Protective effect of bilberry (*Vaccinium myrtillus* L.) extracts on cultured human corneal limbal epithelial cells (HCLEC). *Phytotherapy Research* 24(4): 520-24.

651   Deng S et al. 2006. Serotonergic activity-guided phytochemical investigation of the roots of Angelica sinensis. *J Nat Prod* 69(4):536-41.

652   Turi, C.E. & S.J. Murch. 2013. Targeted and untargeted phytochemistry of Ligusticum canbyi: indoleamines, phthalides, antioxidant potential and use of metabolomics as a hypothesis-generating technique for compound discovery. *Planta Medica* 79: 1370-9.

653   Zhang, Y.T. et al. 2016. (Z)-ligustilide increases ferroportin1 expression and ferritin content in ischemic SH-SY5Y cells. *Eur J Pharmacol* 792:48-53.

654   Tang J. et al. 2009. Pharmacological activities of Z-ligustilide and metabolites in rats. Sichuan Da Xue Xue Bao Yi Xue Ban 40(5): 839-42.

655   Wang Y.H. et al. 2011. Effect and mechanism of senkyunolide 1 as an anti-migraine compound from Ligusticum chuanxiong. *J Pharm Pharmacol* 63(2): 261-6.

656   Kindred, J.H. et al. 2017. Cannabis use in people with Parkinson's disease and Multiple Scerosis: A web-based investigation. *Complement Ther* Med (33): 99-104.

657   Klein, T.W. et al. 2003. The cannabinoid system and immune modulation. *Journal of Leukocyte Biology* 2003 74(4): 486-96.

658 Dale, T. et al. Cannabis for refractory epilepsy in children: a review focusing on CDKL5 Deficiency Disorder. *Epilepsy Research* 151: 31-39.

659 Elliott, J. et al. 2019. Cannabis-based products for pediatric epilepsy: a systematic review. *Epilepsia* 60(1): 6-9.

660 Kozela, E. 2017. Modulation of Astrocyte Activity by Cannabidiol, a Nonpsychactive Cannabinoid. *International Journal of Molecular Science* 18(8).

661 Baron, E.P. 2018. Medicinal Properties of Cannabinoids, Terpenes, and Flavonoids in Cannabis, and Benefits in Migraine, Headache and Pain: An Update on Current Evidence and Cannabis Science. *Headache* 58(7): 1139-1186.

662 Poleszak, E. et al. 2018. Cannabinoids in depressive disorders. *Life Science* 213: 18-24.

663 Aparicio-Blanco, J. et al. 2019. Cannabidiol enhances the passage of lipid nanocapsules across the blood brain barrier both *in vitro* and *in vivo*. *Molecular Pharmaceutics* doi:10.1021/acs.molpharmaceut.8b01344.

664 Krebs, M.O. et al. 2019 Exposure to cannabinoids can lead to persistent cognitive and psychiatric disorders. *European Journal of Pain*. doi: 10.1002/ejp. 1377.

665 Keefe, J.R. et al. 2016. Short-term open-label chamomile (*M. chamomilla*) therapy of moderate to severe generalized anxiety disorder. *Phytomedicine* 23(14): 1699-1705.

666 Amsterdam, J.D. et al. 2012. Chamomile (*Matricaria recutita*) may provide antidepressant activity in anxious, depressed humans: an exploratory study. *Alternative Ther Health Med* 18(5): 44-49.

667 Chang, S.M. & C.H. Chen. 2016. Effects of an intervention with drinking chamomile tea on sleep quality and depression in sleep disturbed postnatal women: a randomized controlled trial. *Journal Adv Nurs* 72(2): 306-15.

668 Amsterdam, J.D. et al. 2009. A randomized, double-blind, placebo-controlled trial of oral Matricaria recutita (Chamomile) extract therapy of generalized anxiety disorder. *British J of Pharmacology* 163: 234-45.

669 Ranasinghe, P. et al. 2013. Medicinal properties of 'true' cinnamon (*Cinnamomum zeylanicum*): a systematic review. *BMC Complement Altern Med* 13: 275

670 Momtaz, S. et al. 2019. Cinnamon, a promising prospect towards Alzheimer's disease. *Pharmacol Research* 130: 241-258.

671 Sartorius, T. et al. 2014. Cinnamon extracts improves insulin sensitivity in the brain and lowers liver fat in mouse models of obesity. *PLoS One* 9(3): e92358.

672 Yang, G. et al. 2013. Huperzine A for Alzheimer's disease: a systematic review and meta-analysis of randomized clinical trials. *PLoS One* 8(9):e74916.

673 Peters, C. et al. 2016. The level of NMDA receptor in the membrane modulates amyloid-beta association and perforation. *J Alzheimer's Disease* 53(1): 197-207.

674 Damar, U et al. 2017. Huperzine A: A promising anticonvulsant, disease modifying and memory enhancing treatment option in Alzheimer's disease. *Med Hypotheses* 99: 57-62.

675 Damar, U. 2016. Huperzine A as a neuroprotective and antiepileptic drug: a review of preclinical research. *Expert Rev Neurother* 16(6): 671-80.

676 Katzenschlager,R. et al. 2004. *J Neurol Neurosurg Psychiatry* 75:12 1672-77.

677 Cilia, R. et al. 2017. Mucuna pruriens in Parkinson disease: A double-blind, randomized, controlled, crossover study. *Neurology* 89(5): 432-38.

678 Rai, S.N. et al. 2017. Immunomodulation of Parkinson's disease using Mucuna pruriens. *Journal Chem Neuroanatomy* 85: 27-35.

679   Aurélie de Rus Jacquet et al. 2017. Lumbee traditional medicine: Neuroprotective activities of medicinal plants used to treat Parkinson's disease-related symptoms. *Journal of Ethnopharmacology* 206: 408-25.

680   Carrera, I. 2017. Neuroprotective Effect of Atremorine in an Experimental Model of Parkinson's Disease. *Curr Pharm Des* 23(18): 2673-84.

681   Carrera, I et al. 2018. Dopaminergic Neuroprotection with Atremorine in Parkinson's Disease. *Curr Med Chem* 25(39): 5372-88.

682   Chiu, S. et al. 2014. Proof of Concept Randomized controlled study of Cognition Effects of the Proprietary Extract *Sceletium tortuosum* (Zembrin) Targeting Phosphodiesterase-4 in Cognitively healthy Subjects: Implications for Alzheimer's Dementia. *Evidence-Based Complementary and Alternative Medicine* 2014:682014.

683   Terburg, D. et al, 2013. Acute effects of *Sceletium tortuosum* (Zembrin), a dual 5-HT reuptake and PDE4 inhibitor, in the human amygdala and its connection to the hypothalamus. *Neuropsychopharmacology* 38(13): 2708-16.

684   Coetzee, D.D et al. High-mesembrine Sceletium extract (Trimesemine™) is a monoamine releasing agent, rather than only a selective serotonin reuptake inhibitor.

685   Bennett, A.C. & C. Smith. 2018. Immunomodulatory effects of *Sceletium tortuosum* elucidated in vitro: Implications for chronic disease. *Journal of Ethnopharmacology* 2124: 134-140.

686   Dimpfel, W. et al. 2018. Effect of Zembrin® and four of its alkaloid constituents on electric excitability of the rat hippocampus. *J Ethnopharmacology* 223: 135-141.

687   Spinelli, M. *The Psychopharmacology of Herbal Medicine* MIT Press Cambridge Mass pages 264-72.

688   Bachinskaya, N. et al. 2011. Alleviating neuropsychiatric symptoms in dementia: the effects of Ginkgo biloba extract EGb 761. Findings from a randomized, controlled trial. *Neuropsychiatr Dis Treat* 2011 7 209-15.

689   Das, A. et al. 2002. A comparative study in rodents of standardized extracts of Bacopa monniera and Ginkgo biloba: anticholinesterase and cognitive enhancing activities. *Pharmacol Biochem Behav* 73(4): 893-900

690   Kandiah, N. et al. 2019. Treatment of dementia and mild cognitive impairment with our without cerebrovascular disease: Expert consensus on the use of Ginkgo biloba extract, EGb 761®. *CNS Neurosci Ther* 25(2): 288-98.

691   Savaskan, E. et al. 2018. Treatment effects of Ginkgo biloba extract EGb 761® on the spectrum of behavioral and psychological symptoms of dementia: meta-analysis of randomized controlled trials. *International Psychogeratrics* 30(3): 285-93.

692   Rapp, M. et al. 2018. Similar treatment outcomes with Ginkgo biloba extract EGb 761 and donepezil in Alzheimer's dementia in very old age: A retrospective observational study. *International Journal of Clin Pharmacol Ther* 56(3): 130-133.

693   Meston, C.M. et al. 2008. Short and long-term effects of Ginkgo biloba extract on sexual dysfunction in women. *Arch Sex Behav* 2008 37(4): 530-547.

694   Cohen A.J. et al. 1998. Ginkgo biloba for anti-depressant-induced sexual dysfunction. *J Sex Marital Ther* 24:2 139-43.

695   Shakibaei, F. et al. 2015. Ginkgo biloba in the treatment of attention-deficit/ hyperactivity disorder in children and adolescents. A randomized, placebo-controlled trial. *Complement Ther Clin Pract* 21(2): 61-7.

696   Jeyam, M. et al. 2012. Molecular understanding and *in silico* validation of traditional medicines for Parkinson's disease. *Asian Journal of Pharm Clin Res* 5: 125-8.

697   Zheng, W. et al. 2016. Extract of Ginkgo biloba for Tardive dyskinesia: meta-analysis of randomized, controlled trials. *Pharmacopsychiatry* 49(3): 107-11.

698 Bent, S. et al. Spontaneous bleeding associated with gingko biloba: a case report and systematic review of the literature. *J Gen Intern Med* 20(7): 657-61.

699 Le Bars P.L. et al. 1997. A placebo-controlled, double-blind, randomized trial of an extract of Ginkgo biloba for dementia. North American EGb Study Group. *JAMA* 278(16): 1327-32.

700 Engelsen, J. et al. 2003. Effect of Coenzyme Q10 and Ginkgo biloba on warfarin dosage in patients on long-term warfarin treatment. A randomized, double-blind, placebo-controlled cross-over trial. *Ugeskr Laeger* 165(18): 1868-71.

701 Woron, J. & M. Siwek. 2018. Unwanted effects of psychotropic drug interactions with medicinal products and diet supplements containing plant extracts. *Psychiatr Poland* 52(6):983-6.

702 Mak, S. et al. 2014. Synergistic inhibition on acetylcholinesterase by the combination of berberine and palmatine originally isolated from Chinese medicinal herbs. *Journal Mol Neuroscience* 53(3): 511-516.

703 Gray, N.E. et al. 2018. Centella asiatica increases hippocampal synaptic density and improves memory and executive function in aged mice. *Brain Behavior* 8(7): e01024.

704 Wattanathorn, J. et al. 2008. Positive modulation of cognition and mood in the healthy elderly volunteer following the administration of Centella asiatica. *Journal of Ethnopharmacology* 116(2): 325-32.

705 Orhan, I.E. et al. 2012. *Centella asiatica* (L.) Urban: From Traditional Medicine to Modern Medicine with Neuroprotective Potential. *Evid Based Complement Altern Med* doi: 10.1155/2012/946259.

706 Hamid, K. et al. 2016. An Investigation of the Differential Effects of Ursane Triterpenoids from *Centella asiatica*, and Their Semisynthetic Analogues, on GABAA Receptors. *Chem Biol Drug Des* 88(3): 386-97.

707 Ahmad, R. M. et al. 2018. Neuroprotective role of Asiatic acid in aluminum chloride induced rat model of Alzheimer's disease. *Front Biosci* (Scholar Edition) 10: 262-275.

708 Gopi, M. & J. V. Arambakkam. 2017. Asiaticoside: Attenuation of rotenone induced oxidative burden in a rat model of hemiparkinsonism by maintaining the phosphoinositide-mediated synaptic integrity. *Pharmaco Biochem Behav* 155: 1-15.

709 Farhana, K.M. et al. 2016. Effectiveness of Gotu Kola Extract 750 mg and 1000 mg Compared with Folic Acid 3 mg in Improving Vascular Cognitive Impairment after Stroke. *Evidence-Based Complementary Alternative Medicine* doi: 10.1155/2016/2795915.

710 Maquart, F.X. et al. 2018. Centella asiatica: entering a new era. *Dermatological Experiences* 20 (1-2):1-3.

711 Umka Welbat, J. et al. 2016. Asiatic Acid Prevent the Deleterious Effects of Valproic Acid on Cognition and Hippocampal Cell Proliferation and Survival. *Nutrients* 8(5).

712 Mandel, S. et al. 2004. Iron and alpha-synuclein in the substantia nigra of MPTP-treated mice: effect of neuroprotective drugs R-apomorphine and green tea polyphenol (-)-epigallocathecin-3-gallate. *Journal of Mol Neuroscience* 24(3): 401-16.

713 Pervin, M. 2017. Blood brain barrier permeability of (-)-epigallocatechin gallate, its proliferation-enhancing activity of human neuroblastoma SH-SY5Y cells, and its preventive effect on age-related cognitive dysfunction in mice. *Biochem Biophys Rep* 9:180-6.

714   Jin, J.S. et al. 2012. Effects of green tea consumption on human fecal microbiota with special reference to *Bifidobacterium* species. *Microbiology and Immunology* 56(11): 729-39.

715   Feng, L. et al. 2016. Tea consumption reduces the incidence of neurocognitive disorders: Findings from the Singapore longitudinal aging study. *Journal of Nutrition Health and Aging* 10: 1002.

716   Bieschke, J. et al. 2010. EGCG remodels mature alpha-synuclein and amyloid-beta fibrils and reduces cellular toxicity. *Proced of the Nat Acad of Sciences of the U.S.A.* 107(17): 7710-5.

717   Liu, X et al. 2017. Association between tea consumption and risk of cognitive disorders: A dose-response meta-analysis of observational studies. *Oncotarget* 8(26): 43306-21.

718   Lardner, A.L. 2014. Neurobiological effects of the green tea constituent theanine and its potential role in the treatment of psychiatric and neurodegenerative disorders. *Nutr Neurosci* 17(4): 145-55.

719   Hidese, S. et al. 2017. Effects of chronic l-theanine administration in patients with majoyr depressive disorder: an open-label study. *Acta Neuropsychiatr* 29(2): 72-9.

720   Sarris, J. et al. 2019. L-theanine in the adjunctive treatment of generalized anxiety disorder: A double-blind, randomized, placebo-controlled trial. *Journal of Psychiatric Research* 110: 31-37.

721   Kim, S. et al. 2019. GABA and l-theanine mixture decreases sleep latency and improves NREM sleep. *Pharm Biol* 57(1): 65-73.

722   Zhu, G. et al. 2018. Synaptic modification by L-theanine, a natural constituent in green tea, rescues the impairment of hippocampal long-term potentiation and memory in AD mice. *Neuropharmacology* 138: 331-40.

723   Carnevale, G. et al. 2011. Anxiolytic-like effect on Griffonia simplicifolia Baill. seed extract in rats. *Phytomedicine* 18(10): 848-51.

724   Birdsall, T.C. 1998. 5-Hydroxytryptophan: A Clinically-Effective Serotonin Precursor. *Altern Med Rev* 3(4): 271-80.

725   Poldinger, W. et al. 1991. A functional-dimensional approach to depression: serotonin deficiency as a target syndrome in a comparison of 5-hydroxytryptophan and fluvoxamine. *Psychopathology* 24: 53-81.

726   Turner, E.H. et al. 2006. Serotonin a la carte: supplement with the serotonin precursor 5-hydroxytryptophan. *Pharmacol Ther* 109(3): 325-38.

727   Bakhtiari, E. et al. 2015. Protective effect of Hibiscus sabdariffa against serum/ glucose deprivation-induced PC12 cells injury. *Avicenna J Phytomed* 5(3): 231-7.

728   Suryanti, S. et al. 2015. Red Sorrel (Hibiscus sabdariffa) prevents the ethanol-induced deficits of purkinje cells in the cerebellum. *Bratisl Lek Listy* 116(2): 109-14.

729   Oboh, G. et al. 2018. Phenolic constituents and inhibitory effects of Hibiscus sabdariffa L. (Sorrel) calyx on cholinergic, monoaminergic and purinergic enzyme activities. *Journal Diet Suppl* 15(6): 910-22.

730   Rival, D. et al. 2009. A Hibiscus abelmoschus seed extract as a protective active ingredient to favour FGF-2 activity in skin. *International Journal of Cosmetic Science* 31(6): 419-426.

731   Jothie, R.E. et al. 2016. Anti-stress activity of *Ocimum sanctum*: Possible effects on Hypothalmic-Pituitary-Adrenal axis. *Phytotherapy Research* 30(5): 805-14.

732   Bhattacharyya, D. et al. 2008. Controlled program trial of *Ocimum sanctum* leaf on generalized anxiety disorders. *Nepal Med Coll Journal* 10(3): 176-79.

733 Siddique, Y.H. et al. 2014. Role of *Ocimum sanctum* leaf extract on dietary supplementation in the transgenic Drosophila model of Parkinson's disease. *Chinese Journal of Natural Medicine* 12(10): 777-81.

734 Kusindarta, D.L. et al. 2018. Ethanol extract of Ocimum sanctum enhances cognitive ability from young adulthood to middle aged mediated by increasing choline acetyl transferase activity in rat model. *Res Vet Sci* 118: 431-438.

735 Sembulingam, K. et al. 2005. Effect of Ocimum sanctum Linn on the changes in central cholinergic system induced by acute noise stress. *Journal of Ethnopharmacology* 96(3): 477-82.

736 Winston, D. & S. Maimes.2007. *Adaptogens: Herbs for Strength, Stamina and Stress Relief.* Healing Arts Press Rochester, VT pages169-170.

737 Jamshidi, N. & M.M. Cohen. 2017. The clinical efficacy and safety of tulsi in humans: a systematic review of the literature. *Evidence-Based Complementary and Alternative Medicine* 2017:9217567.

738 Brattstrom, A. 2007. Scientific evidence for a fixed extract combination (Ze 91019) from valerian and hops traditionally used as a sleep-inducing aid. *Wien Med Wochenscher* 157(13-14): 367-70.

739 Kyrou, I. et al. 2017. Effects of a hops (Humulus lupulus L.) dry extract supplement on self-reported depression, anxiety and stress levels in apparently healthy young adults: a randomized, placebo-controlled, double-blind, crossover pilot study. *Hormones* (Athens) 16(2): 171-80.

740 Brown, T.K. & K. Alper. 2018. Treatment of opioid use disorder with ibogaine: detoxification and drug use outcomes. *Am J Drug Alcohol Abuse* 44(1):24-36

741 Noller, G.E. et al. 2018. Ibogaine treatment outcomes for opioid dependence from a twelve-month follow-up observational study. *Am Journal Drug Alcohol Abuse* 44(1): 37-46.

742 Sershin, H. et al. 1997. Ibogaine and cocaine abuse: pharmacological interactions at dopamine and serotonin receptors. *Brain Res Bull* 42(3): 161-8.

743 Malsh, U. et al. 2001. Efficacy of kava-kava in the treatment of non-psychotic anxiety following pretreatment with benzodiazepines. *Psychopharmacology* 157(3): 277.83.

744 Sarris, J. et al. 2009. The Kava Anxiety Depression Spectrum Study (KADSS): A randomized, placebo-controlled crossover trial using an aqueous extract of Piper methysticum. *Psychopharmacology* 205:399.

745 Chua, H.C. et al. 2016. Kavain, the Major Constituent of the Anxiolytic Kava Extract, Potentiates GABAA Receptors: Functional Characteristics and Molecular Mechanism. *PLoS One* 11(6):e)157700.

746 Jussofie, A. et al. 1994. Kavapryone enriched extract from Piper methysticum as modulator of the GABA binding site in different regions of rat brain. *Psychopharmacology* (Berlin) 116(4): 469-74.

747 Smith, K. & C. Leiras. 2018. The effectiveness and safety of Kava Kava for treating anxiety symptoms: A systematic review and analysis of randomized clinical trials. *Complementary Ther Clin Pract* 33: 107-17.

748 Kruegel, A.C. & O. Grundmann. 2018. The medicinal chemistry and neurpharmacology of kratom: A preliminary discussion of a promising medicinal plant and analysis of its potential for abuse. *Neuropharmacology* 134(pt A):108-120.

749 Penetar, D.M. et al. 2015. A single dose of kudzu extract reduces alcohol consumption in a binge drinking paradigm. *Drug Alcohol Depend* 153: 194-200.

405

750   Lukas, S.E. et al. 2013. A standardized kudzu extract (NPI-031) reduces alcohol consumption in nontreatment-seeking male heavy drinkers. *Psychopharmacology* 226(1): 65-73.

751   Akhondzadeh, S. et al. 2003. *Melissa officinalis* extract in the treatment of patients with mild to moderate Alzheimer's disease: a double blind, randomized, placebo controlled trial. *Journal Neurol Neurosurg Psychiatry* 74(7): 863-6.

752   Cases, J. et al. 2011. Pilot trial of *Melissa officinalis* L. leaf extract in the treatment of volunteers suffering from mild-to-moderate anxiety disorders and sleep disturbances. *Med J Nutrition Metab* 4(3): 211-18.

753   Kennedy, D.O. et al. 2003. Modulation of mood and cognitive performance following acute administration of single doses of *Melissa officinalis* (Lemon balm) with human CNS nicotinic and muscarinic receptor-binding properties. *Neuropsychopharmacology* 28(10): 1871-81.

754   Haybar, H. et al. 2018. The effects of *Melissa officinalis* supplementation on depression, anxiety, stress and sleep disorder in patients with chronic stable angina. *Clin Nutr ESPEN* 26: 47-52.

755   Heydari, N. et al. 2018. Effect of *Melissa officinalis* capsule on the mental health of female adolescents with premenstrual syndrome: a clinical trial study. *International Journal of Adolescent Med Health* doi: 10.1515/ijamh-2017-0015.

756   Halfon, R. 2010. *Gemmotherapy: The Science of Healing with Plant Stem Cells* Healing Arts Press Rochester VT page 74-75.

757   Greaves, M. 2002. *Gemmotherapy and Oligotherapy Regenerators of Dying Intoxicated Cells.* Xlibris Corp pages 96-97

758   Allio, A. 2015. Bud extracts from Tilia tomentosa Moench inhibit hippocampal neuronal firing through GABAA and benzodiazepine receptors activation. *Journal of Ethnopharmacology* 172: 288-96.

759   Ellingwood, F. 1919. *The American Materia Medica, Therapeutics and Pharmacognosy.* Self published

760   Akaike, A. et al. 2010. Mechanisms of neuroprotective effects of nicotine and acetylcholinesterase inhibitors: role of alpha4 and alpha7 receptors in neuroprotection. *Journal of Molecular Neuroscience* 211-16.

761   Baretto, G. et al. 2014. Beneficial effects of nicotine, cotinine and its metabolites as potential agents for Parkinson's disease. *Front Aging Neuroscience* 1-13.

762   Terry, A.V. Jr. et al. 1998. Lobeline and structurally simplified analogs exhibit differential agonist activity and sensitivity to antagonist blockade when compared to nicotine. *Neuropharmacology* 37(1): 93-102.

763   Carradori, S. et al. 2014. Selective MAO-B inhibitors: a lesson from natural products. *Mol Divers* 18: 219-43.

764   Gallardo K.A. & F.M. Leslie. 1998. Nicotine-stimulated release of [3H] norepinephrine from fetal rat locus coeruleus cells in culture. *Journal of Neurochemistry* 70(2): 663-70.

765   Dwoskin,L.P. & P.A. Crooks. 2002. A novel mechanism of action and potential use for lobeline as a treatment for psychostimulant abuse. *Biochem Pharmacol* 63(2): 89-98.

766   Szurpnicka, A. et al. 2019. Therapeutic potential of mistletoe in CNS-related neurological disorders and the chemical composition of Viscum species. *Journal of Ethnopharmacology* 231: 241-252.

767   Von Schoen-Angerer, T. et al. 2015. Viscum album in the treatment of a girl with refractory childhood absence epilepsy. *J Child Neurol* 30(8): 1048-52.

768   Anand, C.L. 1971. Effects of *Avena sativa* on cigarette smoking. *Nature* 1971 233(5320): 496.

769   Jack, R.A. et al. 1971. Treatment of opium addiction. *Brit Med Journal* 4(5778):48.

770   Riederer P. et al. 2004. Clinical applications of MAO-inhibitors. *Curr Med Chem* 11(15): 2033-43.

771   Dimpfel, W. et al. 2011. Ingested oat herb extract (Avena sativa) changes EEG spectral frequencies in healthy subjects. *Journal of Alternative and Complementary Medicine* 17(5): 427-34.

772   Kennedy, D.O. et al. 2017. Acute effects of a wild green-oat (Avena sativa) extract on cognitive function in middle-aged adults: A double-blind, placebo-controlled, within-subjects trial. *Nutr Neurosci* 20(2): 135-51.

773   Wood, M. 2009. *The Earthwise Herbal*. North Atlantic Books. Berekely CA page 262-3.

774   Ngan, A. & R. Conduit. A double-blind, placebo-controlled investigation of the effects of Passiflora incarnata (passionflower) herbal tea on subjective sleep quality. *Phytotherapy Research* 2011 25(8): 1153-9.

775   Akhondzadeh, S. et al. Passionflower in the treatment of opiates withdrawal: a double-blind randomized controlled trial. *Journal Clin Pharm Ther* 2001 26:5 369-73.

776   Faustino, T.T. et al. Medicinal plants for the treatment of generalized anxiety disorder: a review of controlled clinical studies. Brazilian Journal of Psychiatry (*Rev Bras Psiquiatr*) 2010 32:4 429-36.

777   Singh, B. et al. Dual protective effect of Passiflora incarnata in epilepsy and associated post-ictal depression. *Journal of Ethnopharmacology* 2012 139:1 273-9.

778   Appel, K. et al. 2011. Modulation of the gamma-aminobutyric acid (GABA) system by *Passiflora incarnata* L. *Phytotherapy Research* 25(6): 838-43.

779   Dvořáková, M. et al. 2007. Urinary catecholamines in children with attention deficit hyperactivity disorder (ADHD): modulation by a polyphenolic extract from pine bark (pycnogenol). *Nutr Neurosci* 10(3-4): 151-7.

780   Trebaticka, J. et al. 2006. Treatment of ADHD with French maritime pine bark extract, Pycnogenol. *Eur Child Adolesc Psychiatry* 15(6): 329-35.

781   Paarmann, K. et al. 2018. French maritime pine bark treatment decelerates plaque development and improves spatial memory in Alzheimer's disease mice. *Phytomedicine* 57: 39-48.

782   Khan, M.M. et al. 2013. Protection of MPTP-induced neuroinflammation and neurodegeneration by Pycnogenol. *Neurochem* 62(4): 379-88.

783   Rolland, A. et al. 2001. Neurophysiological effects of an extract of *Eschscholzia californica* Cham. (Papaveraceae). *Phytotherapy Research* 15(5): 377-81.

784   Hanus, M. et al. 2004. Double-blind, randomized, placebo-controlled study to evaluate the efficacy and safety of a fixed combination containing two plant extracts (*Crataegus oxyacantha* and *Eschscholtzia californica*) and magnesium in mild-to-moderate anxiety disorders. *Curr Med Res Opin* 20(1): 63-71.

785   Cahlikova, L. et al. 2010. Acetylcholinesterase and butyrylcholinesterase inhibitory compounds from *Eschscholzia californica* (Papaveraceae). *Natural Prod Commun* 5(7): 1035-8.

786   Fedurco, M. et al. 2015. Modulatory Effects of *Eschscholzia californica* Alkaloids on Recombinant GABAA Receptors. *Biochem Research International* doi: 10.1155/2025/617620.

787   Chen, Y.X. et al. 2016. Molecular evaluation of herbal compounds as potent inhibitors of acetylcholinesterase for the treatment of Alzheimer's disease. *Mol Med Rep* 14(1): 446-52.

788   Belcaro, G. et al. 2018. Supplementation with Robuvit in post-traumatic stress disorders associated to high oxidative stress. *Minerva Med* 109(5): 363-368.

789   Ma, P. 2018. *Rhodiola rosea* L. improves learning and memory function: Preclinical evidence and possible mechanisms. *Front Pharmacol* 9:1415.

790   Bangratz M. et al. 2018. A preliminary assessment of a combination of rhodiola and saffron in the management of mild-moderate depression. *Neuropsychiatr Dis Treat* 14: 1821-9.

791   Cropley, M. et al. 2015. The effects of *Rhodiola rosea* L. extract on anxiety, stress, cognition and other mood symptoms. *Phytotherapy Research* 29(12): 1934-9.

792   Amsterdam, J.D. & A.G. Panossian. 2016. *Rhodiola rosea* L. as a putative botanical antidepressant. *Phytomedicine* 23(7):770-83.

793   Mao, J.J. et al. 2015. *Rhodiola rosea* versus sertraline for major depressive disorder: A randomized placebo-controlled trial. *Phytomedicine* 22(3): 394-9.

794   Concerto, C. et al. 2018. Exploring the effect of adaptogenic *Rhodiola rosea* extract on neuroplasticity in humans. *Complement Ther Med* 41: 141-6.

795   Lee, Y. et al. 2013. Anti-inflammatory and Neuroprotective Effects of Constituents isolated from *Rhodiola rosea*. *Evid Based Complement Alternat Medicine* 2013:514049.

796   Akhondzadeh, S. et al. 2010. A 22-week, multicenter, randomized, double-blind controlled trial of *Crocus sativus* in the treatment of mild-to-moderate Alzheimer's disease. *Psychopharmacology* 207(4): 637-43.

797   Farokhnia, M. et al. 2014. Comparing the efficacy and safety of Crocus Sativus L. with memantine in patients with moderate to severe Alzheimer's disease: A double-blind, randomized clinical trial. *Human Psychopharmacology* 29(4): 351-59.

798   Lopresti, A.L. et al, Saffron, a standardized extract from saffron (*Crocus sativus* L.) for the treatment of youth anxiety and depressive symptoms: a randomized, double-blind, placebo-controlled study. *Journal Affect Disord* 232:349-357.

799   Shafiee, M. et al. 2018. Saffron in the treatment of depression, anxiety and other mental disorders: Current evidence and potential mechanisms of action. *Journal Affect Disord* 227: 330-337.

800   Toth, B. et al. 2019. The efficacy of saffron in the treatment of mild to moderate depression: a meta-analysis. *Planta Medica* 85(1): 24-31.

801   Milajerdi, A. et al. 2018. The effects of alcoholic extract of saffron (*Crocus sativus* L.) on mild to moderate comorbid depression-anxiety, sleep quality and life satisfaction in type 2 diabetes mellitus: A double-blind, randomized and placebo-controlled trial. *Complement Ther Med* 41: 196-202.

802   Baziar, S. et al. 2019. *Crocus sativus* L. versus methylphenidate in treatment of children with attention-deficit/hyperactivity disorder: A randomized, double-blind study. *Journal Child Adolesc Psychopharmacol* doi: 10.1089/cap.2018.0146.

803   Bangratz, M. et al. 2018. A preliminary assessment of a combination of rhodiola and saffron in the management of mild-moderate depression. *Neuropsychiatr Dis Treat* 14: 1821-9.

804   Lopresti, A.L. & P.D. Drummond. 2017. Efficacy of Curcumin, and a Saffron/ Curcumin combination for the treatment of major depression: a randomized double-blind, placebo-controlled study. *Journal of Affective Disorders* 207: 188-96.

805   Milajerdi, A. et al. 2018. Saffron extract reduces blood glucose in type 2 diabetes. *J Res Med Sci* 23:16.

806   Schrader, E. 2000. Equivalence of St John's wort extract (Ze 117) and fluoxetine: a randomized, controlled study in mild-moderate depression. *International Clin Psychopharmacol* 15(2): 61-8.

807   Ng, Q.X. et al. 2017. Clinical use of *Hypericum perforatum* (St John's wort) in depression: A meta-analysis. *Journal Affect Disord* 210: 211-21.

808   Neiderhofer, H. 2009. St John's wort treating patients with autistic disorder. *Phytotherapy Research* 23(11): 1521-3.

809   Concerto, C. et al. 2018. Hypericum perforatum extract modulates cortical plasticity in humans. *Psychopharmacology* 235(1): 145-53.

810   Orphan, I.E. et al. 2019. Profiling auspicious butyrylcholinesterase inhibitory activity of two herbal molecules: Hyperforin and Hyuganin C. *Chem Biodivers* doi: 10.1002/cbdv.201900017.

811   Nieminen, T.H. et al. 2010. St John's wort greatly reduces the concentrations of oral oxycodone. *Eur J Pain* 14(8): 854-9.

812   Sowndhararajan, K. et al. 2018. An overview of neuroprotective and cognitive enhancement properties of lignans from *Schisandra chinensis*. *Biomed Pharmacother* 97: 958-68.

813   Li, N. et al. 2018. Sedative and hypnotic effects of Schisandrin B through increasing GABA/Glu ratio and upregulating the expression of GABA$_A$ in mice and rats. *Biomed Pharmacother* 103: 509-16.

814   Liu, Y. et al. 2019. Pharmacodynamic and urinary metabolomics studies on the mechanism of Schisandra polysaccharide in the treatment of Alzheimer's disease. *Food Funct* 10(1): 432-47.

815   Zhang, X. et al. 1995. Isolation and characterization of a cyclic hydroxamic acid from a pollen extract, which inhibits cancerous cell growth in vitro. *Journal of Medicinal Chemistry* 38(4):735-8.

816   Hui, K.M. 2000. Interaction of flavones from the roots of Scutellaria baicalensis with the benzodiazepine site. *Planta Medica* 66(1):91-3.

817   Tao YH, Jiang DY, Xu HB, Yang XL. Inhibitory effect of Erigeron breviscapus extract and its flavonoid components on GABA shunt enzymes. *Phytomedicine* 2008 15(1-2): 92-7.

818   Zhu JT, Choi RC, Li J et al. Estrogenic and neuroprotective properties of scutellarin from Erigeron breviscapus: a drug against postmenopausal symptoms and Alzheimer's disease. *Planta Medica* 2009 75(4):1489-93.

819   Heo JH, Kim DO, Choi SJ, Shin DH, Lee CY. Potent inhibitory effect of flavonoids in Scutellaria baicalensis on Amyloid beta protein-induced Neurotoxicity. *Journal of Agricultural and Food Chemistry*. 2004 52(13):4128-32.

820   Akao T, Kawabata K, Yanagisawa E et al. Baicalin, the predominant flavone glycuronide of scutellariae radix, is absorbed from the rat gastrointestinal tract as the aglycone and restored to its original form. *Journal of Pharmacy and Pharmacology* 2000 52(12):1563-8.

821   Zhou, R. et al. 2015. Baicalin may have therapeutic effect in attention deficit hyperactivity disorder. *Med Hypotheses* 85(6): 761-4.

822   Mu X, He G, Cheng Y, Li X, Xu B, Du G. Baicalein exerts neuroprotective effects in 6-hydroxydopamine-induced experimental parkinsonism *in vivo* and *in vitro*. *Pharmacology Biochemistry and Behavior*. 2009 92(4):642-8.

823   Gu, X.H. et al. 2016. The flavonoid baicalein rescues synaptic plasticity and memory deficits in a mouse model of Alzheimer's disease. *Behav Brain Research* 311: 309-21.

409

824   Tarrago T, Kichik N, Classen B, Prades R, Teixido M, Girait E. Baicalin, a prodrug able to reach the CNS, is a prolyl oligopeptidase inhibitor. *Bioorganic and Medicinal Chemistry* 2008 16(15):7516-24.

825   Fong, Y.K. et al. In vitro and in situ evaluation of herb-drug interactions during intestinal metabolism and absorption of baicalein. *Journal of Ethnopharmacology* 141(12): 742-53.

826   Abbasi, E. et al. 2013. Effects of vitexin on scopolamine-induced memory impairment in rats. *Chin Journal of Physiology* 56(3): 184-9.

827   Patro, G. et al. 2016. Effects of Mimosa pudica L. leaves extract on anxiety, depression and memory. *Avicenna J Phytomed* 6(6): 696-710.

828   Onyije, F.M. et al. 2018. Mimosa pudica protects the testes against cadmium-induced inflammation and oligospermia: Potential benefits in treatment of heavy metal toxicity. *Pathophysiology* 25(4): 293-297.

829   Tasnuva, S.T. et al. 2017. Alpha-glucosidase inhibitors isolated from Mimosa pudica L. *Nat Prod Research* 27: 1-5.

830   Antony, P.J. et al. 2017. Myoinositol ameliorates high-fat diet and streptozotocin-induced diabetes in rats through promoting insulin receptor signaling. *Biomed Pharmacother* 88: 1098-1113.

831   Shergis, J.L. et al. 2017. Ziziphus spinosa seeds for insomnia: A review of chemistry and psychopharmacology. *Phytomedicine* 34: 38-43.

832   Han, H. et al. 2009. Anxiolytic-like effects of sanjoinine A isolated from Ziziphi Spinosi semen: possible involvement of GABAergic transmission. *Pharmacol Biochem Behav* 92(2): 206-13.

833   Park, H.J. et al. 2019. The ethanol extract of Ziziphus jujuba var. spinosa seeds ameliorates the memory deficits in Alzheimer's disease model mice. *Journal of Ethnopharmacology* 233: 73-79.

834   Chen, C. et al. 2018. The prodrug of 7,8-dihydroxyflavone development and therapeutic efficacy for treating Alzheimer's disease. *Proc Natl Acad Sci U S A* 115(3):578-83.

835   Yang, Y.J. et al. 2014. Small molecule TrkB agonist 7,8-dihydroxyflavone reverses cognitive and synaptic plasticity deficits in a rat model of schizophrenia. *Pharmacol Biochem Behav* 122: 30-36.

836   Nie, S. et al. 2019. 7,8-dihydroxyflavone protects nigrostriatal dopaminergic neurons from rotenone-induced neurotoxicity in rodents. *Parkinsons Disease* 2019:9193534.

837   Garcia-Diaz B.G. et al. 2017. 7,8-dihydroxyflavone ameliorates cognitive and motor deficits in a Huntington's disease mouse model through specific activation of the PLC_y1 pathway. *Hum Mol Genet* 26(16): 3144-3160.

838   Kang, M.S. et al. 2017. Autism-like behavior caused by deletion of vaccinia-related kinase 3 is improved by TrkB stimulation. *Journal Exp Med* 214(10): 2947-66.

839   Aydin-Abidin, S. & I. Abidin. 2019. 7,8-dihydroxyflavone potentiates ongoing epileptiform activity in mice brain slices. *Neurosci Lett* 703: 25-31.

840   Korkmaz, O.T. et al. 2014. 7,8-hydroxyflavone improves motor performance and enhances lower motor neuronal survival in a mouse model of amyotrophic lateral sclerosis. *Neurosci Lett* 566: 286-91.

841   Cho, S.J. et al. 2019. 7,8-dihydroxyflavone protects high glucose-damaged neuronal cells against oxidative stress. *Biomol Ther* (Seoul) 27(1): 85-91.

842   Zhang, X.L. et al. 2018. From the cover: 7,8-dihydroxyflavone rescues lead-induced impairment of vesicular release: A novel therapeutic approach to lead intoxicated children. *Toxicol Sci* 161(1): 186-195.

410

843   Chen, J. et al. 2011. Antioxidant activity of 7,8-dihydroxyflavone provides neuroprotection against glutamate-induced toxicity. *Neurosci Lett* 499(3): 181-5.

844   Ren, Q. et al. 2014. 7,8-dihydroxyflavone, a TrkB agonist, attenuates behavioral abnormalities and neurotoxicity in mice after administration of methamphetamine. *Psychopharmacology* 231(1): 159-166.

845   Small, G.W. et al. 2018. Memory and Brain Amyloid and tau effects of a bioavailable form of curcumin in non-demented adults: A double-blind, placebo-controlled 18 month trial. *Am J Geriatr Psychiatry* 26(3): 266-77.

846   Tang, M. & C. Taghibiglou. 2017. The mechanisms of action of curcumin in Alzheimer's disease. *J Alzheimers Disease* 58(4): 1003-1016.

847   Giri, R. et al. 2004. Curcumin, the active constituents of tumeric, inhibits amyloid peptide-induced cythchemokine gene expression and CCR5-mediated chemotaxis of THP-1 monocytes by modulating early growth response-1 transcription factor. *Journal of Neurochemistry* 91(5): 1199-210.

848   Wynn, J et al. 2018. The effects of curcumin on brain-derived neurotrophic factor and cognition in schizophrenia: a randomized, controlled study. *Schizophrenia Research* 195: 572-3.

849   Fanaei, H. et al. 2016. Effect of curcumin on serum brain-derived neurotrophic factor levels in women with premenstrual syndrome: A randomized, double-blind, placebo-controlled trial. *Neuropeptides* 56: 25-31.

850   Smith, T.J. & B. Ashar. 2019. Iron deficiency anemia due to high-dose turmeric. *Cureus* 11(1).

851   Del Valle-Mojica, L.M. et al. 2011. Aqueous and ethanolic *Valeriana officinalis* extracts change the binding of ligands to glutamate receptors. *Evid Based Complement Alternat Medicine* 2011:891819.

852   Mineo, L. et al. 2017. Valeriana officinalis root extract modulates cortical excitatory circuits in humans. *Neuropsychobiology* 75(1): 46-51.

853   Pakseresht, S. et al. 2011. Extract of valerian root (*Valeriana officinalis* L.) vs. placebo in treatment of obsessive-compulsive disorder: a randomized double-blind study. *J Complement Integr Med* 8.issue-1/1553-3840.

854   Samaei, A. et al. 2018. Effect of valerian on cognitive disorders and electroencephalography in hemodialysis patients: a randomized, cross over, double-blind clinical trial. *BMC Nephrology* 19(1): 379.

855   Okubo, H. et al. 2012. Dietary patterns and risk of Parkinson's disease: a case-control study in Japan. *European Journal of Neurology* 19(5): 681-8.

856   Phan, C.W. et al. 2017. Edible and medicinal mushrooms: Emerging brain food for the mitigation of neurodegenerative diseases. *Journal Med Food* 20(1): 1-10.

857   Feng, Lee et al. 2019. The association between mushroom consumption and mild cognitive impairment: A community-based cross-sectional study in Singapore. *Journal of Alzheimer's Disease* 68(1): 197-203.

858   Rogers, R. 2011. *The Fungal Pharmacy: The Complete Guide to Medicinal Mushrooms and Lichens of North America.* North Atlantic Books Berkeley, CA.

859   Chandra, L.C. et al. 2013. White button, Portabella and shiitake mushroom supplementation up-regulates interleukin-23 secretion in acute dextran sodium sulphate colitis C57BL/6 mice and murine macrophage J.744.1 cell line. *Nutrition Research* 33(5): 388-96.

860   Wong K.H., M. Naidu, P. David, R. Bakar, S.Vikineswary. 2012. Neuroregenerative potential of Lion's Mane mushroom, *Hericium erinaceus*, in the treatment of peripheral nerve injury (Review). *International Journal of Medicinal Mushrooms.* 14: 427-46.

861   Mori, K. et al. 2009. Improving effects of the mushroom Yamabushitake (Hericium erinaceus) on mild cognitive impairment: a double-blind placebo-controlled clinical trial. *Phytotherapy Research* 23(3): 367-72.

862   Nagano, M. et al. 2010. Reduction of depression and anxiety by 4 weeks *Hericium erinaceus* intake. *Biomed Research* 31(4): 231-7.

863   Tseng, T.T. et al. 2018. The cyanthin diterpenoid and sesterterpene constituents of *Hericium erinaceus* mycelium ameliorate Alzheimer's disease-related pathologies in APP/PS1 transgenic mice. *International Journal of Molecular Science* 19(2).

864   Cheung W.M., W.S. Hu, P.W. Chu, S.W. Chiu, N.Y. Ip. 2000. Ganoderma extract activates MAP kinases and induces neuronal differentiation in rat pheochromocytoma PC12 cells. *FEBS Letters* 486: 291-296.

865   Phan CW, P. David, M. Naidu, K.H.Wong, V. Sabaratnam. 2013. Neurite outgrowth stimulatory effects of culinary-medicinal mushrooms and their toxicity assessment using differentiating Neuro-2a and embryonic fibroblast BALB/3T3. *BMC Complementary and Alternative Medicine.* 13:261.

866   Ling-Sing S.S., M. Naidu, P. David, K.H. Wong, V. Sabaratnam. 2013. Potentiation of neuritogenic activity of medicinal mushrooms in rat pheochromocytoma cells. *BMC Complementary and Alternative Medicine* 13(157): 13-15.

867   Henao, S.L.D. et al. 2018. Randomized clinical trial for the evaluation of immune modulation by yogurt enriched with beta-glucans from Lingzhi or reishi medicinal mushroom, Ganoderma lucidum (Agaricomycetes), in children from Medelllin, Columbia. *International Journal of Medicinal Mushrooms* 20(8): 705-16.

868   Li, Z. et al. 2019. Protective role of Amanita caesarea polysaccharides against Alzheimer's disease via Nrf2 pathway. *International Journal of Biological Macromolecules* 121: 29-37.

869   An, S. 2017. Pharmacological basis for use of *Armillaria mellea* polysaccharides in Alzheimer's disease: Antiapoptosis and antioxidation. *Oxid Med Cell Longevity* 2017:4184562.

870   Ojemann, L.M. et al. 2006. Tian ma, an ancient Chinese herb, offers new options for the treatment of epilepsy and other conditions. *Epilepsy Behav* 8(2): 376-83.

871   Lo, Y.C. et al. 2012. Comparative study of contents of several bioactive components in fruiting bodies and mycelia of culinary-medicinal mushrooms. *International Journal of Medicinal Mushrooms* 14(4): 357-63.

872   Karaman, M. et al. 2018. *Coprinus comatus* filtrate extract, a novel neuroprotective agent of natural origin. *Nat Prod Res* 17:1-5.

873   Li, B. et al. 2016. 3'-deoxyadenosine (cordycepin) produces a rapid and robust antidepressant effect via enhancing prefrontal AMPA receptor signaling pathway. *International Journal of Neuropsychopharmacol* 19(4).

874   Olatunji, O.J. et al. 2016. Neuroprotective effects of adenosine isolated from Cordyceps cicadea against oxidative and ER stress damages induced by glutamate in PC12 cells. *Environ Toxicol Pharmacol* 44: 53-61.

875   Zhang, Y. et al. 2018. Structural characteristics and bioactive properties of a novel polysaccharide from Flammulina velutipes. *Carbohydr Polym* 197: 147-56.

876   Sulkowska-Ziaja, K. et al. Chemical composition and biological activity of extracts from fruiting bodies and mycelial cultures of *Fomitopsis betulina*. *Mol Biol Rep* 45(6): 2535-44.

877   Giridharan, V.V. et al. 2011. Amelioration of scopolamine induced cognitive dysfunction and oxidative stress by *Inonotus obliquus*- a medicinal mushroom. *Food Funct* 2(6): 320-7.

412

878   Han, Y. et al. Inonotus obliquus polysaccharides protect against Alzheimer's disease by regulating Nrf2 signaling and exerting anti-oxidative and anti-apoptotic effects. *Int J Biol Macromol* 131: 769-778.

879   Zhang, Y. et al. 2016. Polysaccharides from *Pleurotus ostreatus* alleviate cognitive impairment in a rat model of Alzheimer's disease. *Int J Biol Macromol* 92: 935-941.

880   Griffiths, R.R. et al. 2006. Psilocybin can occasion mystical-type experiences having substantial and sustained personal meaning and spiritual significance. *Psychopharmacology* 187(3): 268-83.

881   Grob, C.S. et al. 2011. Pilot study of psilocybin treatment for anxiety in patients with advanced-stage cancer. *Archives of General Psychiatry* 68(1): 71-8.

882   Cathart-Harris, Robin L. et al. 2012. Neural Correlates of the Psychedelic State as determined by fMRI studies with Psilocybin. *Proceedings of the National Academy of Sciences of the United States of America.* 109(6): 2138-43.

883   Psychedelic Research Group. 2018. More realistic forecasting of future life events after Psilocybin for treatment-resistant depression. *Front Psychol* doi: org/10.3389/fpsyg.2018.01721.

884   Wang, K. et al. 2018. Polysaccharopeptide from Trametes versicolor blocks inflammatory osteoarthritis pain-morphine tolerance effects via activating cannabinoid type 2 receptor. *International Journal Biol Macromol* doi: 10.10116/ijbiomac.2018.12.212.

885   Gupta, G. et al. 2019. Aqueous extract of Wood Ear mushroom Auricularia polytricha (Agaricomycetes), demonstrated antiepileptic activity against seizure induced by maximal electroshock and isoniaszid in experimental animals. *International Journal of Medicinal Mushrooms* 21(1): 29-35.

886   Milgrom, L.R. 2008. Homeopathy and the new fundamentalism: a critique of the critics. *Journal Altern Complement Med* 14(5): 589-94.

887   Emoto, M. 1999. *The Message from Water.* 2nd Ed. Hado Pub

888   Grimaldi-Bensouda, L. et al. 2016. Homeopathic medical practice for anxiety and depression in primary care: The EP13 cohort study. *BMC Complement Altern Med* 16: 125.

889   Danno, K. et al. 2018. Management of anxiety and depressive disorders in patients > 65 years of age by homeopath general practitioners versus conventional general practitioners, with overview of the EP12-LASER study results. *Homeopathy* 107(2): 81-89.

890   Macias-Cortés, E.C. et al. 2015. Individualized homeopathic treatment and fluoxetine for moderate to severe depression in peri- and postmenopausal women (HOMDEP-MENOP study): a randomized, double-dummy, double-blind, placebo-controlled trial. *PLoS One* 2015 10(3).

891   Hock, N. & G. Juckel. 2018. Homeopathy for psychiatric patients-for and against. *Nervenarzt* 89(9): 1014-9.

892   Adler, U. et al. 2011. Homeopathic individualized Q-potencies versus fluoxetine for moderate to severe depression: double-blind, randomized, non-inferiority trial. *Evid Based Complement Alternat Med* 2011:520182.

893   Boericke, Wm. 1927. *Pocket Manual of Homeopathic Materia Medica and Repertory.* 9th Ed. B. Jain Pub. India.

894   Rogers, Laurie Szott & R. Rogers. *Praire Deva Flower Essences* Prairie Deva Press Edmonton AB Canada

895   Rogers, R. 2016. *Mushroom Essences: Vibrational Healing from the Kingdom Fungi.* North Atlantic Berkeley CA.

413

896   Masuda, A. et al. 2005. Repeated thermal therapy diminishes appetite loss and subject complaints in mildly depressed patients. *Psychosomatic Medicine* 67(4): 643-7.

897   Moncrieff, R. 1977. Emotional response to odors. *Soap, Perfumery and Cosmetics* 50: 24-25.

898   Kusumawardani, S.R. et al. 2017. Theta brainwave activity as the reponse to Lavender (Lavendula angustifolia) aromatherapy inhalation of postgraduate students with academic stress condition. *IOP Conference Series: Material Science and Engineering* 180 012271.

899   Elisabetsky, E. 1997. *Anticonvulsant properties of linalool and gamma-decanolactone in mice.* WOCMAP II- Abstracts, Mendoza Argentina.

900   Balacs, T. 1995. The psychopharmacology of essential oils. Aroma '95 Conference Proceedings: Brighton: Aromatherapy Publications.

901   Wang, Z.J. & T. Heinbockel. 2018. Essential Oils and their constituents targeting the GABAergic system and sodium channels as treatment of Neurological Diseases. *Molecules* 23(5).

902   Lofan, M. & C. Gold. 2009. Meta-analysis of the effectivenss of individual intervention in the controlled multisensory environment (Snoezelen) for individuals with intellectual disability. *J Intellect Dev Disabil* 34(3): 207-15.

903   Berg, A. et al. 2010. Snoezelen, structured reminiscence therapy and 10-minutes activation in long term care residents with dementia (WISDE): study protocol of a cluster randomized controlled trial. *BMC Geriatr* 31(10):5.

904   Szott-Rogers, Laurie. 2014. *Scents of Wonder: Aromatic Solutions for Health, Beauty and Pleasure.* Second Ed. Prairie Deva Press. Edmonton Alberta.

905   Sánchez-Viana, D.I. et al. 2017. The effectiveness of aromatherapy for depressive symptoms: A systematic review. *Evid Based Complement Alternat Med* doi: 10.1155/2017/5869315.

906   Buckle, J. 2015. *Clinical Aromatherapy: Essential Oils in Healthcare.* Third Ed. Elsevier page 228.

907   Green, A. 2013. Age and apolipoprotein E e4 effects on neural correlates of odor memory. *Behav Neurosci* 127(3): 339-49.

908   Liu, B.J. et al. 2019. Relationship between poor olfaction and mortality among community-dwelling older adults: A cohort study. *Annals of Internal Medicine* doi: 10.7326/M18-0775.

909   Schecklmann, M. et al. 2013. A systematic review on olfaction in child and adolescent psychiatric disorders. *J Neural Transm* 120(1): 121-30.

910   Buckle, J. 2015. *Clinical Aromatherapy: Essential Oils in Healthcare.* Third Ed. Elsevier page 290-1.

911   Sowndhararajan, K et al. 2017. Effect of the essential oil and supercritical carbon dioxide extract from the root of Angelica gigas on human EEG activity. *Complement Ther Clin Pract* 28: 161-8.

912   Zhao, R.J. et al. 2005. The essential oil of Angelica gigas NAKAI suppresses nicotine sensitization. *Biol Pharm Bull* 28(12): 2323-6.

913   Ayuob, N.N. et al. 2018. Ocimum basilicum improves chronic stress-induced neurodegenerative changes in mice hippocampus. *Metab Brain Dis* 33(3): 795-804.

914   Watanabe, E. et al. 2015. Effects of bergamot (Citrus bergamia) essential oil aromatherapy on mood states, parasympathetic nervous system activity, and salivary cortisol levels in 41 healthy women. *Forsch Komplementmed* 22(1): 43-9.

915   Han, X. et al. Bergamot (Citrus bergamia) essential oil inhalation improves positive feelings in the waiting room of a mental health treatment centre: A pilot study. *Phytotherapy Research* 31(5): 812-16.

916   Bagetta, G. et al. 2010. Neuropharmacology of the essential oil of bergamot. *Fitoterapia* 81: 453-461.

917   Rose, J. & F. Behm. 1994. Inhalation of vapor from black pepper extract reduces smoking withdrawal symptoms. *Drug and Alcohol Dependence* 34(3): 225-9

918   Fajemiroye, J.O. et al. 2014. Anxiolytic and antidepressant like effects of a natural food flavour (E)-methyl isoeugenol. *Food Funct* 5(8): 1819-28.

919   Bagci, E. et al. 2016. Anthriscus nemorosa essential oil inhalation prevents memory impairment, anxiety and depression in scopolamine-treated rats. *Biomed Pharmacother* 84: 1313-20.

920   Chen, H.M. & H.W. Chen. 2008. The effect of applying cinnamon aromatherapy for children with attention deficit hyperactivity disorder. *Journal of Chinese Medicine* 19(112): 27-34.

921   Tao, G. et al. 2005. Eugenol and its structural analogs inhibit monoamine oxidase A and exhibit antidepressant-like activity. *Bioorg Med Chem* 13(15): 4777-4788

922   Farisa, B.S. et al. 2018. Effects of patchouli and cinnamon essential oils on biofilms and hyphae formation by Candida species. *J Mycol Med* 28(2): 332-339.

923   Cioanca, O. et al. 2013. Cognitive-enhancing and antioxidant activity of inhaled coriander volatile oil in amyloid-B rat model of Alzheimer's disease. *Physiol Behav* 120: 193-202.

924   Liu, B.B. et al. 2015. Essential oil of Syzygium aromaticum reverses the deficits of stress-induced behaviors and hippocampal p-ERK/p-CREB/brain-derived neurotrophic factor expression. *Planta Medica* 81(3): 185-93.

925   Morshedi, D et al. 2015. Cuminaldehyde as the major component of *Cuminum cyminum*, a natural aldehyde with inhibitory effect on alpha-synuclein fibrillation and cytotoxicity. *Journal Food Science* 80(10): H2336-45.

926   Matthew, T. 2017. Eucalyptus oil inhalation-induced seizure: a novel, underregcognized, preventable cause of acute symptomatic seizure. *Epilepsia Open* 2(3): 350-4.

927   Skalli, S. 2011. Epileptic seizure induced by fennel essential oil. *Epileptic Disord* 13(3): 345-7.

928   Al-Harrasi, A. et al. 2019. Distribution of the anti-inflammatory and anti-depressant compounds: incensole and incensole acetate in genus Boswellia. *Phytochemistry* 161: 28-40.

929   Riva, A et al. 2019. Oral administration of a lecithin-based delivery form of boswellic acid (Casperome®) for the prevention of symptoms of irritable bowel syndrom: a randomized clinical study. *Minerva Gastroenterol Dietol* 65(1): 30-35.

930   Pellegrini, L. et al. 2016. Managing ulcerative colitis in remission phase: usefulness of Casperome®, an innovative lecithin-based delivery system of *Boswellia serrata* extract. *Eur Rev Med Pharmacol Sci* 20(12): 2695-2700.

931   Lee, C. et al. –Gingerol attenuates beta amyloid induced oxidative cell death via fortifying cellular antioxidant defense system. *Food Chem Toxicol* 49: 1261-9.

932   Cioanca, O. et al. 2015. Anti-acetylcholinesterase and antioxidant activity of inhaled juniper oil on amyloid beta (1-42) induced oxidative stress. *Neurochem Research* 40: 953-960.

933   Bradley, B. et al. Effects of orally administered lavender essential oil on responses to anxiety-provoking film clips. *Human Psychopharmacology* 24: 319-330.

415

934 Woelk, H, & S. Schlafke. 2010. A multi-center, double-blind, randomized study of the lavender oil preparation Silexan in comparison to Lorazepam for generalized anxiety disorder. *Phytomedicine* 17: 94-99.

935 Buckle, J. 2015. *Clinical Aromatherapy: Essential Oils in Healthcare*. Third Ed. Elsevier page 171.

936 Ibid page 172-175.

937 Johannessen, B. 2013. Nurses experience of aromatherapy use with dementia patients experiencing disturbed sleep patterns. An action research project. *Comp Ther Clinical Practice* 19(4): 2009-13.

938 Blyth. 2011. *Effect of lavender on the sleep of autistic children*. Unpublished RJBA dissertation.

939 Hynson, B. & J. Gilbert. 2009. Unpublished dissertation. RJ Buckle Ass.

940 Fujii, M. 2013. Lavender aroma therapy for behavioral and psychological symptoms in dementia patients. *Geriatr Gerontol Int* 8(2): 136-8.

941 Jimbo, D. et al. Effect of aromatherapy on patients with Alzheimer's disease. *Psychogeriatrics* 9: 173-179.

942 Curran, P. 2003. *Effect of diffusing lavender at sunset on patients with dementia*. Unpublished dissertation for RJBA.

943 Gu, S.M. et al. 2019. Limonene inhibits methamphetamine-induced sensitizations via the regulation of dopamine receptor supersensitivity. *Biomol Ther* (Seoul) doi: 10.4062.biomolther.2018.213.

944 Jimbo, D. et al. 2011. Effect of aromatherapy on patients with Alzheimer's disease. *Psychogeriatrics* 9: 73-7.

945 Elliott, M. et al. 2007. The essential oils from Melissa officinalis L. and Lavandula angustifolia Mill. as potential treatment for agitation in people with severe dementia. *International J Essential Oil Ther* 1: 143-152.

946 Ballard, C.G. et al. 2002. Aromatherapy as a safe and effective treatment for the management of agitation in severe dementia: the results of a double-blind, placebo-controlled trial with Melissa. *Journal Clin Psychiatry* 63: 553-558.

947 Dolara, P. et al. 1996. Characterization of the action on central opioid receptors of furaneudesma-1,3-diene, a sesquiterpene from myrrh. *Phytotherapy Research* 10(supp 1): 81-83.

948 Chen, Y. et al. 2008. Inhalation of neroli oil and its anxiolytic effects. *J Complement Integrative Med* 5(1).

949 Igarashi, M. et al. 2014. Effects of olfactory stimulation with rose and orange oil on prefrontal cortex activity. *Complement Ther Med* 22(6): 1027-31.

950 Farisa, B.S. et al. 2018. Effects of patchouli and cinnamon essential oils on biofilms and hyphae formation by Candida species. *J Mycol Med* 28(2): 332-339.

951 Chalifour, M. *Peppermint in opiate-withdrawal in a locked hospital unit*. Unpublished dissertation for RJ Buckle Assoc.

952 Kennedy, D. et al. 2018. Volatile terpenes and brain function: investigation of the cognitive and mood effects of Mentha x piperata L. essential oil with in vitro properties relevant to central nervous system function. *Nutrients* 10(8) doi: 10.3390/nu10081029.

953 Anis, E. et al. 2018. Evaluation of phytomedicinal potential of perillyl alcohol in an in vitro Parkinson's disease model. *Drug Dev Research* 79(5): 218-224.

954 Yang, H. et al. 2016. Alpha pinene, a major constituent of pine tree oils, enhances non-rapid eye movement sleep in mice through GABAA-benzodiazepine receptors. *Mol Pharmacol* 90: 530-9.

955   Hongratanaworakit, T. 2009. Simultaneous aromatherapy massage with rosemary oil on humans. *Sci Pharm* 77: 375-387.

956   Sorenson, K. et al. 1999. Effects of aroma with poor attention span in music lessons. Unpublished dissertation RJ Buckle Associates.

957   Filiptsova, O.V. et al. 2018. The effect of the essential oils of lavender and rosemary on the human short-term memory. *Alexandria Journal Medicine* 54: 41-44.

958   Moss, M. & L. Oliver. 2012. Plasma 1,8-cineole correlates with cognitive performance following exposure to rosemary essential oil aroma. *Ther Adv Psychopharmacology* 2: 103-13.

959   Pathan, S. 2009. Anti-convulsant evaluation of safranal in pentylenetetrazole-induced status epilepticus in mice. *International Journal of Essential Oil Ther* 3:106-8.

960   Moss, L. et al. 2010. Differential effects of the aromas of Salvia species on memory and mood. *Human Psycho Pharmacol Clin Exp* 25: 388-96.

961   Perry, N.S. et al. 2013. Salvia for dementia therapy: review of pharmacological activity and pilot tolerability clinical trial. *Pharmacol Biochem Behav* 75: 651-659.

962   Kennedy, D.O. et al. 2010. Monoterpenoid extract of sage (Salvia lavandulaefolia) with cholinesterinase-inhibiting properties improves cognitive performance and mood in healthy adults. Journal of *Psychopharmacology* 25: 1088.

963   Aydin, E. et al. 2016. The effects of inhaled Pimpinella peregrina essential oil on scopolamine-induced memory impairment, anxiety and depression in laboratory rats. *Mol Neurobiol* 53: 6557-67.

964   Azizi, Z. et al. 2012. Cognitive-enhancing activity of thymol and carvacrol in two rat models of dementia. *Behav Pharmacol* 23: 241-49.

965   Erreira, F. et al. 1996. Effects of Valeriana officinalis on [3H] GABA. Release in synaptosomes: further evidence for the involvement of free GABA in the valerian-induced release. *Rev Port Farm* 46(2): 74-77.

966   Houghton, P.J. 1999. The scientific basis for the reputed activity of Valerian. *J Pharm Pharmacol* 51(1): 505-12.

967   Dobetsberger, C. & G. Buchbauer. 2011. Actions of essential oils on the central nervous system: an updated review. *Flavour and Fragrance Journal* 26(5): 300-316.

968   Benny, A. & J. Thomas. 2019. Essential oils as treatment strategy for Alzheimer's disease: current and future perspectives. *Planta Medica* 85(3): 239-48.

969   Friedmann, Terry S. http://files.meetup.com/1481956/ADHD%20Research%20by%20Dr.%20Terry%20Friedmann.pdf

970   Caldwell, N. 2001. *Effects of ylang ylang on cravings of women with substance abuse.* RJBA unpublished dissertation.

971   Buckle, J. 2015. *Clinical Aromatherapy: Essential Oils in Healthcare.* Third Ed. Elsevier page 301.

972   Barrett, D. 2002. Aromatherapy to alleviate addiction withdrawal in hospitalized patients. RJBA unpublished dissertation.

973   Kunz, S. et al. 2007. Ear acupuncture for alcohol withdrawal in comparison with aromatherapy: a randomized, controlled trial. *Alcoholism: Clin Exp Research* 31(3): 436-42.

974   Lyu, R.M. et al. 2018. Phoenixin: a novel brain-gut-skin peptide with multiple bioactivity. *Acta Pharmacol Sinica* 39(5): 770-3.

975   Jiang, J.H. et al. 2015. Phoenixin-14 enhances memory and mitigates memory impairment induced by Abeta1-42 and scopolamine in mice. *Brain Research* 1629: 298-308.

976   McIlwraith, E.K. et al. 2019. Regulation of Gpr173 expression, a putative phoenixin receptor, by saturated fat acid palmitate and endocrine-disrupting chemical bisphenol A through a p38-mediated mechanism in immortalized hypothalamic neurons. *Mol Cell Endocrinol* 485: 54-60.

977   Ohbuchi, K. et al. 2016. Ignavine: a novel allosteric modulator of the mu opioid receptor. *Sci Rep* 6: 31748.

978   Olsen, E.K. et al. 2016. Marine AChE inhibitors isolated from *Geodia barretti*: natural compounds and their synthetic analogs. *Org Biomol Chem* 14(5): 1629-40.

979   Di, X. et al. 2018. 6-bromoindole derivatives from the Icelandic marine sponge *Geodia barretti*: isolation and anti-inflammatory activity. *Mar Drugs* 16(11):

980   Sun, Q. 2019. 9-methylfascaplysin is a more potent beta amyloid aggregation inhibitor than the marine derived alkaloid, fascaplysin, and produces nanomolar neuroprotective effects in SH-SY5Y cells. *Mar Drugs* 17(2).

981   Doidge, N. 2015. *The Brain's Way of Healing*. Penguin page 157

982   Lipsman, N. et al. 2018. Blood-brain barrier opening in Alzheimer's disease using MR-guided focused ultrasound. *Nat Commun* 9(1): 2336.

983   Doidge,N. pages 226-279.

984   Zhongyi Chen et al. 2014. Incorporation of therapeutically modified bacteria into gut microbiota inhibits obesity. *J of Clin Invest* 124(8): 3391-3406.

985   Ackerman, J. 2016. U.S. Navy recruits gut microbes to fight obesity and disease. *Scientific American* October 19.

986   Tiwari, S. et al. 2019. Biosensors for epilepsy management: State of Art and Future Aspects. *Sensors* (Basel) 19(7).

987   Fischbach, G.D. & R.L. Fischbach. 2004. Stem Cells: Science Policy and Ethics. *Journal of Clinical Investigation* 114: 1364-70.

988   Politis, M. et al. 2010. Serotonergic neurons mediate dyskinesia side effects in Parkinson's patients with neural transplants. *Science Translational Medicine* 238ra doi: 10.1126/scitranslmed.30000976.

Made in the USA
Columbia, SC
16 December 2020

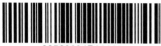